T0297082

The Breathless Heart

Michele Emdin • Alberto Giannoni
Claudio Passino
Editors

The Breathless Heart

Apneas in Heart Failure

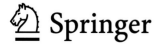 Springer

Editors
Michele Emdin
Institute of Life Sciences
Scuola Superiore Sant'Anna and
Fondazione Toscana Gabriele Monasterio
Pisa
Italy

Claudio Passino
Institute of Life Sciences
Scuola Superiore Sant'Anna and
Fondazione Toscana Gabriele Monasterio
Pisa
Italy

Alberto Giannoni
Fondazione Toscana Gabrielle Monasterio
Pisa
Italy

ISBN 978-3-319-26352-6   ISBN 978-3-319-26354-0   (eBook)
DOI 10.1007/978-3-319-26354-0

Library of Congress Control Number: 2016959210

Printed on acid-free paper

This Springer imprint is published by Springer Nature
The registered company is Springer International Publishing AG
The registered company is Gewerbestrasse 11, 6330 Cham, Switzerland

Preface

Heart failure is a major cause of hospitalization and mortality, despite recent advancements in diagnosis and treatment. The search for hidden pathophysiological triggers of disease evolution and potential targets of therapy has rediscovered an old, forgotten feature of the heart failure syndrome: apnea. Apneas may present themselves either as a sign or a symptom in the individual patient, but are often overlooked by clinicians, though they are both a marker of severity and a mediator of risk. Apneas are invariably associated with cyclic hyperpneas both in the asleep and in the awake subject with heart failure, possibly as an initial compensatory response.

Apnea/hyperpnea phenomena oblige the clinician to reevaluate the physiology of respiration and cardiovascular function. However, is there still place for physiology in the decision-making for patients with cardiovascular diseases in the era of imaging, genetics, and molecular biology?

The answer is in the affirmative, as demonstrated by the clinical value of periodic breathing/Cheyne-Stokes respiration (PB/CSR) [1, 2] in patients with heart failure (Fig. 1). This abnormal breathing pattern has been known for centuries, but it is only during the last decades that its pathophysiology and its clinical meaning have been adequately investigated.

In particular, the underlying derangement of neural control of respiratory centers, its impact on prognosis, and the relevance of the phenomenon as a therapeutic target have been the object of an increase of interest and literature during the last decades, yet with diverse experimental findings and contradictory opinions.

The recent failure of two large trials testing the effectiveness of noninvasive mechanical ventilation (CANPAP and SERVE-HF) [3, 4] in improving the outcome of heart failure patients has confirmed the need to summarize the current knowledge on this topic. For this purpose, this book has been thought for all researchers and clinicians interested in the field. An international faculty has collaborated in furnishing a complete overview touching all aspects of the apnea phenomenon in heart failure patients.

The historical background of pathophysiological alterations determining the occurrence of central apneas in different disorders will be presented. A thorough description of the visceral feedbacks and in particular of the chemoreflex system, whose deregulation plays a key role in central apnea origin and maintenance, and the mathematical models proposed to describe PB/CSR will be presented. The role

Fig. 1 "Record showing
Cheyne-Stokes respiration
(from a case of aortic and
mitral insufficiency with
atherosclerosis). The time
record gives second."
Original legend in Ref. [5]

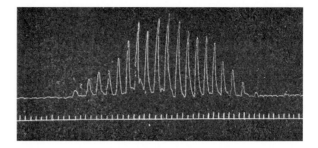

and feasibility of different diagnostic approaches, including the modern recording
of apneas by the implanted device, will be the object of analysis.

Finally, the authors will try to define the significance of apneas during sleep and
during wakefulness, the different pathophysiology of obstructive and central apneas,
and the most advanced tools for the treatment of central apneas, including the novel
technique of phrenic nerve stimulation, presented by a principal investigator of the
clinical trial addressing its efficacy.

The whole matter, two thousand years after the Hippocrates' description and two
centuries after the brilliant description by the Irish physician Cheyne, is still largely
debated: this book can be considered a companion for all interested in increasing their
knowledge on its significance, in order to improve clinical care of heart failure patients.

Michele Emdin
Alberto Giannoni
Pisa, Italy   Claudio Passino

References

1. Cheyne J. Dublin hospital reports. 1818;2:216.
2. Stokes W. The diseases of the heart and the aorta. Dublin: Hodges and Smith;
   1854. p. 323–6.
3. Bradley TD, Logan AG, Kimoff RJ, Sériès F, Morrison D, Ferguson K, Belenkie I,
   Pfeifer M, Fleetham J, Hanly P, Smilovitch M, Tomlinson G, Floras JS; CANPAP
   Investigators. Continuous positive airway pressure for central sleep apnea and
   heart failure. N Engl J Med. 2005;353:2025–33.
4. Cowie MR, Woehrle H, Wegscheider K, Angermann C, d'Ortho MP, Erdmann E,
   Levy P, Simonds AK, Somers VK, Zannad F, Teschler H. Adaptive servo-
   ventilation for central sleep apnea in systolic heart failure. N Engl J Med. 2015;
   373:1095–105.
5. Howell WH. Influence of various conditions on respiration. Modified respiratory
   movements. In: A text book of physiology for medical students and physicians.
   Philadelphia/London: WB Saunders Cop; 1919. p. 717.

Contents

Historical Background and Glossary of the Apnea Phenomenon

1

Apneas and Heart Disease

Michele Emdin and Alberto Aimo

Abbreviations

AHI	Apnea-hypopnea index
CSR	Cheyne-Stokes respiration
EEG	Electroencephalogram/electroencephalography
HF	Heart failure
OSAS	Obstructive sleep apnea syndrome
PB	Periodic breathing
PSG	Polysomnography
RDI	Respiratory disturbance index

1.1   Introduction

"A remarkable abnormal rhythm of respiration, first observed by Cheyne but afterwards more fully studied by Stokes and hence called by their combined names, occurs in certain pathological cases. The respiratory movements gradually decrease both in extent and rapidity until they cease altogether, and a condition of apnoea, lasting it may be for several seconds, ensues. This is followed by a feeble

M. Emdin (✉)
Institute of Life Sciences, Scuola Superiore Sant'Anna, Pisa, Italy

Division of Cardiology and Cardiovascular Medicine, Fondazione Toscana Gabriele Monasterio, Pisa, Italy
e-mail: emdin@ftgm.it

A. Aimo
Institute of Life Sciences, Scuola Superiore Sant'Anna, Pisa, Italy
e-mail: a.aimo@sssup.it

© Springer International Publishing Switzerland 2017
M. Emdin et al. (eds.), *The Breathless Heart*,
DOI 10.1007/978-3-319-26354-0_1

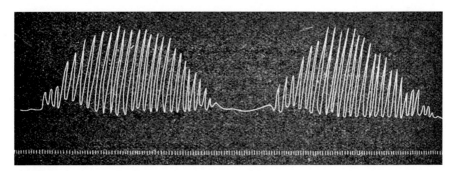

Fig. 1.1 Typical example of Cheyne-Stokes respiration (Source: Hartridge H, 1940 [6])

respiration, succeeded in turn by a somewhat stronger one, and thus the respiration returns gradually to the normal, or may even rise to hyperpnoea or slight dyspnea after which it again declines in a similar manner (Fig. 1.1). The cause of the phenomena is not thoroughly understood. Stokes connected it with a fatty condition of the heart, but it has been met with in various maladies. Schiff observed it as the result of compression of the medulla oblongata; and closely similar phenomena have been observed during sleep, under perfectly normal conditions" [1].

This report summarizes the state of the art about Cheyne-Stokes respiration (CSR) in 1879. The oscillatory respiratory pattern named CSR or periodic breathing (PB) (according to the presence or absence of apneas, respectively) has stimulated the curiosity of physicians for centuries.

1.2   From Hippocrates to Hunter, Cheyne and Stokes: Watching the Ill Breathing

Interestingly, the condition now known as obstructive sleep apnea syndrome (OSAS) was described only in 1889, while PB/CSR was noted long before, being easily recognizable and most of all occurring also during wakefulness. The very same father of medicine Hippocrates (460–379 BC) is thought to have provided the first account of PB/CSR: "His respiration was rare and large, *like a person who forgot for a time the need of breathing and then suddenly remembered*" [2].

We must wait until 1781 to find another account of PB/CSR. Describing the case history of a Mr. Boyed, who apparently suffered from atrial fibrillation and congestive heart failure, the British surgeon John Hunter wrote: "The pulse was irregular, as usual, and quick; but *his breathing was very particular: he would cease breathing for twenty or thirty seconds, and then begin to breathe softly, which increased until he breathed extremely strong, or rather with violent strength, which gradually died away till we could not observe that he breathed at all.* He could not lie down without running the risk of being suffocated, therefore he was obliged to sit up in his chair" [3].

However, the accounts by two Irish physicians were to achieve more relevance, giving also the name to this breathing pattern. In 1818, John Cheyne published in the *Dublin Hospital Reports* "A case of Apoplexy, in which the fleshy part of the heart was converted into fat". In the course of his description of a patient with probable cardiac asthma he stated: "The only peculiarity in the last period of his illness, which lasted eight or nine days, was in the state of the respiration. For several days *his breathing was irregular; it would entirely cease for a quarter of a minute, then it would become perceptible, though very low, then by degrees it became heaving and quick and then it would gradually cease again*: this revolution in the state of his breathing occupied about a minute, during which there were about thirty acts of respiration" [4].

In 1854, William Stokes published another report of the so-called "fatty degeneration of the heart" (corresponding to adverse ventricular remodeling with extensive fibrosis). In his account, he wrote: "But there is a *symptom which appears to belong to a weakened state of the heart* and which therefore may be looked for in many cases of fatty degeneration. I have never seen it except in examples of that disease. The symptom in question was observed by Dr. Cheyne […]. It consists in *the occurrence of a series of inspirations, increasing to a maximum and then declining in force and length until a state of apparent apnoea is established*. In this condition the patient may remain for such a length of time as to make his attendants believe that he is dead when a low inspiration, followed by one more decided marks the commencement of a new ascending and then descending series of inspirations. The decline in the length and force of the respirations is as regular and remarkable as their progressions increase. *The inspirations become each one less deep than the preceding, until they are all but imperceptible, and then the state of apparent apnoea occurs*. This is *at last broken by the faintest possible inspiration*; *the next effort is a little stronger, until* so to speak *the paroxysm of breathing is at its height, again to subside by a descending scale*" [5].

Of note, the descriptions by Hunter, Cheyne, and Stokes all refer to patients with severe heart failure (HF), outlining the strong association between this breathing pattern and HF [6]. Furthermore, all these reports refer to awake patients, but the fact that PB/CSR can be a diurnal phenomenon in HF was curiously overlooked for around 150 years, possibly because of the development of sleep medicine from the last decades of the nineteenth century and the subsequent assessment of PB/CSR only in the setting of breathing disturbances occurring during sleep.

The original descriptions report on periodicities characterized by rhythmic changes of respiratory phases and respiratory pauses in a relation of 60:15 s. The duration of respiratory cycles varies between 12 and 130 s. The relation of the hyperpnea and apnea phase is between 6:4 and 75:70 s, and the number of breaths ranges between 3 and 30 during one hyperpnea phase.

Less common is "Biot's breathing", accompanied by repetitive "runs" of several normal respirations—up to 4 or more at a time—followed suddenly by a period of apnea. The duration of the cycle is very variable, occasionally as short as 10 s and sometimes as long as a minute. This is a clinical rarity and is found in meningitis, brain compression, and brain destruction. Originally, this breathing pattern was called *rhythme meningitique* as it was in the nineteenth century routinely used by physicians as a diagnostic tool for meningitis [7].

1.3   Between Nineteenth and Twentieth Century: The Golden Age of Physiology

As stated by the Italian physiologist Luciani in 1923, "PB/CSR is not necessarily a manifestation of illness. It can be remarked in animals during lethargy; it sometimes occurs during sleep in healthy subjects, especially children and elderly; it is often remarked at high altitude (2,500–4,500 m over sea level), more frequently during sleep, but also during wakefulness" [8].

The occurrence of PB/CSR at high altitude was particularly fascinating for scientists. The first report of this phenomenon probably dates back to 1857. In that year, the famous physician John Tyndall made his first ascent of Mont Blanc (4,807 m), and when he was near the summit he was so exhausted that he laid down on the snow and immediately fell asleep. A Mr. Hirst, who accompanied him, woke him up saying: "You quite frightened me. *I have listened for some minutes and have not heard you breathe once*" [9]. Thirty-three years later, the Observatoire Vallot was installed on Mont Blanc; working there, the Swiss physician Egli-Sinclair noted: "Concerning the respiration, *I distinctly observed that it had the Stokes character*, that is it seemed regular during a certain time, after which a few rapid and profound breaths were drawn, suspension of a few seconds following" [10]. This preliminary observation was extended by Angelo Mosso, who carried out a series of physiological experiments at the Capanna Regina Margherita, at 4,560 m on Monte Rosa. Speaking of the respiration of his brother during sleep, he wrote in 1894: "The breathing sometimes continued for hours with this rhythm, *three descending movements* of which the first is forcible, and the other two or three weak, being followed by a *pause* which lasted regularly 12 s before the *return of another series of three descending respirations*" [11]. The keeper of the Capanna Regina Margherita displayed a different, more typical PB/CSR pattern, with periodical waxing and waning of respiration and shorter apneic periods [10]. Mosso performed also the first recordings of PB/CSR (Fig. 1.2), [12] and correctly recognized that PB/CSR at high altitude is not a temporary phenomenon, being detectable "even after 2–3 months at the Capanna" [12]. The observation—that periodic breathing continues for a long period at high altitude—has been confirmed amongst members of the Mount Everest Expedition of 1953 and also during the Himalayan Scientific Expedition of 1960–61 [13].

Of note, Mosso failed to interpret correctly the phenomenon, as he proposed that ventilation was globally depressed (and not increased) and not ascribing PB/CSR to hypoxic conditions but to hypocapnia (which was instead a consequence of overall hyperventilation) [13].

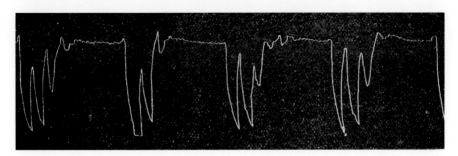

Fig. 1.2 High-altitude Cheyne-Stokes respiration recorded by Angelo Mosso in his brother (Source: Luciani L, 1923. [8])

Fig. 1.3 Induction of Cheyne-Stokes respiration by hyperventilation in a healthy subject (the Haldane experiment) (Source: Hartridge H, 1940 [6])

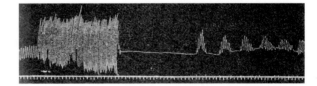

In the first decade of the twentieth century, the relationship between PB/CSR and variations in arterial blood gases attracted a lot of interest [14]. The discoveries on this topic are brilliantly summarized in the following extract from a 1910 textbook of physiology:

> If [a normal subject] is caused to breathe deeply and frequently for about two minutes, so as to produce a prolonged apnoea, the respiration, when it is resumed spontaneously, is of the Cheyne-Stokes type (Haldane) (Fig. 1.3). The explanation given by Haldane is that the fail in the partial pressure of the oxygen in the pulmonary alveoli during the primary apnoea, with the consequent fall of oxygen pressure in the arterial blood and respiratory centres, leads to the production of lactic acid in the respiratory centre and elsewhere, which stimulates the centre in the same way as carbon dioxide, and thus permits it to be excited by a smaller partial pressure of carbon dioxide than that normally necessary. As soon as the pressure of carbon dioxide, which is increasing during the period of apnoea, has reached the exciting value breathing is resumed. The respiration, beginning as very feeble movements, rapidly increase in strength till the breathing becomes quite deep or actually dyspnoeic. The store of oxygen is replenished by this thorough ventilation of the lungs, the changes in the excitability of the respiratory centre due to lack of oxygen disappear, and the centre relapses in a period of repose. During the period of apnoea the oxygen pressure sinks once more to the point at which the change in the excitability of the respiratory centre by carbon dioxide occurs, and the breathing again starts. In pathological cases, the want of oxygen may be associated either with deficient circulation through the bulb-centre or with deficient intake by the lungs. The administration of oxygen through a mask has been shown in such cases to abolish the periodicity in the respiration, and to render it more normal [15].

A crucial role of brain hypoperfusion and hypoxia was suggested through original experiments on animals. For example, it was noted that turtles continued to survive for some time after heart extraction, developing an oscillatory breathing pattern; frogs were subjected to the ligature of the aorta, cats to intermittent occlusions of cerebro-afferent vessels, dogs to systemic asphyxia, and so on [8, 16]. Also a depression of breathing centers could evoke PB/CSR, as suggested by the finding that PB/CSR could be induced or exacerbated in HF patients through hypodermic injections of morphine [8] and that the administration of other sedatives and hypnotics, such as chloral hydrate, induced ventilatory oscillations in healthy dogs and rabbits [8]. Even severe brain damage, such as brain hemorrhage with intracranial hypertension or decerebration with bilateral vagotomy, could induce an oscillatory breathing pattern [8]. Finally, a typical example of CSR was reported in a patient with end-stage chronic kidney disease, and an oscillatory breathing pattern was experimentally reproduced through intravenous injections of creatine and ammonium carbonate, suggesting a link between uremic state and PB/CSR [8].

In the attempt to provide a unitary explanation of PB/CSR, in 1923, Luciani interpreted PB/CSR as the product of "periodic oscillations in the excitability of centres controlling ventilation" [8]. Such "oscillations in excitability" could be triggered by an initial variation in respiratory gases (as in the experiment by Haldane), being then sustained by the periodical changes in arterial oxygen and carbon dioxide contents. The first perturbation of the system could also be represented by systemic or local hypoxia, inducing hyperventilation, which inhibited respiration, and so on. It was more difficult to explain how a depression of breathing centers (produced by drugs or brain damage) could result in PB/CSR, but such depression might impair the fine modulation of breathing in order to buffer the changes in arterial gas content, causing ventilation to become oscillatory.

In the present book, the history of research about PB/CSR will be somehow recapitulated by discussing our current interpretation of PB/CSR in different disease conditions (Chap. 3), providing a unitary theory of PB/CSR pathogenesis (Chaps. 4 and 5), and finally assessing the opportunity to treat it and the current therapeutic options (Chaps. 12 and 13).

1.4 From the Birth of Sleep Medicine to the Rediscovery of PB/CSR in Heart Failure

Chapters 9 and 10 will explore the diagnostic techniques for PB/CSR (and for other respiratory disturbances). These techniques have been developed in the twentieth century and have allowed the development of sleep medicine, which for some decades held the monopoly of research about PB/CSR.

In 1925, the first sleep laboratory was founded at the University of Chicago [17]. Four years later, electroencephalography (EEG) was introduced by Hans Berger; the potentialities of this techniques were not understood for some decades (probably accounting in part for Berger's depression and final suicide, in 1941) [17]. However, with regard to the sole setting of sleep medicine, EEG proved an essential

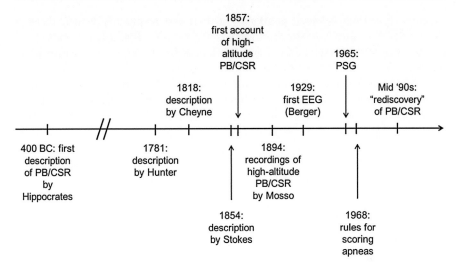

Fig. 1.4 Twenty-five hundred years of breathlessness. The main events in the history of research about periodic breathing/Cheyne-Stokes respiration are indicated on a time-line

instrument to dissect the structure of sleep and was included in a comprehensive tool for assessing sleep disturbances (including sleep apneas). This tool was named polysomnography (PSG) and was introduced in 1965 by French neurologist Henri Gastaut [17]. It promoted the development of sleep medicine into an autonomous field of research, a status consecrated for example by the first international conference on sleep disorders in 1967 and the development of the first manual for scoring apneas in 1968 [17]. In the following decades, the study of apneas remained the prerogative of the burgeoning field of sleep medicine, which focused mostly on the pathophysiology, diagnosis, and management of obstructive sleep apnea syndrome (OSAS) [17].

It was not until the mid-1990s that a new interest for central apneas/hypopneas became to emerge, this time among cardiologists [18]. The abnormalities of respiratory control mechanisms producing PB/CSR were explored up to the molecular level [18]. The prevalence of PB/CSR among HF patients was assessed; this breathing pattern was associated with worse prognosis, because of its association with a more severe HF status, and possibly because it contributes to HF progression [18]. The controversies about PB/CSR treatment and the "rediscovery" of PB/CSR as a diurnal phenomenon are the current frontiers of research in this field [19, 20].

The landmark events in the history of PB/CSR are summarized in Fig. 1.4.

Conclusions

The review of the literature on CSR discloses an enormous variance of the opinions expressed. CSR was observed in healthy subjects, as well as in patients with HF, while other forms of PB were observed in neurosurgical, cardiac, pulmonary, and pediatric diseases. CSR was explained as sequel of prolongation of circulation time between pulmonary alveoli and respiratory center, through increased sensitivity of the respiratory center to CO2, diminished sensitivity of the respiratory center to CO2 and O2-deficit, local blood flow disturbances. Other forms of PB may rise from lesion of pathways in the brain stem with disinhibition of basic rhythms, brain immaturity, alterations of consciousness, and respiratory obstructions. Rhythmic changes of the heart rhythm, of excitability of the heart muscle, of blood pressure, of EEG, and of neurological and mental signs may accompany PB/CSR.

1.5 Appendix: A Brief Dictionary of Breathlessness

Herein, the current definitions of the main terms pertaining to PB/CSR will be provided. For the sake of clarity, these definitions will be repeated in Chap. 9, dealing with the techniques used to diagnose and classify breathing disturbances in HF.

A reduction $\geq 90\%$ of airflow, compared to baseline, and lasting for ≥ 10 s is named *apnea*. The apneas can be *central* (in case of the contextual absence of airflow and respiratory movements), *obstructive* (when the absence of airflow is coupled to the presence of thoracic and abdominal movements), or *mixed* (usually starting as central apnea and ending as obstructive) [21].

A hypopnea is defined as a reduction of airflow $\geq 30\%$ for ≥ 10 s, together with either $\geq 3\%$ arterial oxygen desaturation or an arousal; a distinction between central and obstructive hypopneas is not usually performed, albeit being relevant from a pathophysiological point of view [21].

The *respiratory disturbance index (RDI)* corresponds to the average number of apneas, hypopneas, and respiratory event-related arousals per hour of sleep; its calculation requires an EEG recording and then the use of PSG. The diagnosis of OSAS is made when a RDI cut-off (usually ≥ 10) is reached [21].

The *apnea-hypopnea index (AHI)* is calculated as the number of apneas and hypopneas per hour of estimated sleep time. AHI values are categorized as normal (0–4), mild sleep apnea (5–14), moderate sleep apnea (15–29), and severe sleep apnea (≥ 30) [21].

PB is a pattern of periodical waxing and waning of tidal volume characterized by hypopneas and an AHI ≥ 15. As stated above, when central apneas are present, the proper definition is *CSR* [22].

References

1. Foster M. A text book of physiology. 3rd ed. London: Macmillan; 1879.
2. Gibson GA. Cheyne-Stokes respiration. Edinburgh: Oliver and Boyd; 1982.
3. Hunter J. Original cases. Library of Royal College Surgeons of England; 1781.
4. Cheyne J. A case of apoplexy, in which the fleshy part of the heart was converted into fat. Dublin Hosp Rep. 1818;2:216–23.
5. Stokes W. The diseases of the heart and the Aorta. Dublin: Hodges and Smith; 1854. p. 323–6.

6. Hartridge H, editor. Bainbridge and Menzies's essentials of physiology. 9th ed. London: Longmans; 1940.
7. Biot MC. Contribution a l'étude du phenomene respiratoire de Cheyne-Stokes. Lyon: Lyon Med; 1876.
8. Luciani L. Fisiologia dell'uomo (Human physiology). 6th ed. Milan: Società editrice libraria; 1923.
9. Tyndall J. In: Rhys E, editor. Glaciers of the alps and mountaineering in 1861, Everyman's library. London: Dent; 1906.
10. Sinclair E. Annales de l'Observatoire Meteorologique du Mont Blanc. Paris: G. Steinheil; 1893.
11. Mosso A. Life of man in the high Alps. London: T. Fisher Unwin; 1894.
12. Clarke A. Harper's practical genetic counselling. 8th ed. Boca Raton: CRC Press; 2014.
13. Ward M. Periodic respiration. A short historical note. Ann R Coll Surg Engl. 1973;52:330–4.
14. Pitt GN, Pembrey MS, Allen RW. Observations upon Cheyne-Stokes' respiration. Med Chir Trans. 1907;90:49–82.15.
15. Stewart GN, Edin MD. A manual of physiology with practical exercises. 6th ed. New York: Wood W & Co; 1910.
16. Howell WH. A text-book of physiology for medical students and physicians. 7th ed. Philadelphia: Saunders; 1919.
17. Chokroverty S. Atlas of sleep medicine. 2nd ed. Philadelphia: Elsevier; 2014.
18. Tomita Y, Kasai T, Kisaka T, Rossiter HB, Kihara Y, Wasserman K, Daida H. Altered breathing syndrome in heart failure: newer insights and treatment options. Curr Heart Fail Rep. 2015;12:158–65.
19. Naughton MT. Cheyne-Stokes respiration: friend or foe? Thorax. 2012;67:357–60.
20. Naughton MT. Respiratory sleep disorders in patients with congestive heart failure. J Thorac Dis. 2015;7:1298–310.
21. Berry RB, Budhiraja R, Gottlieb DJ, Gozal D, Iber C, Kapur VK, Marcus CL, Mehra R, Parthasarathy S, Quan SF, Redline S, Strohl KP, Davidson Ward SL, Tangredi MM, American Academy of Sleep Medicine. Rules for scoring respiratory events in sleep: update of the 2007 AASM manual for the scoring of sleep and associated events. Deliberations of the Sleep Apnea Definitions Task Force of the American Academy of Sleep Medicine. J Clin Sleep Med. 2012;8:597–619.
22. Lorenz R, Ito A. The definition of "Cheyne-Stokes rhythms". Acta Neurochir (Wien). 1978;43:61–76.

Mechanics and Chemistry of Respiration in Health

2

A Synopsis of the Regulation of Breathing

Claudio Passino, Elisabetta Cacace, Daniele Caratozzolo, Federico Rossari, and Luigi Francesco Saccaro

Abbreviations

ATP	Adenosine triphosphate
CCHS	Congenital central hypoventilation syndrome
CNS	Central nervous system
C_P	Transpulmonary compliance
C_T	Thoracic compliance
C_{TP}	Thoracopulmonary compliance
DPG	Diphosphoglycerate
DRG	Dorsal respiratory group
E1	First phase of expiration
E2	Second phase of expiration
early-I	Early inspiratory
Eaug	Expiratory augmenting
ERV	Expiratory reserve volume

C. Passino (✉)
Institute of Life Sciences, Scuola Superiore Sant'Anna, Pisa, Italy

Division of Cardiology and Cardiovascular Medicine, Fondazione Toscana Gabriele Monasterio, Pisa, Italy
e-mail: passino@ftgm.it

E. Cacace • D. Caratozzolo • F. Rossari • L.F. Saccaro
Institute of Life Sciences, Scuola Superiore Sant'Anna, Pisa, Italy
e-mail: e.cacace@sssup.it; d.caratozzolo@sssup.it; f.rossari@sssup.it; l.saccaro@sssup.it

© Springer International Publishing Switzerland 2017
M. Emdin et al. (eds.), *The Breathless Heart*,
DOI 10.1007/978-3-319-26354-0_2

FEV1	Forced expiratory volume in 1 s
FRC	Functional residual capacity
GABA	Gamma-amino butyric acid
GPR4	G-protein coupled receptor 4
HbA	Haemoglobin A
HCVR	Hypercapnic ventilatory response
HVR	Hypoxic ventilatory response
Iaug	Inspiratory augmenting
IRV	Inspiratory reserve volume
J receptor	Juxtacapillary receptors
late-I	Late inspiratory
NBCe	Electrogenic sodium/bicarbonate cotransporters
NO	Nitric oxide
nNOS	Neural nitric oxide synthase
NTS	Nucleus tractus solitarii
P_{ao}	Alveolar pressure
P_{BS}	Pressure at body surface
P_L	Transpulmonary pressure
P_{pl}	Intrapleural pressure
PCs	Peripheral chemoreceptors
P_{TT}	Transthoracic pressure
post-I	Post-inspiratory
pre-I	Pre-inspiratory
PRG	Pontine respiratory group
R	Relaxed
RARs	Rapidly adapting receptors
RTN	Retrotrapezoid nucleus
RV	Residual volume
SIDS	Sudden infant death syndrome
T	Tense
TASK	TWIK-related acid-sensitive K^+ channel
TEA	Tetraethylammonium
VC	Vital capacity
V_T	Tidal volume

2.1   Introduction

The aim of this chapter is to review the structure and function of the human respiratory system and to outline its key regulatory components. We further describe how ventilation is modulated by neural and chemical cues under physiological conditions, focusing on the interplay between central and peripheral chemoreceptors.

By respiration, we refer to its physiological concept, which encompasses the uptake of oxygen from the air and its transport to the cells and the transport of carbon dioxide from tissues to lungs. Physiological respiration comprises breathing, which is called ventilation in organisms with lungs and includes inspiration (inhalation) and expiration (exhalation).

Pulmonary ventilation corresponds to the so-called tidal volume multiplied by the respiratory rate, thus equalling roughly 6 l per min at rest (500 ml multiplied by 12 breaths per minute). Alveolar ventilation equals the air volume that flows in and out of the alveoli participating to gas exchanges in 1 min. Thence, it corresponds to the difference between the tidal volume and the anatomic dead space (i.e. the volume of the airways that are not involved in gas exchanges) multiplied by the respiratory rate.

The main function of the respiratory system is gas exchange between the external environment and blood, but the features of the respiratory system also perform immunitary and endocrine functions, notably by producing the angiotensin-converting enzyme. Furthermore, the air passage through the upper airways is responsible for vocalization.

2.2   Functional Pulmonary Anatomy and Mechanics of Ventilation

2.2.1   Functional Pulmonary Anatomy

Ventilation is ensured by the air passage from the nasal cavity or the mouth to the lungs, through the airways, i.e. the pharynx, the larynx, the trachea, the bronchi and the bronchioles [1, 2]. The tracheobronchial tree can be considered as a series of 23 generations of airway branches that undergo a dichotomic division at each generation, starting from the trachea (generation 0) until the alveolar sacs (generation 23). From a functional point of view, airways can be divided into a conducting zone, which contributes to moisten, filter and warm the inspired air; and a respiratory zone, where gas exchange occurs. The conducting zone comprises the nose, the mouth, the pharynx, the larynx, the trachea and the first 16 generations of bronchi and bronchioles (until terminal bronchioles). Here, pathogens and potentially irritating particles are removed by the mucociliary clearance system, i.e. the rhythmic beating waves of epithelial cilia and the mucus that is secreted by epithelial goblet cells and submucosal glands. The conducting zone is thus filled with gas that never reaches the exchange areas, i.e. the alveoli, and is called dead space air (about 150 ml).

The respiratory zone includes the respiratory bronchioles, the alveolar ducts, the alveolar sacs and roughly 300–400 million alveoli. The total surface responsible for gas exchange equals approximately 75 m^2.

2.2.1.1 Pulmonary Volumes

Airflow is determined by volumetric variations of the thoracic cavity, with the deepest inspiration corresponding to maximum lung expansion. The main pulmonary volumes are:

1. Tidal volume (V_T), i.e. the amount of air, on average 500 mL, that is inspired or expired during quiet breathing
2. Inspiratory reserve volume (IRV), about 3,000 mL, that can be added to V_T with forced inspiration
3. Expiratory reserve volume (ERV), usually 1,000–1,500 mL, i.e. the maximum volume of expired air, besides V_T
4. Residual volume (RV), which equals to about 1,000 mL that cannot be displaced even with forced expiration

Other pulmonary volumes have been defined, such as FEV1 (forced expiratory volume in 1 s), a widely used proxy measurement of airway narrowing, being typically low in patients with bronchoconstriction.

Pulmonary capacities are defined as the sum of two or more pulmonary volumes. The most widely considered ones are:

1. The inspiratory capacity, which equals the V_T plus the IRV. This capacity is the amount of air that a person can breathe in starting from a normal expiration and reaching the maximum amount of lung distension upon inspiration. Its approximate value is 3,500 ml.
2. The functional residual capacity corresponds to the sum of the ERV and the RV. It is defined as the quantity of air in the lungs at the end of a normal expiration (around 2,300 ml)
3. The vital capacity (VC) equals the IRV plus the V_T plus the ERV. This capacity corresponds to the greatest amount of air that can be exhaled from the lungs after a maximum inspiration and a maximum expiration (approximately 4,500 ml)
4. The total lung capacity is the amount of air contained in the lungs at the end of a maximum inhalation. It equals the VC plus the RV.

2.2.1.2 Respiratory Muscles

Every ventilatory act comprises two phases: inspiration and expiration. Inspiration is relatively short (about 2 s) and is determined by the contraction of principal inspiratory muscles, i.e. the *intercostales externi* and the diaphragm. The first ones are located in each intercostal space and run obliquely downward and forward from the upper to lower ribs. They are innervated by the intercostal nerves, branches of the thoracic spinal nerves. Their concerted action lifts the rib cage and increases the anteroposterior diameter of the chest cavity [2, 3].

However, the expansion of the thoracic cavity at rest is mostly due to the longitudinal expansion caused by the diaphragm. This is a dome-shaped muscle that separates the thoracic and the abdominal cavities. A trefoil leaf-shaped central tendinous aponeurosis offers insertion to lumbar and costal diaphragm components that respectively originate from the lumbar vertebrae and the arcuate ligaments and from the last ribs and the xiphisternum. The diaphragm is innervated by the phrenic nerve that originates from the 4th cervical nerve, but also receives contributions from the 3rd and 5th cervical nerves in humans. When contracted, the diaphragm lowers (1–10 cm) and lengthens transversally, with a behaviour described as that of a piston in an expanding cylinder. Therefore, it synergizes with the movement of the rib cage, enabling lung expansion.

Upon forced inspiration the load on principal inspiratory muscles increases and accessory muscles are recruited. Under hyperventilation conditions of about 50 l/min, muscles such as the *sternocleidomastoideus*, the *trapezius*, the *serratus*, the vertebral column extensors and the *pectoralis minor* collaborate in expanding the thoracic cavity, usually reversing their normal insertions and origins. Upward movement of the rib cage is supported by the *scalenes*, three symmetric muscles (middle, anterior, posterior) which arise from the cervical vertebrae and insert onto the first two ribs. Other accessory muscles are found in the back, such as the *levatores costarum* muscles, as well as in the head and neck. During inspiration, negative pressure would cause the collapse of the laryngopharynx if *genioglossi, geniohyoidei, sternohyoidei* and *sternothyreoidei* muscles were not active in keeping the pharynx patent.

During quiet breathing, expiration is prompted by the relaxation of inspiratory muscles, which lets the elastic recoil of lungs and rib cage shrink the thoracic cavity. Expiration is usually longer than inspiration, but can be shortened in heavy breathing. In this case, expiratory and abdominal muscles contraction reduces the thoracic volume through compression of the viscera, thus accelerating air expulsion. Expiratory muscles, i.e. the *intercostales interni*, the *subcostales* and the *transversus thoracis* muscles lower and pull back the ribs and the sternum, reducing the thoracic volume.

2.2.1.3 Pulmonary Circulation

The pulmonary circulation comprises two systems: the functional pulmonary circulation (*vasa publica*) and the trophic pulmonary circulation (*vasa privata*).

The functional pulmonary circulation is defined as a low-resistance, high-volume and low-pressure circulatory system. Pulmonary arteries divide into branches in a parallel fashion to the airways: deoxygenated blood flows from the right ventricle in the pulmonary trunk, which branches into two pulmonary arteries. Once in the lungs, pulmonary arteries undergo a series of tree-like divisions, until the alveolar capillary bed where gas exchange occurs. Since pulmonary arteries receive the whole cardiac output, they are characterized by a large compliance (about 7 ml/mmHg), due to their short length, large diameters and extensible walls. Pulmonary veins are also thin walled and highly compliant. Both pulmonary arteries and veins display a much smaller amount of smooth muscle than their counterparts in the systemic circulation. Oxygenated blood flows back to the left atrium through the four pulmonary veins.

The nutritive pulmonary circulation is represented by the bronchial vessels. The bronchial arteries, branches of the thoracic aorta, accompany and perfuse bronchi and bronchioles, together with lung connective tissue, visceral pleurae and the walls of pulmonary vessels. Small bronchial veins are affluents of the azygos vein on the right, while the left side may drain into the left superior intercostal vein or into the accessory hemiazygos vein. However, part of the bronchial venous blood mixes with the oxygenated blood that flows in the pulmonary veins, thus contributing to the so-called "anatomical shunt", together with the Thebesian veins, i.e. small coronary vessels that drain in the left ventricle. The main consequence of this shunting is that the arterial pO_2 is slightly lower than the alveolar pO_2.

2.2.2 The Mechanical Substrate of Respiration

2.2.2.1 Resistances
Respiratory muscles exert physical work against elastic and non-elastic resistances [3].

Inspiration is an active action, where respiratory muscles must overcome just the lung elastic resistances, performing a positive work. During expiration, in contrast, the work of respiratory muscles is negative, as restful expiration is based on elastic recoil only.

During exercise, the increase in ventilation produces an increase in the tidal volume and in the respiratory rate. In addition to elastic resistances, also viscous and inertial resistances must be faced in this condition, increasing the energy consumption.

In fact, high tidal volumes and low respiratory rates enhance the elastic components of resistances, while non-elastic ones are increased at higher respiratory rates. The physiological respiratory rate at rest (12 breaths per minute) is an optimal trade-off between these two extremes.

Elastic Resistances
During inspiration, the energy employed to win elastic resistances is stored as potential energy and released during expiration. The elastic resistances include the elastic recoil due to elastin fibres of the lung stroma and the surface tension at the air-surfactant interface in the alveoli, discussed later. Upon forced ventilation, the work of expiratory muscles contributes to a quick increase in pressure.

Non-elastic Resistances
Non-elastic resistances comprise inertia, viscous tissue deformation and airways frictional resistance. Inertia is due to the considerable mass of air and of rib cage components, all of which have an inertia, collectively defined as *inertance*, which increases with respiratory rate. Viscous tissue deformation is a viscoelastic form of resistance, which is traditionally modelled as a dashpot: in addition to normal elastic deformations, almost all biological tissues show a time-dependent response to a force; the faster the deformation rate, the higher the resistance. Quick and intense forces are thus slowed down and dampened as by a dashpot. The last component of non-elastic resistance is due to airways conformation: according to Poiseuille's law for a straight and non-branched pipe, considering airways length and air viscosity as constant, airways resistance depends on the fourth power of the radius. Therefore,

approximating each airway segment as an ideal tube, at distal branchings, where airways total surface is at its highest, resistance and laminar flux velocity are low, while in the trachea air velocity is higher and pressure is concurrently reduced, keeping the flow rate constant.

Turbulent Flux Resistances
While the laminar flux previously considered exists mainly in smaller bronchioles, the air flow in the trachea and in the bigger bronchi is predominantly turbulent, because of the length and the irregular lining of airways. Hence, friction against the walls becomes a major resistance component, and mucus is a crucial factor in smoothing out irregularities.

2.2.2.2 Pulmonary, Thoracic and Thoracopulmonary Compliances
The whole thoracopulmonary system can be considered as composed by three spaces (alveolar, intrapleural, atmospheric) and two limiting structures or containers (lungs and rib cage, each one having its own elastic properties).

Referring to these spaces, we can define three pressures: (1) the *transpulmonary pressure* (P_L), which equals the difference between the alveolar (P_{ao}) and the intrapleural pressure (P_{pl}); (2) the *transthoracic pressure* (P_{TT}), that corresponds to the difference between the intrapleural and the atmospheric pressure at the body surface (P_{BS}); (3) the *transmural pressure*, which equals the algebraic sum of transpulmonary and transthoracic pressure [1].

The P_L equals 4 mmHg at the end of a quiet expiration, when the alveolar pressure is 0 mmHg and the intrapleural pressure is −4 mmHg: at this pulmonary volume (equivalent to the FRC) no force is acting on the alveolar or the pulmonary tissue, so this is the pulmonary equilibrium volume. When external forces produce a change in intrapleural pressure, P_L increases or decreases, ensuring alveolar distension. P_L is the expression of pulmonary elastic recoil: the effectiveness of P_L in determining volumetric variations in response to external forces is defined as compliance, i.e. the change in volume (ΔV) of a structure for each unit change in pressure (ΔP). When referred to the isolated lung specifically, it is called *transpulmonary compliance* (C_P).

An analogous *thoracic compliance* (C_T) can be defined as well, considering volumetric variations in response to P_{TT} variations. The P_{TT} is responsible for the expansion of the rib cage and is equivalent to the P_{pl} if thoracic wall muscles are relaxed, being P_{BS} normally equal to 0. Upon inspiration, the pressure exerted by muscles is negative, thus reducing P_{TT}, while the opposite occurs during expiration.

The transmural pressure is the pressure exerted by the whole thoracopulmonary complex on the air volume contained in the lung, i.e. the difference between P_{ao} and P_{BS}. Being P_{BS} normally equal to 0, the transmural pressure should correspond to the pressure that would be measured inside the alveoli. The elastic forces of the rib cage and the pulmonary tissues limit extreme volumetric variations for minimum and maximum values of VC. This results into a variation of *total* (i.e. *thoracopulmonary*) *compliance* (C_{TP}) depending on different volumes: C_{TP} is at its highest for volumes ranging between FRC and RV, and is very low at extreme volumes [1].

2.2.2.3 The Intrapleural Pressure

Volumetric changes of the rib cage produce negative or positive pressures, depending on the ventilatory phase [4]. The pressure is uniformly transmitted to the lungs thanks to the parietal and visceral pleural leaflets. Without the pleurae, uneven expansions or contractions would rupture the lungs. The intrapleural cavity is located between the two leaflets: it is a virtual space (10 µm) normally filled with a serous fluid that is filtered by the capillaries of the parietal leaflet and reabsorbed by the parietal leaflet stomata and by the visceral leaflet. This fluid reduces the friction between the membranes and maintains the negative pressure that keeps lungs expanded. The space between parietal and visceral pleurae is at subatmospheric pressure (-5 cmH$_2$O), i.e. a relative vacuum. The intrapleural pressure (P_{pl}) is maintained by osmotic and lymphatic reabsorption of interstitial fluid and by the elastic structure of rib cage and lungs.

2.3   Pulmonary Gas Exchange

2.3.1   Alveolar Structure, Surfactant and Alveolar Gas Exchange

In one second, about 80 ml of blood undergo gas exchange with atmosphere. In order to achieve this, the blood-atmosphere barrier must fulfil two requirements: a wide overall surface and a negligible thickness (about 0.5 µm). The human blood-atmosphere barrier is located at the interface between the alveoli and the pulmonary capillaries. The alveolocapillary membrane comprises 6 layers: (1) the alveolar liquid lining given by the surfactant; (2) the alveolar epithelium (made of type I and II pneumocytes); (3) the epithelial basal membrane; (4) a virtual interstitial space; (5) the capillary endothelial basal membrane and (6) the endothelium itself. The two basal membranes and the interstial space are virtually fused together.

Gas exchange occurs by diffusion. The gas displacement across the membrane is dependent on Fick's law, which states $Q = D*A/T * \Delta P$, where Q equals the gas flow across the membrane, D is a diffusion coefficient specific for each gas, A is the exchange surface area, T is the thickness of the interface and ΔP is the difference between the gas partial tensions in the alveoli and in the lumina of capillaries [2]. Another important factor is the time of contact between blood and air at the alveolocapillary interface: at rest the time that blood takes to flow through a pulmonary capillary is 0.75 s, which is redundant if compared to the time required for O_2 and CO_2 diffusion (0.25 s for oxygen, even less for carbon dioxide, whose D is 20 times higher).

The A/T ratio cannot be directly measured, but it is usually inferred in clinical practice by applying Fick's law to CO administration and diffusion across the alveolocapillary membrane. This is possible given that the CO capillary partial tension is normally 0 and its alveolar amount is known, thus reducing the ΔP component of the equation to the CO administered amount that can be found in the alveoli.

An essential component of the alveolocapillary membrane is the surfactant layer: the surfactant is a proteolipidic tensioactive fluid that is produced by type II pneumocytes. When the air enters the alveoli, alveolar pressure increases: according to Laplace's law, such a rise in the alveolar ΔP would cause a steep reduction in the radius of the alveoli, if superficial tension were constant. Surfactant lipidic components instead reduce the superficial tension, thereby avoiding alveolar collapse [2].

2.3.2   The Ventilation to Perfusion Ratio in Physiological and Pathological Conditions

The ventilation to perfusion ratio (V/Q) is defined as the ratio between the amount of air that reaches the alveoli in 1 min and the blood flow through the pulmonary circulation expressed in l/min (which is equivalent to the cardiac output). In normal conditions, V is equal to 4 l of air per minute and Q to 5 l of blood per minute, their ratio is 0.8.

The V/Q ratio increases from lung bases to the apices: three zones can be identified considering different V/Q ratio values. Zone 1 corresponds to alveoli that are located in the pulmonary apices: in a standing subject, the gravity force counterbalances the blood flow to the upper alveoli, until the apex, where the blood pressure may not be sufficient to keep capillaries patent (although this does not normally occur in healthy lungs). Indeed, for every centimetre of distance in height from the heart level, the pressure in pulmonary arterial vessels decreases by 0.74 mmHg.

Zone 2 extends to those alveoli with a sufficient blood pressure to avoid a capillary stenosis on the arterial side but not on the venous one, resulting in a temporary interruption of the blood flow until the pressure on the arterial side overcomes the alveolar pressure and restores capillary blood flow.

Finally, most alveoli are efficiently perfused and ventilated, with a continuous blood flow, pertaining to zone 3.

As perfusion rises from zone 1 to zone 3, the most prominent contribution in blood efflux to pulmonary veins comes from zone 3. On the other hand, more oxygenated blood flows from zone 1 and zone 2. The ventilation to perfusion ratio (V/Q) has been conceived as a quantitative parameter to describe this phenomenon.

2.3.3   Modulation of Gas Transport by Haemoglobin

Approximately 98 % of blood oxygen is combined with haemoglobin, while 2 % is freely dissolved in plasma. Oxygen solubility in water is low, but it can be increased by transport proteins, such as haemoglobin (HbA). Deoxyhaemoglobin has low affinity for oxygen and a compact structure due to many loose electrostatic interactions. This is defined as *tense* (T) conformation, in contrast to the *relaxed* (R) conformation of oxyhaemoglobin. In fact, when oxygen binds the iron atom of one haeme, it partially displaces a valine residue, causing the breakage of some weak interactions of haemoglobin subunits. Hence, binding of each oxygen molecule loosens the whole tetramer structure, exposing other haeme groups to further linkage with oxygen. This property is defined as *cooperative effect*: the sigmoid shape of the curve that plots oxyhaemoglobin percentage against pO_2, i.e. the haemoglobin dissociation curve, is due to this mechanism [3, 5].

The haemoglobin dissociation curve is rightward shifted by low pH values, higher temperature, increased 2,3 biphosphoglycerate (2,3 DPG) and high CO_2 concentration (Bohr effect). Protons bind to haemoglobin inducing new hydrogen bonds that stabilize T conformation. The curve is rightward shifted in tissues, where pH is lower, pCO_2 is higher: haemoglobin affinity to oxygen thus drops down in tissues, where a greater release of oxygen is usually required. Conversely, in lungs, where pH is higher and pCO_2 is lower, haemoglobin affinity to oxygen is higher, promoting the formation of oxyhaemoglobin.

The haemoglobin dissociation curve is also leftward shifted by hypothermia, which increases haemoglobin affinity for oxygen, and by low CO_2 concentration and 2,3 DPG. To modulate haemoglobin affinity to oxygen, haemoglobin is allosterically regulated by 2,3 DPG. The enzyme DPG mutase catalyses the formation of 2,3 DPG from 1,2 DPG, a glycolysis intermediate, while DPG phosphatase catalyses the inverse reaction. Higher pH values enhance mutase activity and inhibit the phosphatase, ultimately increasing oxygen release. Regulation of DPG synthesis is crucial, for instance, for adaptation to pO_2 variations at different altitudes.

2.3.3.1 CO_2 Transportation

Haemoglobin also carries CO_2 and H^+. However, a finer mechanism indirectly involves haemoglobin also in CO_2 transport in blood, as acid bicarbonate. As a matter of fact, deoxyhaemoglobin easily binds protons. Hence in tissues, where oxygen concentration is low, deoxyhaemoglobin removes from blood 40 % of total protons. Since these are ultimately a product of carbonic anhydrase reaction, the equilibrium shifts towards the production of bicarbonate and higher concentration of CO_2 are stored in blood. The opposite is true in the lungs, where CO_2 is released to be expired.

Since CO_2 is more soluble in water than oxygen, a small portion of total CO_2 (about 5 %) is dissolved in blood, even though only about 10 % of exhaled CO_2 comes from this source.

About 90 % of total blood CO_2 is found as carbamino compounds with aminic groups of haemoglobin or plasma proteins.

2.4   Central Control of Ventilation

Ventilation is controlled by an automatic rhythm generated within the brainstem to accomplish the main task of keeping arterial blood PO_2, PCO_2 and pH approximately constant. Although the specific site harbouring the central pattern generator is still unknown, the firing rates of some neurons seem related to precise phases of the respiratory cycle. Inspiratory neurons are those showing increased firing frequency of action potential during inspiration, whereas expiratory ones fire primarily during expiration. Functionally, they represent a heterogeneous population of interneurons, upper motor neurons (premotor neurons) and lower motor neurons that control respiratory muscles. Those neurons are grouped into three main subdivisions: dorsal and ventral respiratory groups within the *medulla oblongata* and pontine respiratory one.

Dorsal respiratory group (DRG) is bilateral and consists of a specific portion of *nucleus tractus solitarii* (NTS) and other neurons in adjacent areas of the posterior medulla. Mainly premotor inspiratory neurons, which project to contralateral lower motor neurons of inspiratory muscles, compose this group. In particular, DRG provides the main contribute to the generation of basic respiratory rhythm. Moreover, it represents the visceral sensory termination of cranial nerves IX and X, which convey afferent signals from peripheral receptors for respiratory reflexes [6].

Ventral respiratory group (VRG), instead, is located anterolaterally to the dorsal one in both sides of the medulla. It contains interneurons, upper and lower motor neurons, both inspiratory and expiratory, which are organized into three regions with specific functions: rostral, intermediate and caudal [1, 6].

The rostral portion consists of the majority of Bötzinger complex, which governs the expiratory activity of the caudal VRG [1, 3, 6].

The intermediate region comprises the *nuclei ambiguus* and *para-ambigualis*, which contain somatic motor neurons that reach musculature of the upper airways via cranial nerves IX and X to dilate them during inspiration. In addition, Bötzinger complex projects into the intermediate region with the so-called pre-Bötzinger complex, whose pacemaker neurons contribute to the generation of the respiratory rhythm [1, 3, 6].

The caudal section, instead, is represented by premotor neurons grouped within *nucleus retroambigualis*. Their axons leave the brainstem to contact spinal motor neurons that innervate expiratory muscles. Signals from the Bötzinger complex control caudal VRG and thus expiration as well [1, 3, 6].

Pontine respiratory group (PRG) is a pivotal modulator of respiratory outputs, but it is not involved in their generation. It is located in the posterior *pons*, consisting of neurons interspersed within reticular formation magnocellular nuclei, caudally, and *nuclei parabrachialis medialis* and Köllinker-Fuse, rostrally. Since a *midpons* transection leads to increased pulmonary volume after inspiration and decreased respiratory rate, the caudal PRG is also known as apneustic centre, meaning that it can cause apneusis. On the other hand, apneusis is prevented by signals from the rostral PRG, which is hence named pneumotaxic centre as it coordinates respiration [1, 6].

Each of the above groups contains neurons showing characteristic firing patterns that are interrelated with the others to establish the respiratory cycle. These include early inspiratory, inspiratory augmenting, late inspiratory, post-inspiratory, expiratory augmenting and pre-inspiratory (or post-expiratory) neurons (Fig. 2.1) [1, 3].

They have specific distribution within respiratory *nuclei* and are functionally different, carrying out specific tasks:

- Inspiratory augmenting (Iaug) neurons show an increasingly higher firing rate during inspiration, followed by a sudden and progressive decrease in the first phase of expiration (E1) to definitively cease during its second phase (E2). This

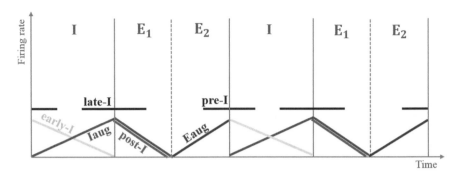

Fig. 2.1 Characteristic firing patterns of respiratory neurons within two consecutive breathing cycles. Each cycle is subdivided into inspiration (*I*), first (*E1*) and second (*E2*) part of expiration. Legend: *Iaug* inspiratory augmenting (*grey*), *early-I* early inspiratory (*yellow*), *late-I* late inspiratory (*purple*), *post-I* post-inspiratory (*green*), *Eaug* expiratory augmenting (*red*), *pre-I* pre-inspiratory (*brown*)

peculiar pattern of action potential is transferred to the phrenic nerve, so that also the diaphragm can show a contraction profile that traces that of Iaug neurons.

Nuclei para-ambigualis and *tractus solitarii* contain mainly premotor Iaug neurons. Their firing rate is modulated by chemoreceptors that respond to partial pressure variations of arterial blood gases and pH.

- Early inspiratory (early-I) neurons maximally fire at the beginning of inspiration, and then progressively slow down, becoming resting in both E1 and E2. Early-I are primarily located in *nucleus para-ambigualis* and seem to be premotor neurons of upper airway dilators or to control them.
- Late inspiratory (late-I) neurons are located in the same *nuclei* of Iaug ones and act as "switch-off" neurons. Actually, the former show constant firing rate across the end of inspiration and the start of E1, switching off Iaug neurons.
- Post-inspiratory (post-I) neurons show decrementing frequency of action potential during E1, whereas are silent during the rest of the cycle. They are "switch-off" neurons as well, but inhibit also expiratory augmenting neurons, which start firing only when post-Is cease their activity. Post-I neurons are dispersed in DRG, receive from peripheral receptors and project to various *nuclei*.
- Expiratory augmenting (Eaug) neurons fire with a ramp pattern only during E2, both in quiet and forced expiration. They are mainly localized in *nucleus retroambigualis* and act as both interneurons, to keep Iaug silent and premotor neurons, reaching the contralateral anterior horn of the spinal cord to synapse with lower motor neurons of expiratory muscles.
- Pre-inspiratory (pre-I) neurons, harboured in the Bötzinger and pre-Bötzinger complex, show an approximately constant firing rate over E2 and inspiration, so as to cease Eaug discharge.

As shown, specific firing rates of two different neural populations set the pace for as many expiratory phases, E1 and E2. The muscular counterpart adapts to this staging as a consequence.

The central pattern generation of breathing relies on mutual and mainly inhibitory connections among different classes of respiratory neurons. Neuronal populations connected one another with inhibitory synapses bring about alternating firing rates thanks to adaptation to their reciprocal discharges. The latter is due to specific calcium and calcium-activated potassium channels found on the cell surface of the above neurons. However, also rebound depolarization and tonic excitatory inputs from reticular formation of the brainstem and peripheral receptors contribute to the pattern generation [1, 6, 7].

After the generation of the central pattern of breathing, excitation is transferred to the respiratory muscles with peculiar pattern of activation and a short delay: upper airway dilator muscles are the first to be recruited in inspiration, showing a constant or decrementing pattern of activation. 50 to 100 ms later, the phrenic nerve activates the diaphragm with a ramp profile. Immediately after, intercostal muscles start to contract cranio-caudally with a similar ramp pattern. In normal breathing, muscular activity in expiration is confined in E1: a residual contraction of the diaphragm counteracts lung elastic recoil, and recruitment of upper airway constrictor muscles increases resistance against the airflow and slows down the efflux. In forced expiration, instead, expiratory muscles contract during E2 to speed up the air outflow.

When the airway resistance increases because of an obstructive state, the contraction of the upper airways dilators abnormally anticipates diaphragm contraction, which is strengthened if compared to normal breathing. Air inflow becomes oral rather than nasal, and the outflow is facilitated by the recruitment of dilators also in expiration. Finally, inspiratory accessory muscles and expiratory muscles are engaged within the respiratory cycle.

The bulbo-pontine generator of the respiratory rhythm is involved in several reflex pathways rising from peripheral receptors.

Pulmonary and respiratory tract receptors exert a feedback regulation via vagal afferents on final inspiratory volume, to optimize pulmonary compliance and respond to irritation. These receptors are classified into:

• Pulmonary stretch receptors
• Rapidly adapting receptors (RARs)
• Juxtacapillary (J) receptors

The first ones, located into bronchial smooth musculature, are slowly adapting and innervated by large myelinated fibers with high speed of conduction. These receptors mediate the Hering-Breuer reflex: their firing rate increases with pulmonary volume, usually when this exceeds 500 mL, to activate brainstem "switch-off" neurons, which block inspiration and reduce respiratory rate. As corollary functions, stretch receptors make expiratory motor neurons more excitable, inhibit upper airway dilators and cause bronchodilation and tachycardia. However, this reflex shows a triggering threshold modifiable by other afferents: hypercapnia, hypoxia and acidosis revealed by chemoreceptors, in addition to signals from proprioceptors, can decrease the sensibility of the above mechanism, so that both respiratory rate and volume increase [2, 3].

RARs, instead, are polymodal receptors within the tracheobronchial epithelium that fire bursts of action potentials, characterized by fast adaptation, in response to several mechanical and chemical *stimuli*: rapid airflow, irritant chemicals, such as particulates or inflammatory mediators, and local oedema. The signal is conveyed at low speed by vagal myelinated fibers to the NTS, where it triggers reflexes such as coughing, sighing, bronchoconstriction and abundant mucus secretion in the airways [1, 3].

Finally, J receptors represent nervous terminations of unmyelinated C fibers around pulmonary capillaries. These receptors also respond to chemical and mechanical *stimuli* by releasing tachykinin. This neuropeptide has two main functions: first, it induces local irritation, and second it activates RARs causing cough. J receptors convey the above information to the brain medulla to activate reflexes aimed at inducing broncho- and laryngo-constriction and tonic contraction of inspiratory muscles, resulting in inspiratory apnoea. This seems to be a protective reflex against potential dangers for the respiratory tract [1, 3].

Other key peripheral receptors involved in reflex control of breathing are chemoreceptors, whose function will be described in further details in next section, and proprioceptors of respiratory muscles, namely muscle spindles and Golgi tendon organs, both innervated by fibers of the phrenic nerve. These proprioceptors prevent respiratory muscles from being excessively contracted or stretched. In addition, muscle metaboreceptors sensible to tissue PO_2, PCO_2, pH and potassium ion concentration can block inspiration in response to muscle fatigue. All these reflexes preserve integrity of respiratory musculature.

Furthermore, other peripheral receptors exert a mild regulation on respiratory rhythm. As a case in point, the vagus nerve conveys information from the gastrointestinal tract to NTS to modify the diaphragm contraction in particular conditions, such as deglutition and vomiting. Other regulatory afferents to the central generator of respiration arise from baroreceptors: substantial risings in arterial blood pressure cause an earlier block of inspiration, thus apnoea, whereas its collapse results in hyperventilation.

The central pattern generation of breathing can also be controlled by descending fibers from upper nervous structures that are mainly connected to PRG. The motor cortex adapts breathing to specific tasks, i.e. phonation, singing and voluntary hyper or hypoventilation, whereas the locomotor pattern generation to rhythmic actions such as running and swimming. Besides, the hypothalamus is responsible for changes in ventilation that naturally occur after physical and emotional perturbations. [1, 3, 6, 7].

2.5 Functional Architecture of Chemoreceptive Control of Ventilation

Among the different cues that modulate ventilation, chemical modifications play an essential role in breathing regulation, in the homeostasis of blood acid–base balance, in cardiorespiratory integration and in the autonomic regulation of heart function (Fig. 2.2).

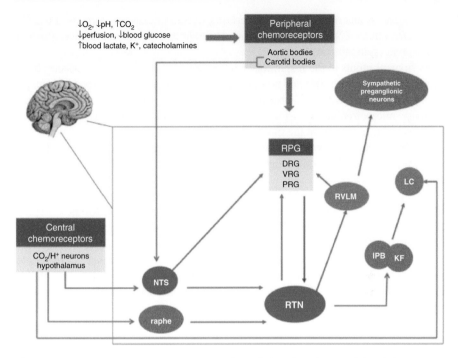

Fig. 2.2 Architecture of the chemical control of ventilation. Cues from peripheral chemoreceptors are conveyed via the chemoreflexes to the respiratory centre. Peripheral chemoreceptors are located in the aortic bodies and carotid bodies. Central chemoreception likely relies both on CO_2-sensitive neurons spread all over the brain and on the retrotrapezoid nucleus (RTN) in the brainstem, which can sense pH and CO_2 changes either directly or indirectly via glial cells. The RTN receives inputs from carotid bodies through the NTS (nucleus of the solitary tract), from the raphe and from the hypothalamus, where $CO_2/H+$ sensitive neurons are located. Efferent projections from the RTN include those directed to the RPG (respiratory pattern generator), which are ultimately responsible for respiratory rate adjustments in response to CO_2 modifications. This effect can also be mediated by RTN projections to the RVLM (rostral ventrolateral medulla), which modulate the activity of RPG neurons and the sympathetic tone on cardiovascular system. A feedback circuit holds between the RTN and the RPG, which in turn sends projections back onto the RTN. Arousal reactions to hypercapnia are probably mediated by the projections of RTN to the lPB (lateral parabrachial nucleus) and to the KF (Kölliker-Fuse nucleus), which further forward signals to the LC (locus coeruleus). Many projections connect the lateral hypothalamus to other chemosensitive areas, such as the LC, the NTS, the RPG, the RTN and the rMR (rostral median raphe). These projections might be responsible for a tonic stimulation during wakefulness. Caudal raphe in turn sends projections to the pre-Bötzinger complex (pBC)
KF Kölliker-Fuse nucleus, *LC* locus coeruleus, *lPB* lateral parabrachial nucleus, *NTS* nucleus of the solitary tract, *pBC* pre-Bötzinger complex, *rMR* rostral median raphe, *RTN* retrotrapezoid nucleus, *RPG* respiratory pattern generator, *RVLM* rostral ventrolateral medulla

Chemical modifications are sensed by chemoreceptors and conveyed by chemoreflexes. An increase in $PaCO_2$ or H^+ concentration or a decrease in PaO_2 elicit an increase in the level of the respiratory neuron activity in the medulla, while opposite changes trigger a slight decrease in the level of activation of these neurons.

The general anatomical circuit underlying chemoreflexes are composed by: (1) sensors/receptors; (2) afferent (parasympathetic) fibers; (3) an integrative centre and (4) efferent (sympathetic) fibers.

Peripheral inputs to the respiratory centre comprise chemoreflexes, arising from peripheral chemoreceptors, and non-chemical reflexes, arising from the upper respiratory tract, from the lung, C-fibre endings related to bronchial circulation and pulmonary microcirculation (J-receptors), phrenic nerve afferents, baroreceptor reflexes and afferents from the musculoskeletal system.

During normal unlaboured breathing (eupnoea), the concerted action of chemoreflexes keeps $PaCO_2$ within a tight range, centred on a physiological set-point of about 40 mmHg [8].

Chemoreceptors provide a tonic stimulus to breathe, continuously adjusting ventilation to $PaCO_2$ fluctuations [9, 10]. Reciprocal interactions control the interplay between chemoreflexes, arousal and sleep: in fact, chemoreflexes are state-dependent and, conversely, chemoreceptor stimulation produces arousal. Small fluctuations around the $PaCO_2$ set-point have no impact on the state of vigilance. Large acute increases in $PaCO_2$ (from diving, sleep apnoea, bronchial disease or airway blockade), instead, elicit arousal from sleep and noxious sensations in awake subjects (i.e. dyspnoea, urge to breathe, panic) [11, 12].

Conversely, arousal and negative emotions can stimulate breathing and support the hypercapnic ventilatory response [11, 13, 14].

Many questions on the integration of peripheral and central chemical inputs are still open, especially on the location and features of central chemoreception circuits.

2.5.1 Peripheral Chemoreceptors

Peripheral chemoreceptors (PCs) are located bilaterally in the carotid bodies and in the aortic bodies. However, aortic bodies do not play a substantial role in the hypoxic ventilatory responses, only producing a slight increase in the respiratory rate upon hypoxic stimuli.

Carotid bodies are about 6 mm^3 in volume and can be found close to the bifurcation of the common carotid artery. Accordingly to their role, their perfusion rate is very high – about 10 times the level that would be proportional to their metabolic rate, which is itself quite high, and 20 times the perfusion of the brain. The arterial/venous pO_2 difference is thus very small, and the outgoing blood can be considered as arterial.

The cell types that can be found in the carotid bodies are type 1 cells (glomus cells), of neuroectodermal origin, and type II cells (sustanticular, sheath or glomoid cells), whose function is unknown.

Every type 1 cell is in contact with the synaptic endings of neurons located in the petrosal ganglion of the glossopharyngeal nerve. The nerve branch that transports these afferent inputs is the carotid sinus nerve or Hering's nerve. Efferent nerves only account for 5 % of the nerve endings on glomus cells: they modulate receptor-afferent discharge and comprise preganglionic sympathetic fibers from the superior cervical ganglion.

Discharge rate in the afferent nerves from the carotid bodies increases in response to a decrease in PaO_2 or pH, a rise in $PaCO_2$, a perfusion drop-down, a decrease in blood glucose concentration or an increased blood concentration of lactate, potassium, and catecholamines [15]. The response is rapid (1–3 s) and consists in an increase in both the respiratory rate and the depth of breathing.

The whole hypoxic ventilatory response and about 1/3 of the hypercapnic ventilatory response upon normoxia conditions are controlled by PCs [16].

The way hypoxia triggers the release of neurotransmitters from glomus cells is not fully elucidated: two theories respectively postulate the presence of a K^+ channel which is at the same time an O_2 sensor, and a haeme or related protein (cytosolic or mitochondrial) which acts as an O_2 sensor, thus eliciting the activation of the glomus cells upon modifications of the redox state [17].

The glomus cells express many neurotransmitters, notably ATP, acetylcholine, dopamine, adenosine, serotonin, GABA and histamine [18]. In particular ATP and acetylcholine have been proposed as putative transmitters for carotid sinus nerve chemoexcitation, the first one acting on P2X2/3 postsynaptic ionotropic receptors and the second one binding post- and pre-synaptic nicotinic receptors.

Efferent pathways comprise inhibitory stimuli triggered by NO released by nNOS-positive glossopharyngeal fibers.

The chemoexcitation of Hering's nerve is then integrated in the nucleus of the solitary tract, which also relays inputs from pulmonary mechanoceptors, coordinating them with other areas of the brainstem respiratory network. The efferent component of this chemoreflex circuit is the phrenic nerve and nerves arising from the cervical, thoracic and lumbar plexus that rhythmically activate the respiratory musculature.

2.5.2   Central Chemoreceptors

Current opinion on the architecture of central chemoreception is recently undergoing a reinterpretation, where two views are currently accepted: according to the first model, central chemoreception is based on direct effects of H^+ distributed throughout the CNS. Many evidences support such a picture, which can explain the non-respiratory effects of CO_2 (i.e. aversive, behavioural and arousal effects) [11, 14, 19].

However, according to another emerging model, the hyperventilation response triggered by slight increase in CO_2 is instead mediated by a direct effect of protons on the carotid bodies, that are centrally integrated, and few brainstem structures, such as the retrotrapezoid nucleus (RTN) and a subset of serotoninergic neurons [20]. Early studies mapped central chemoreceptor location bilaterally on the rostral, intermediate and caudal zones of the ventrolateral surface of the medulla oblongata [21], distinct from VRG and DRG. Targeted inhibition approaches have recently identified more precise neuronal phenotypes within the medullary region, i.e.

glutamatergic neurons in the retrotrapezoid nucleus, noradrenergic neurons of the locus coeruleus, serotoninergic neurons within the medullary raphe and purinergic receptors responding to ATP near the ventral surface. Among these populations, glutamatergic neurons in the retrotrapezoid nucleus are the most likely candidates for the role of key chemoreceptive components: in fact genetic lesion of the RTN or deletion of two proton detectors expressed by RTN neurons (TASK-2 and GPR4) nearly abolishes the hypercapnic ventilatory response [20, 22, 23].

RTN role is further supported by the induction of congenital central hypoventilation syndrome (CCHS) upon mutations of the homeodomain transcription factor Phox2b, which is expressed by all CO_2-responsive RTN neurons.

In contrast, locus coeruleus and orexin neurons of the lateral hypothalamus are rather involved in aversive sensation and arousal from sleep following large acute increases in CO_2 [24] .

Probably both views can hold, with a more prominent role for RTN neurons in central chemoreception coexisting with a large network of pH, CO_2 and HCO_3^--sensing sites spread all over the brain.

This is consistent with the evidence that ventilation cannot be considered as a unique function of extracellular pH, thus suggesting that other cues, such as CO_2, act as independent inputs [25].

Cellular targets for these factors have been identified as TWIK-related acid-sensitive K^+ (TASK) for extracellular pH and tetraethylammonium (TEA)-sensitive K^+ channels for intracellular pH. A putative CO_2 sensor has been postulated, but not demonstrated in central chemoreceptors (while in carotid bodies it activates L-type calcium channels [26]).

Serotoninergic neurons within the medullary raphe magnus probably play a major role as chemoreceptors as well. Many evidences are supporting this hypothesis: (1) the activation of such neuron populations stimulates ventilation; (2) the hypercapnic ventilatory response is depressed when serotoninergic neuron development is impaired, when serotoninergic neurons are globally pharmacogenetically inhibited; (3) these neurons exhibit a pronounced state dependence, with higher discharge rate during active waking and silencing during REM sleep.

It remains unclear how serotonin actually modulates chemoreflexes: although CO_2-responsive neurons are diffusely present in various raphe nuclei, serotonin might act on CO_2 sensors located elsewhere, facilitating respiratory reflexes triggered in other areas than the raphe. This hypothesis is supported by the evidence that serotonin can fully rescue the ventilatory impairment caused by inhibition of lesions of such serotoninergic neurons [27].

CO_2-sensitive astrocytes in the medulla oblongata might also play a role in central chemosensitivity. In fact, these astrocytes display CO_2-induced ATP release and acid-induced depolarization. ATP released by pH-sensitive astrocytes could further activate RTN neurons via ATP P2Y receptors and possibly an electrogenic sodium-bicarbonate transporter (NBCe) that moves bicarbonate into the cells, further enhancing extracellular acidification and RTN neuron depolarization [28].

Central chemoreceptors are responsible for approximately 2/3 of the hypercapnic ventilator response upon normoxia conditions [24]. Rises of 1 mmHg in $PaCO_2$

determine an increase in ventilation of about 2 l per min (40%). Other cues that stimulate central chemoreceptors are falls in pH of the cerebrospinal fluid.

2.5.3 Key Features of Chemoreflexes

2.5.3.1 Hypoxic Ventilatory Response (Fig. 2.3)

Respiratory rate increases upon drops in O_2 concentration in the inspired air. This effect is more striking at pO_2 values lower than 60 mmHg and paradoxically depressed during severe hypoxia (pO_2 <20 mmHg). However, hyperventilation increases pH and reduces pCO_2, which in turn counteracts the HVR. Therefore, the increase in the respiratory rate occurs only when the hypoxic stimulus is strong enough to overcome the inhibitory effect of increased pH and reduced pCO_2. Deoxygenated haemoglobin is also a weaker acid than HbO_2, so falls in Hb saturation determine an increase in blood pH, which also counteracts the HVR [29–31] .

Severe CNS hypoxia can also elicit a powerful stimulation of breathing called autoresuscitation, whose hallmark is gasping. Gasping is constituted by a short sequence of intense inspiratory efforts that either restores normal breathing and oxygenation or precedes death. Its physiological substrate is an increased INaP (persistent sodium current) in lower brainstem respiratory

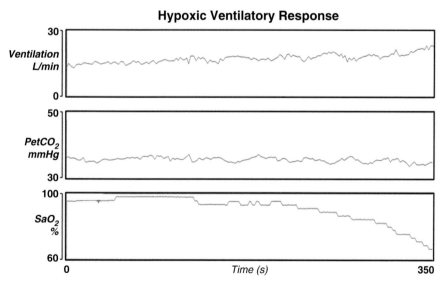

Fig. 2.3 Example of a hypoxic ventilator response (*HVR*) performed using the rebreathing technique. From *top to bottom*: breath-by-breath minute ventilation end tidal partial pressure of carbon dioxide signal and oxygen saturation. The subject is connected to a rebreathing circuit through a mouthpiece and experiences progressive isocapnic hypoxia (from resting oxygen saturation values to 70–80%, according to individual tolerance), end-tidal CO_2 being kept at baseline value, by passing a portion of the expired air into a scrubbing circuit before returning it to the rebreathing bag. The linear regression slope between minute ventilation and SaO_2 expresses the HVR

neurons, possibly facilitated by serotonin [32, 33] and ATP release from astrocytes [34]. The gasping response might be compromised in the sudden infant death syndrome (SIDS) [35].

Exercise enhances the response to hypoxia even when the pCO_2 is not increased, probably through lactic acidosis, afferent inputs from muscles or catecholamine secretion. Indeed, this hyperventilation induces a fall in $PaCO_2$ that is highly beneficial in curbing lactic acidosis [36].

2.5.3.2 Hypercapnic Ventilatory Response (Fig. 2.4)

The normal response to $PaCO_2$ rises is hyperventilation that ceases when the $PaCO_2$ is brought back to normal levels as a result of the increased rate of CO_2 pulmonary extraction. This mechanism ensures that $PaCO_2$ levels are maintained at around 40 mmHg. However, set-points of ventilatory equilibrium can be established around different values: this is what happens for instance in case of CO_2 inhalation, when prominent rises in the pCO_2 of the inspired air lead to slight changes in the alveolar pCO_2. In this case, the $PaCO_2$ does not fall to normal values and stands at a new, higher set-point. Yet when the CO_2 content of the inspired air is more than 7%, hyperventilation response is not adequate to maintain alveolar and arterial pCO_2 in a range compatible with life, thus inducing central nervous system depression and CO_2 narcosis [29, 31].

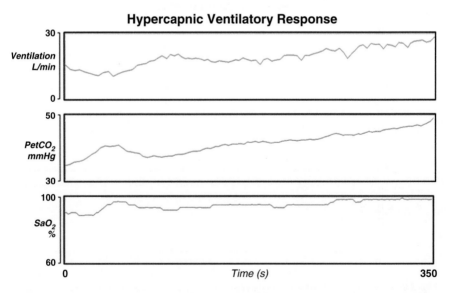

Fig. 2.4 Example of a hypercapnic ventilator response (*HCVR*) performed using the rebreathing technique. Same signals and setting as in Fig. 2.2. The subject undergoes progressive normoxic hypercapnia (from resting end-tidal CO_2 values until 50 mmHg or an increase ≥ 10 mmHg from the basal values, according to individual tolerance), inspired partial pressure of O_2 being kept at baseline value by adding oxygen to the circuit. The linear regression slope between minute ventilation and end-tidal pressure of CO_2 expresses the HCVR

2.5.3.3 Integration of Central and Peripheral Chemoreflexes

Although peripheral chemoreceptors mostly respond to hypoxia and central chemo-receptors mainly sense hypercapnia, such a segregation between the functions of different chemoreceptors would surely be limiting. Indeed, it has been demonstrated that respiratory responses cannot be considered as the mere algebraic sum of the individual effects produced by $PaCO_2$, PaO_2 and pH [20].

The HVR is modulated by CO_2 levels and HCVR is conversely regulated by pO_2 levels: for higher alveolar pCO_2, the pO_2 threshold for hyperventilation elicitation is lower, i.e. the HVR is enhanced by elevated pCO_2 and triggered at values lower than 60 mmHg.

Likewise, in case of lower alveolar pO_2, the HCVR is more abrupt in its onset, i.e. the respiratory rate undergoes a more prominent increase in response to pCO_2 increases. HCVR is also influenced by the pH, being anticipated at lower pCO_2 thresholds in case of metabolic acidosis, and deferred to higher pCO_2 values in case of alkalosis.

These considerations justify the evidence that ventilatory responses in asphyxia are greater than the sum of expected responses to pCO_2 rises or pO_2 falls when considered separately.

During hypoxia, the increase in respiratory rate elicited by carotid body stimulation is counterbalanced by a reduction in RTN neuronal activity produced by the concomitant alkalosis.

Conversely, the RTN neuron impact to breathing is more prominent when carotid bodies are not stimulated, such as in hyperoxia, thus reducing the respiratory deficits.

References

1. Conti F, Battaglia-Mayer A. Section 4: Sistema Respiratorio. In: Fisiologia medica, Vol. 2, Milano: Ed. Ermes; 2010. pp. 239–79; 381–405.
2. Hall J, Guyton A. Chapter 38: Pulmonary ventilation. In: Textbook of medical physiology. Philadelphia: Saunders; 2011. pp. 497–502; 539–45.
3. Lumb AB, Pearl RG. Part 1: Basic principles. In: Nunn's applied respiratory physiology, 6th ed. Edinburgh: Elsevier Health Sciences; 2005. pp. 12–4; 25–79; 174–80.
4. Charalampidis C, Youroukou A, Lazaridis G, Baka S, Mpoukovinas I, Karavasilis V, et al. Physiology of the pleural space. J Thorac Dis. 2015;7 Suppl 1:S33–7.
5. Nelson D, Lehninger A, Cox M. Chapter 5.1: Reversible binding of a protein to a ligand: oxygen-binding proteins. In: Lehninger principles of biochemistry. 5th ed. New York: W.H. Freeman; 2008. p. 158–72.
6. Boron WF, Boulpaep EL. Chapter 32: Control of ventilation. In: Medical physiology. 2nd updated ed. St. Louis: Elsevier Health Sciences; 2012, pp. 725–45.
7. Kandel ER, Schwartz JH, Jessell TM, Siegelbaum SA, Hudspeth J. Principles of neural science. 5th ed. New York: McGraw Hill Professional; 2013. p. 1031–6.
8. Duffin J, Bechbache RR, Goode RC, Chung SA. The ventilatory response to carbon dioxide in hypoxic exercise. Respir Physiol. 1980;40:93–105.
9. Blain GM, Smith CA, Henderson KS, Dempsey JA. Contribution of the carotid body chemo-receptors to eupneic ventilation in the intact, unanesthetized dog. J Appl Physiol. 2009;106:1564–73.

10. Dempsey JA, Smith CA, Blain GM, Xie A, Gong Y, Teodorescu M. Role of central/peripheral chemoreceptors and their interdependence in the pathophysiology of sleep apnea. Adv Exp Med Biol. 2012;758:343–9.

11. Kaur S, Pedersen NP, Yokota S, Hur EE, Fuller PM, Lazarus M, et al. Glutamatergic signaling from the parabrachial nucleus plays a critical role in hypercapnic arousal. J Neurosci. 2013;33:7627–40.

12. Parshall MB, Schwartzstein RM, Adams L, Banzett RB, Manning HL, Bourbeau J, et al. American Thoracic Society Committee on Dyspnea. An official American Thoracic Society statement: update on the mechanisms, assessment, and management of dyspnea. Am J Respir Crit Care Med. 2012;185:435–52.

13. Hu J, Zhong C, Ding C, Chi Q, Walz A, Mombaerts P, et al. Detection of near-atmospheric concentrations of CO_2 by an olfactory subsystem in the mouse. Science. 2007;317:953–7.

14. Taugher RJ, Lu Y, Wang Y, Kreple CJ, Ghobbeh A, Fan R, et al. The bed nucleus of the stria terminalis is critical for anxiety-related behavior evoked by CO_2 and acidosis. J Neurosci. 2014;34:10247–55.

15. Kumar P, Prabhakar NR. Peripheral chemoreceptors: function and plasticity of the carotid body. Compr Physiol. 2012;2:141–219.

16. Gonzalez C, Almaraz L, Obeso A, Rigual R. Carotid body chemoreceptors: from natural stimuli to sensory discharges. Physiol Rev. 1994;74:829–98.

17. Prabhakar NR, Peng YJ. Peripheral chemoreceptors in health and disease. J Appl Physiol. 2004;96:359–66.

18. Nurse CA. Neurotransmitter and neuromodulatory mechanisms at peripheral arterial chemoreceptors. Exp Physiol. 2010;95:657–67.

19. Nattie E, Comroe Jr JH. Distinguished lecture: central chemoreception: then … and now. J Appl Physiol. 2011;110:1–8.

20. Guyenet PG, Bayliss DA. Neural control of breathing and CO_2 homeostasis. Neuron. 2015;87:946–61.

21. Loeschcke HH. Central chemosensitivity and the reaction theory. J Physiol. 1982;332:1–24.

22. Kumar NN, Velic A, Soliz J, Shi Y, Li K, Wang S, et al. Regulation of breathing by CO_2 requires the proton-activated receptor GPR4 in retrotrapezoid nucleus neurons. Science. 2015;348/6240:1255–60.

23. Ruffault PL, D'Autréaux F, Hayes JA, Nomaksteinsky M, Autran S, Fujiyama T, et al. The retrotrapezoid nucleus neurons expressing Atoh1 and Phox2b are essential for the respiratory response to CO_2. eLIFE. 2015;4:e07051.

24. Nattie E, Li A. Central chemoreception 2005: a brief review. Auton Neurosci. 2006;126–127:332–8.

25. Lassen NA. Is central chemoreceptor sensitive to intracellular rather than extracellular pH? Clin Physiol. 1990;10:311–9.

26. Summers BA, Overholt JL, Prabhakar N. CO_2 and pH independently modulate L-type Ca2+ current in rabbit carotid body glomus cells. J Neurophysiol. 2002;88:604–12.

27. Hodges MR, Tattersall GJ, Harris MB, McEvoy SD, Richerson DN, Deneris ES, et al. Defects in breathing and thermoregulation in mice with near-complete absence of central serotonin neurons. J Neurosci. 2008;28:2495–505.

28. Erlichman JS, Leiter JC. Glia modulation of the extracellular milieu as a factor in central CO_2 chemosensitivity and respiratory control. J Appl Physiol. 2010;108:1803–11.

29. Ganong WF. Review of medical physiology, vol. 36. 21st ed. New York: Lange Medical Books/ McGraw- Hill; 2003. p. 675–85.

30. Duffin J. Measuring the ventilatory response to hypoxia. J Physiol. 2007;584:285–93.

31. Duffin J. The chemoreflex control of breathing and its measurement. Can J Anaesth. 1990;37:933–42.

32. Peña F, Parkis MA, Tryba AK, Ramirez JM. Differential contribution of pacemaker properties to the generation of respiratory rhythms during normoxia and hypoxia. Neuron. 2004;43:105–17.

33. Tryba AK, Peña F, Ramirez JM. Gasping activity in vitro: a rhythm dependent on 5-HT2A receptors. J Neurosci. 2006;26:2623–34.
34. Marina N, Tang F, Figueiredo M, Mastitskaya S, Kasimov V, Mohamed-Ali V, et al. Purinergic signalling in the rostral ventro-lateral medulla controls sympathetic drive and contributes to the progression of heart failure following myocardial infarction in rats. Basic Res Cardiol. 2013;108:317.
35. Darnall RA. The carotid body and arousal in the fetus and neonate. Respir Physiol Neurobiol. 2013;185:132–43.
36. Forster HV, Haouzi P, Dempsey JA. Control of breathing during exercise. Compr Physiol. 2012;2:743–77.

Hypopneas and Apneas as Physiological and Pathological Phenomena Throughout the Life Span

3

Pediatric Apneas, Diverse Central Apneas, and Obstructive Apneas

Alberto Giannoni, Chiara Borrelli, and Valentina Raglianti

Abbreviations

AD	Alzheimer's disease
AF	Atrial fibrillation
AHI	Apnea/hypopnea index
AHVR	Acute hypoxic ventilatory response
ALS	Amyotrophic lateral sclerosis
ALTE	Apparent life-threatening event
ANP	Atrial natriuretic peptide
AOP	Apnea of prematurity
ASV	Adaptive servo ventilation
BIPAP	Bilevel positive airway pressure
BMI	Body mass index
CA	Carbonic anhydrase
CAI	Central apnea index
CB	Carotid body
CBS	Cerebral blood flow
CHF	Chronic heart failure
CIH	Chronic intermittent hypoxia
CKD	Chronic kidney disease

A. Giannoni (✉) • V. Raglianti
Division of Cardiology and Cardiovascular Medicine,
Fondazione Toscana Gabriele Monasterio, Pisa, PI, Italy
e-mail: alberto.giannoni@ftgm.it; v.raglianti@outlook.it

C. Borrelli
Life Science Institute, Scuola Superiore Sant'Anna, Pisa, Italy
e-mail: c.borrelli@sssup.it

© Springer International Publishing Switzerland 2017
M. Emdin et al. (eds.), *The Breathless Heart*,
DOI 10.1007/978-3-319-26354-0_3

CM	Chari malformation
CLF	Cerebrospinal fluid
CNS	Central nervous system
COPD	Chronic obstructive pulmonary disease
CPAP	Continuous positive airway pressure
CRP	C reactive protein
CSA	Central sleep apnea
CSF	Cerebrospinal fluid
CSR	Cheyne-Stokes respiration
CTEPH	Chronic thromboembolic pulmonary hypertension
DTI-MRI	Diffusion tensor imaging-magnetic resonance imaging
EEG	Electroencephalography
eICA	Extracranial internal carotid artery
ESRD	End stage renal disease
FD	Fabry disease
GABA	Gamma-aminobutyric acid
GFR	Glomerular filtration rate
GG	Genioglossus
HCVR	Hypercapnic ventilatory response
HF	Heart failure
HVD	Hypoxic ventilatory depression
HVR	Hypoxic ventilatory response
ICSA	Idiopathic central sleep apnea
IL6	Inteleukin 6
KT	Kidney transplant
LC	Locus coeruleus
LG	Loop gain
LV	Left ventricle
MAD	Mandibular advancing device
MCI	Mild cognitive impairment
MRI	Magnetic resonance imaging
MSA	Multisystem atrophy
MRSA	Muscle-related sleep apnea
MS	Multiple sclerosis
NFT	Neurofibrillary tangles
NHD	Nocturnal hemodialysis
NIV	Noninvasive ventilation
NOT	Nocturnal oxygen therapy
NREM	Sleep nonrapid eye movement
NSVT	Nonsustained ventricular tachycardia
OSA	Obstructive sleep apnea
$PaCO_2$	Arterial partial pressure of carbon dioxide
PaO_2	Arterial partial pressure of oxygen
AP	Positive atrial pressure
PAP	Pulmonary arterial pressure
PB	Periodic breathing
PH	Pulmonary hypertension

PPH	Precapillary pulmonary hypertension
PVR	Pulmonary vascular resistance
PWP	Precapillary wedge pressure
REM	Rapid eye movement
ROS	Reactive oxygen species
RTN	Retrotrapezoid nucleus
RVLM	Rostro ventrolateral medulla
RVSP	Right ventricular systolic pressure
SDB	Sleep disordered breathing
SIDS	Sudden infant death syndrome
SUDEP	Sudden unexpected death in epilepsy
TNFa	Tumor necrosis factor alpha
UA	Upper airway
UPPP	Uvulopalatopharyngoplasty
VA	Ventilatory acclimatization
VE	Ventilation
VE/VO$_2$ slope	Ventilation/oxygen output slope
WHO	World Health Organization

3.1 Introduction

Central and obstructive apneas are respiratory disturbances that may affect patients with different underlying conditions, from cardiac and pulmonary to neurological affections. In this chapter, we will discuss the principal clinical scenarios associated with hypopneas and apneas throughout the life span, and we will mainly focus on the physiology/pathophysiology of these respiratory disturbances.

Apparently, different physiologic states and pathologies are associated with different mechanisms of disease, and thus the relationship between each background condition and hypopneas/apneas may vary from one case to the other. This has led to a fragmented view of the pathology and to a tendency to iteratively look at apneas from the same angle, depending on the expertise and field of interest of every single clinician. Indeed, a cardiologist with a specific interest on Cheyne-Stokes respiration (CSR) of heart failure patients would preferentially focus on chemoreflex overactivity and prolonged circulatory delay, with little attention to the acid-base balance, to possible concomitant neurological disorders, or changes in pulmonary function/hemodynamics. However, it is possible that some key mechanisms may be concealed in different clinical scenarios and determine the onset and maintenance of ventilatory instability, despite being apparently unrelated to the main patient pathology.

Therefore, the aim of the present chapter is to avoid the short-sightedness related to a monotonous perspective by cardiologists, neurologists, neonatologists, nephrologists, sleep specialists, and high-altitude physicians, recapitulating and integrating their different experiences to stimulate a synergistic and open approach of researchers in the field of apneas/hypopneas. A comprehensive view of all the apneas that could occur throughout the life span is summarized in Table 3.1.

Table 3.1 Comprehensive view of the pathophysiological mechanisms, clinical complications, and available treatment options for different types of apneas throughout the life span

Type of apnea	Age of onset	Clinical complications	Pathophysiological mechanisms	Therapy
AOP	Preterm Newborns	Cerebral damage due to intermittent hypoxia	Persistence of fetal breathing responses (e.g., biphasic response to hypoxia) ↓ Chemosensitivity to CO_2 ↑ Laryngeal chemoreflex	A2 agonists (methylxanthines, caffeine, theophylline) Bicuculline CPAP
PB of childhood	Newborns prior than 4 weeks of age	Considered almost benign	Peripheral chemoreceptor immaturity, ↑ sensitivity to hypoxia, narrow CO_2 apneic threshold	Usually untreated
SIDS	Infants within 6 months of age	Sudden death	Triple risk model[a]	Quit smoking during pregnancy Sleeping supine Treating AOP
Apnea at high altitude	Whenever ascending to high altitude	↓ Sleep quality ↑ Daytime sleepiness Memory loss, confusion ↑ Acute Mountain Sickness	Hyperventilation due to ↓ PaO_2 ↑ Chemosensitivity to CO_2 and O_2 ↓ Cerebrovascular flow and reactivity Pulmonary J receptors stimulation	O_2, CO_2 Acetazolamide Theophylline BDZ (less useful) CPAP Yoga
ICSA	Throughout the life span	Generally benign ↓ Quality of sleep	Chronic hyperventilation due to ↑ peripheral and central chemosensitivity	CO_2 Hypnoinducers (zolpidem)
CSA-CSR in neurologic conditions	Age of onset depends on the underlying pathology	↓ Quality of sleep and life hemodynamic consequences Brain damage	White matter changes Hypoxia and relative ischemia Brainstem infarction Cerebral edema AD and MS plaques in the brainstem	CPAP ASV Donepezil
OSA/MSA in neurologic conditions	Age of onset depends on the underlying pathology	↓ Quality of sleep and life hemodynamic consequences ↑ Brain damage	Damage of neuronal fibers of UA dilator muscles or weakness of UA dilators muscles in OSA Peripheral muscle weakness and dependency from diaphragmatic activity in MSA	CPAP Inspiratory/expiratory muscle training

CSA-CSR in kidney failure	Usually elderly	Negative hemodynamic consequences leading to hypertension or secondary CHF, arrhytmias and accelerated glomerulosclerosis	↑ Chemosensitivity to CO_2 and O_2 ↑ Brain damage ↓ Clearance of toxic molecules Volume overload/rostral fluid shift Uremia Inflammation	NHD KT CPAP
CSA-CSR in pulmonary hypertension	Early in group 1, late in group 2 and 3, variable in group 4 and 5	Worsening of pulmonary vascular reactivity and remodeling, further hypoxia, detrimental effects on RV overload and failure	Hypoxemia, RV overload and reduced cardiac output in all groups HF-related mechanisms (see Chaps. 4 and 5) for group 2	O_2 CPAP HF treatment in group 2
OSA	Childhood	Hyperactivity, reduced sleep quality, reduced school performance	Adenotonsillary hypertrophy and craniofacial abnormalities ↑ Adipose and lymphoid tissue around the neck Obesity	CPAP Weight loss Surgery for cranial abnormalities
	Elderly	CHF, hemodynamic consequences, increased sympathetic tone, reduced sleep quality, daytime sleepiness, increased risk of car accidents, increased incidence of metabolic syndrome and diabetes	Craniofacial abnormalities Obesity Inflammation Volume overload/rostral fluid shift Increased loop gain (chemosensitivity)	CPAP Surgery Oral appliance therapy O_2 Acetazolamide Eszopiclone Paroxetine

[a]Triple risk model: risk factors, autonomic imbalance (mainly depending on the serotonergic system), additional triggers (i.e., sleeping prone)

AD Alzheimer disease, *AOP* apnea of prematurity, *ASV* adaptive servoventilation, *BDZ* benzodiazepines, *CHF* chronic heart failure, *CPAP* continuous positive airway pressure, *CSA* central sleep apnea, *CSR* Cheyne-Stokes respiration, *ICSA* idiopathic central sleep apnea, *KT* kidney transplantation, *MS* multiple sclerosis, *MSA* Muscle related sleep apnea, *NHD* nocturnal hemodialysis, *OSA* obstructive sleep apnea, *PB* periodic breathing, *SIDS* sudden infant death syndrome

3.2   Pediatric Apneas and Sudden Infant Death Syndrome

3.2.1   Definition

Children may experience two types of breathing abnormalities of central origin: apnea of prematurity (AOP) and periodic breathing (PB). AOP is defined by the American Academy of Pediatrics as "an unexplained episode of cessation of breathing for 20 s or longer, or a shorter respiratory pause associated with bradycardia (in preterms heart rate <30 bpm), desaturation ($SpO_2 < 85\%$), cyanosis, pallor, and/or marked hypotonia." PB, instead, is defined as periods of regular respiration for as long as 20 s followed by apneic episodes of at least 10 s or less occurring at least three times in succession [1]. In addition, as in adults, children may also experience obstructive apneas (OSA).

3.2.2   Epidemiology

The prevalence of clinically overt AOP in infants in the United States is 0.5–0.6% of all newborns, while it reaches 2.3% in hospitalized children [2]. On the other hand, PB is very common in preterm babies born less than 28 weeks' gestation (75%), and it lowers as gestational time increases (down to 7% in babies born at 34–35 weeks) [3, 4]. PB cannot be observed in the 2–4 weeks after birth, a period in which the maturation of peripheral chemoreceptors happens [5]. Lastly, OSA show a bimodal pattern of presentation, with an increased prevalence in early childhood (2–6 years) and during adulthood [3].

3.2.3   Clinical Presentation, Risk Factors, and Complications

In general, the clinical manifestation of an apneic event in children is dramatic; therefore, in 1986, the National Institutes of Health Consensus Development Conference on Infantile Apnea and Home Monitoring created the term ALTE (apparent life-threatening event) to describe "an episode that is frightening to the observer and is characterized by some combination of apnea (central or occasionally obstructive), color change (usually cyanotic or pallid, but occasionally erythematous or plethoric), marked change in muscle tone (usually marked limpness), choking or gagging. In some cases, the observer fears that the infant has died" [6].

AOP babies that present with ALTE should be treated to prevent the risk for further neurological damage sustained by chronic intermittent hypoxia (CIH). Those infants, in fact, may already have comorbidities related to prematurity, such as infections and intracranial hemorrhages, and CIH may be an additive factor for damage progression [7]. However, longer-term complications of AOP have not been extensively studied.

ALTE episodes are also associated with sudden infant death syndrome (SIDS): 4–13% of SIDS patients had a history of apnea, even though there is no plain demonstration of the correlation between the two, and no appreciable reduction of ALTEs was found with the advent of "Back to Sleep Program" [8], a program that encouraged parents to put their babies to sleep supine, and not prone [9, 10]. This association could be due to the common risk factors shared between AOP and SIDS: reduced gestational age and weight at birth [11], alongside with immaturity of central respiratory controllers and lung physiology are by far the most studied ones [12]. However, other risk factors for SIDS were found that complicate its pathogenesis (low socioeconomical status, maternal history of smoking during pregnancy, abnormalities of the proinflammatory system and channelopathies that lead to prolonged QT syndrome) [13].

PB, on the other hand, is not generally clinically manifest and can be sometimes witnessed and/or documented by polysomography [14]. This phenomenon is thought to be almost benign and related to carotid body (CB) maturational process, low birth weight and prematurity (risk factors shared with SIDS and AOP, as explained above), and most of the times it wears off spontaneously with no known sequelae [15]. However, long-term consequences of pediatric PB have not been investigated, and nowadays it is not known whether it can account as a risk factor for future PB development in adults; even fewer data are available on the connection between AOP and PB even though, as stated above, some risk factors are shared between the two conditions.

Finally, OSA in children usually manifests with snoring, restless sleep, diaphoresis, enuresis, cyanosis, excessive daytime sleepiness, and behavior or learning problems; furthermore, witnessed apneas can be referred. In addition, signs of adenotonsillary breathing and/or facial abnormalities can be noted, which lead to mouth breathing, nasal obstruction, adenoidal facies, and hyponasal speech. Anatomical abnormalities (e.g., Down syndrome, palatoschisis) and adenotonsillary hypertrophy account for most of the risk factors for OSA in children, along with hypertension and obesity, the latter being responsible for the increased prevalence of OSA in children (from 2 % up to 5–10 %) [16]. As we will further explain in Sect. 3.3, obesity and hypertension play a major role in both inducing and maintaining a complex inflammatory status that is responsible for the perpetuation of the abnormality [17]. Long-term complications of untreated OSA are considerably better studied in the field of pediatric apneas; hemodynamic consequences, metabolic syndrome, increased insulin resistance, increased sympathetic activation, increased risk for type 2 diabetes mellitus, cor pulmonale, and loss of intellectual quotient are the ones that occur more frequently [18].

3.2.4 Pathophysiology

Preterm babies have reduced lung volume, hypoxemia, impaired respiratory reflexes and impaired response to hypoxia and hypercapnia due to immature central development, which are thought to be the major pathophysiological determinants of *AOP* [17]. Those babies demonstrate a particular response to hypoxia, called "biphasic response to hypoxia," which persists longer in life in preterm infants [19] (Fig. 3.1, panel a). When exposed to a hypoxic stimulus (FiO_2 from 21 % to 15 %),

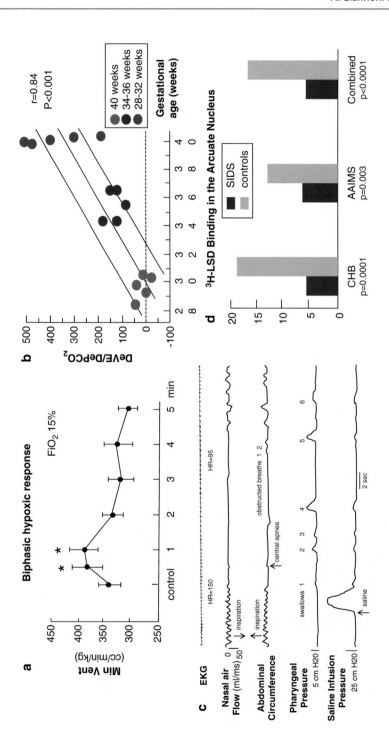

Fig. 3.1 Comprehensive mechanisms of Apnea of Prematurity (AOP) and Sudden Infant Death Syndrome (SIDS)

Panel a: Biphasic response to hypoxia is one of the main physiopathological determinants of apnea of prematurity (AOP). Preterm infants, in fact, demonstrate initially an increased response in ventilation in hypoxic conditions, and then a reduction due to persistence of fetal ventilatory responses (with permission from Martin et al., *J Pediatr*, 1998 [19])

Panel b: Reduced response to carbon dioxide is another key pathophysiological mechanisms for AOP development (with permission from Krauss et al., *Pediat Res*, 1975 [20]). Due to lung hypoplasia during uterine life, fetuses tend to reduce metabolism to prevent excessive O_2 consumption. In turn, decreased metabolism and/or decreased cerebral blood flow can be responsible for reduced CO_2 production and/or central responsiveness to CO_2

Panel c: Exaggerated laryngeal chemoreflex may also lead to apnea. In this panel, an apneic event in response to saline administration (*arrow; last row*) leads to central apnea (*arrow; second row*; with permission from Thach, *Am J Med*, 1997 [230]).

Panel d: Impaired serotonergic system is one of the main physiopathological determinants of AOP and SIDS. Reduced binding to the serotonergic receptor of the radioligand in the arcuate nucleus, coupled with immaturity of serotonergic neurons (not shown) is an index of underdevelopment of this system (with permission from Kinney, *Ped Develop Path*, 2005 [29]). CHB Children's Hospital Boston dataset, AAIMS Aberdeen Area Infant Mortality Study dataset, Combined CHB and AAIMS datasets combined there is first an increase and then a decrease in minute ventilation, which leads to further hypoxemia and apnea [1]. This response is thought to be for the first part due to CB stimulation, and then related to central inhibition of respiration in response to hypoxia. Central chemoception to CO_2 is also decreased in babies born preterm, prolonging the apneic period [20] (Fig. 3.1, panel b). These phenomena are thought to be due to the persistence of fetal responses to hypoxia and hypercapnia. In fact, due to lung hypoplasia during uterine life, fetuses tend to reduce metabolism to prevent excessive O_2 consumption [12]. In turn, decreased metabolism and/or decreased cerebral blood flow can be responsible for reduced CO_2 production and/or central responsiveness to CO_2. The reduced CO_2 production can in turn explain the extremely narrow gap between eupneic and apneic CO_2 threshold (1.3 mmHg vs. 3–4 mmHg in normal adults) [21], which can than be responsible for perpetuated unstable breathing. It is possible to speculate that those detrimental responses wear off with age due to lungs' development and maturation of central controllers [12].

Another important mechanism in the genesis of AOP is an exaggerated laryngeal chemoreflex response, which determines a decrease in ventilation up to apnea after the stimulation of the laryngeal mucosa [22] (Fig. 3.1, panel c). This exaggerated response is likely centrally based too, since no modification of laryngeal receptors or central connections have been described [7], while a decrease of the apneic response after utilization of central agents as theophylline has been shown [23]. Among the various neurotransmitters responsible for central integration of laryngeal chemoreflex information, GABA and adenosine are by far the most studied ones. GABA mediates respiratory inhibition in babies, a result confirmed by the finding that GABA-A receptors inhibition with bicuculline reverses GABA-induced apnea [24]. Adenosine too induces respiratory depression in newborn rabbits [25] and piglets [26], as opposed as what happens in adults. The physiological reason of this phenomenon is unknown; however, respiratory immaturity may be the cause. Adenosine and GABA pathways are extremely interconnected with each other. Wilson et al. demonstrated that adenosine-induced ventilatory depression can be reversed by the injection of either intraventricular or intramedullary GABA-A antagonist bicuculline. Moreover, adenosine receptors and GABA receptors are coexpressed in diverse medullary regions (raphé pallidus, rostro ventrolateral medulla, and gigantocellularis nucleus). These findings suggest that adenosine receptors are located on GABA neurons, thereby contributing to GABA-induced ventilatory depression. Furthermore, these findings are the pathophysiological correlates of antagonists (methylxanthines) employement in the treatment of neonatal respiratory disturbances [27].

Prematurity and central chemoreceptors impairment are also risk factors for the development of SIDS. However, according to the "triple risk model" proposed by Kinney and Filiano in 1994, the contextual imbalance of the autonomic and cardiovascular systems, coupled with the presence of triggering factors (i.e., infections, sleeping prone) are required for SIDS to happen.

The role of the autonomic system was first theorized because of demonstrated bradycardia and increased apnea time before the fatal event; many theories have been postulated to explain this phenomena, but the most compelling one is related to the impairment of the serotonergic system of the brainstem, because of its role in sleep, breathing, and autonomic regulation [28]. At least 50 % of SIDS cases show impairment in the serotonergic system as both nucleus arcuatus and the nuclei of the midline raphé are hypoplasic in SIDS children; neuronal loss has been described, along with cellular immaturity and reduced expression and/or binding to the serotonergic receptors 5HT1A [29] (Fig. 3.1, panel d). As those regions are involved in central sensitivity to carbon dioxide (CO_2), and since those regions are connected to effector nuclei of the sympatho-vagal system that play a major role in the arousal responses, especially to increased CO_2, it is reasonable to postulate that underdevelopment of this system plays a major role in the pathophysiology of SIDS [30, 31]. Hypoplasia and underdevelopment of the autonomic system, particularly the serotonergic system, determine reduced protective responses to stressors such as hypoxia or hypercapnia, leading to death. Moreover, it is interesting to notice how smoking during pregnancy is coupled with impairment of the medullary serotonergic system, thus contributing to the reduced chemosensitivity [28].

In PB pathophysiology, differently from AOP, a prominent role of peripheral chemoreceptors has been described [32]. Babies with PB, in fact, have lower PaO_2 compared to healthy controls, and breathe on the steep portion of the PaO_2/VE curve. Chronic intermittent hypoxia has been associated with inflammation [33], hyperplasia of CB [34] and, in turn, with increased sensitivity to hypoxia of the peripheral chemoreceptors. In addition, taking into consideration the narrow difference between apneic and eupneic CO_2 threshold (as explained above), it is possible to assume that increased ventilation in response to hypoxia and then relative hypocapnia can perpetuate unstable breathing and generate PB [32]. Differently from AOP, no modifications in the chemoreflex response to hypercapnia have been described in PB babies to our notice, making central chemoreceptors involvement unlikely [32].

On the other hand, the pathophysiology of OSA has been more thoroughly unraveled. There are three main pathophysiological actors of OSA development in children and adults alike (see also Sect. 3.3): anatomical malformations, metabolic conditions, and ventilatory instability. Children with OSA generally have craniofacial abnormalities and adenotonsillary hypertrophy, which play a pivotal role in airway occlusion [35]; however, recent data on surgical outcomes of adenotonsillectomy showed that 20 % of nonobese and 50 % of obese patients still manifest OSA despite surgery [36], suggesting that other mechanisms of disease are involved. Children with OSA are generally obese (especially visceral obesity) [37], and have increased parapharyngeal fat pads that mechanically occludes upper airways [38, 39]; moreover, they have higher adipokine levels and increased oxidative stress and inflammation (augmented NF-kB, IL-6, TNFa, PCR, HIFa expression), which can impact on retropharyngeal lymphoid tissue thus worsening UA occlusion [40]. Intermittent hypoxia due to intermittent UA occlusion may, in turn, impair cognitive and cardiovascular performances and increase sympathetic drive, leading to hypertension and impaired hemodynamics.

Moreover, the inflammatory status associated with hypoxia and obesity may itself impact on cardiovascular balance, inducing endothelial dysfunction and increasing sympathetic drive (for more details, please refer to Sect. 3.3) [41]. Finally, the ventilatory responses to both hypoxia ad hypercapnia have not been extensively studied. Although a trend to a decreased response to hypercapnia and hypoxia was found, together with impaired sleep arousal to hypercapnia [42], no definite statement can be made due to the small population recruited.

3.2.5 Treatment

In light of *AOP* pathophysiology, different therapeutical approaches have been investigated, by means of pharmacological and nonpharmacological treatments. Among different pharmacological agents used for AOP therapy, methylxanthines, namely theophylline and caffeine are the most used ones, as they reduce the apneic events in preterms [43] by stimulating the central respiratory centers [30] (possibly due to A2 receptors antagonism) and diaphragmatic contractility [44], according to the pathophysiological circuit we have previously described.

GABA antagonists such as bicuculline were also investigated in premature piglets after laryngeal stimulation and administration of CGS, an adenosine agonist. Bicuculline prevented laryngeal stimulation-induced apnea after CGS administration towards pre-CGS values and prevented phrenic frequency, inspiratory and expiratory time reduction. However, there was still a trend towards phrenic area and frequency reduction after laryngeal stimulation - even though to a lesser extent when compared to post-CGS administration – suggesting the need of further evaluation of bicuculline activity before testing the drug in humans [31]. In another study, bicuculline was administrated intracisternally in newborn piglets exposed to intermittent hypoxia, reversing hypocapnic ventilatory depression [26].

Among nonpharmacological treatments CPAP has been proposed in infants with AOP as it increases pulmonary volumes and functional residual capacity, thus decreasing loop gain (expression of ventilator instability) [17, 30]. Moreover, preterm babies often exhibit an occlusive component in their apneic episodes, making CPAP more efficient.

Finally, it is crucial that babies are put to sleep in a supine position, so as to decrease the risk of SIDS in those already particularly fragile infants [13].

With regard to *PB*, as we have previously reported, it is generally considered a benign condition and therefore it is not treated.

Finally, according to the American Academy of Pediatrics on Childhood, OSA children exhibiting signs of adenotonsillary hypertrophy should undergo surgical treatment with adenotonsillectomy. In addition to that, CPAP treatment is recommended for OSA children that either do not have adenotonsillary hypertrophy or cannot undergo surgery. Moreover, CPAP treatment is also recommended in case of OSA persistence after adenotonsillectomy. Weight loss should be strongly recommended to all children who are overweight or obese. Finally, intranasal corticosteroids are recommended in children with adenotonsillary hypertrophy in which surgery is contraindicated [17].

3.3 Diverse Central Apneas in Physiological and Pathological Conditions

3.3.1 Idiopathic Central Sleep Apnea

3.3.1.1 Definition

Idiopathic central sleep apnea (ICSA) is a respiratory disorder characterized by repetitive apneas during nighttime in absence of an identified underlying cause. The apneas must be of at least 10 s and they must be 85 % central in nature, according to the definition given by Xie et al. in 1994 [45]. The respiratory cycle length (apnea/hypopnea + hyperventilation) is lower in ICSA as compared to the Cheyne-Stokes respiration of heart failure (HF) (on average 35 s vs. around 70 s), with only a trend toward a reduced apnea length in ICSA (17.6 ± 1.1 versus 25.8 ± 2.1 s, p = 0.071), with similar time spent with $SaO_2 < 90$ %, but reduced maximal SaO_2 desaturation again in ICSA (minimum SpO_2: 88.3 ± 1.4 in ICSA vs. 83.1 ± 1.7 in HF, $p < 0.05$) [46].

3.3.1.2 Epidemiology and Clinical Presentation

Symptoms of ICSA include: nocturnal awakenings and insomnia, nocturnal choking, restless sleep, snoring, or excessive daytime sleepiness [45]. As previously stated, Xie et al. defined ICSA as nighttime apneas. However, considering the pathophysiology of the phenomenon (see also Sect. 3.2.1.3), it is likely that apneas may occur also during the daytime.

3.3.1.3 Pathophysiology

In ICSA subjects, a higher responsiveness to carbon dioxide has been documented [47] and it is generally believed to be responsible for the chronic hyperventilation observed in ICSA subjects have lower arterial partial pressure of carbon dioxide ($PaCO_2$) throughout the 24 h. However, ICSA has only been documented during the nighttime, when the withdrawal of nonchemical control of respiration may favour respiratory periodicity (see also Chap. 4). However, it is reasonable to speculate that the disturbance extends during daytime as well; in fact, chronic hyperventilation and lower $PaCO_2$ may narrow the gap from the eupneic and the apneic threshold, thus resulting in daytime ICSA [47].

The chronic hyperventilation of ICSA subjects has been shown to be due to an increased chemosensitivity to carbon dioxide. Xie et al. found an increased sensitivity to CO_2, both with the single breath technique (0.51 ± 0.10 vs. 0.25 ± 0.004 L/min/mmHg, $p < 0.005$), which is used to assess the peripheral chemosensitivity to hypercapnia, and the rebreathing technique (3.14 ± 0.34 vs. 1.60 ± 0.32 L/min/mmHg, $p < 0.05$), which is used instead to assess the central chemosensitivity to hypercapnia [47]. Similarly, Solin et al. found an increased sensitivity to CO_2 in ICSA subjects as compared to controls, with the single breath technique (0.58 ± 0.07 vs. 0.27 ± 0.02,

$p=0.024$), but not with rebreathing technique (3.53 ± 0.29 vs. 2.14 ± 0.22 L/min/mmHg, $p=0.002$) [46]. Interestingly, there was no difference in peripheral chemosensitivity to CO_2 between ICSA and HF patients with central sleep apnea (CSA), while HF patients with CSA showed a trend to higher central chemosensitivity to CO_2, though not significant ($p=0.084$). Furthermore, peripheral and central chemosensitivity to CO_2 showed a good correlation with AHI in HF patients with CSA r = 0.65, p < 0.001), but not in ICSA ($r=0.39, p=0.238$) or normal subjects ($r=-0.15, p=0.73$).

During nighttime, a deep breath or a sudden increase in minute ventilation generally triggers ICSA, driving $PaCO_2$ below the apneic threshold; during apnea $PaCO_2$ increases up to the chemoreflex threshold inducing hyperventilation, due to overactive chemoreceptors, and sustaining the periodicity. A relative degree of hypocapnia and hyperventilation persists during ICSA cycles, maintaining respiratory instability. ICSA ceases either with sudden increase in ventilation, which leads to either EEG or movement arousal, or with ventilatory changes that increase $PaCO_2$, ceasing breathing periodicity [45].

The pathophysiological bases of the increased chemoreflex response to carbon dioxide and the subsequent hyperventilation observed in ICSA are not known yet, differently from the setting of HF (see also Chap. 5). It is tempting to speculate that genetic clusters may be found in ICSA subjects, keeping them in an underdamping condition (see also Chap. 4) and predisposing them to an easier shift toward ventilatory instability.

3.3.1.4 Treatment

Although generally considered benign, ICSA can be associated with decreased quality of sleep, excessive daytime sleepiness, and overall reduced quality of life. Inhaled CO_2 at night, in addition to added dead space via a facial mask, was shown to reduce the AHI from 43.7 ± 7.3 to 5.8 ± 0.9 ($p<0.005$), because of the increased gap between eupneic and apneic CO_2 thresholds [48]. Treatment with sleep inducers, such as zolpidem, has been tried. Zolpidem increased sleep time and reduced arousals, reducing both the AHI (from 24.0 ± 11.6 to 15.1 ± 7.7 ($p<0.001$) and daytime sleepiness [49]. Another potential treatment approach in ICSA patients may be yoga training. Yoga trainers, during spontaneous breathing, demonstrate lower responses to hypoxia and hypercapnia, as well as lower breathing frequency and minute ventilation [50]. Therefore, yoga could be an interesting and potentially functional alternative to less suitable pharmacologic treatments in ICSA patients that chronically hyperventilate due to increased response to CO_2.

3.3.2   Apneas at High Altitude

3.3.2.1 Definition

A characteristic waxing and waning breathing pattern known as PB accompanies sleep at high altitude. Typically, PB occurs at altitudes above 2000 m with different degree of severity, partly depending on individual characteristics; however, above 4000 m altitude, the majority of subjects usually experience PB.

3.3.2.2 Clinical Presentation

Sojourners to high altitudes frequently experience sleep disturbances, often reporting restless and sleepless nights, sometimes describing a feeling of suffocation on awakening from sleep. PB usually consists of 2–4 breaths, separated by an apnea of 5–15 s duration from the next burst of 2–4 breaths, closely resembling the PB of the premature infant. During PB also arterial SaO_2 oscillates and, depending on the altitude, it does it dangerously on the steep part of the oxygen dissociation curve. PB at high altitude during sleep was first described by Mosso in 1886 (Fig. 3.2, panel a) [51]. The role of PB at high altitudes has not been fully clarified. If at relatively lower altitudes (3000–3500 m) PB may be an adaptive response because of increased oxygenation, at higher altitudes it may be detrimental because of sleep disturbances and arousal up to full wakefulness, which leads to morning sleepiness and memory and cognitive impairment [52].

3.3.2.3 Pathophysiology

At high altitudes, subjects are exposed to a reduced oxygen tension, with a subsequent reduction in PaO_2 in the bloodstream. This fall induces rapid (within minutes) peripheral chemoreflex stimulation with an increase in ventilation and PaO_2 restoration, a response called acute hypoxia ventilatory response (AHVR). However, this response soon wears off, determining hypoxic ventilatory decline (HVD). The reason of this phenomenon is not clear, but it is probably due to decreased chemoreceptor sensitivity. Within days, a ventilatory acclimatization (VA) takes place with progressive increase in ventilation and PaO_2 [52]. In the phase of VA, PB may occur. The increase in ventilation occurring during VA is not sufficient to determine PB. Indeed, with increased ventilation (VE) and lower $PaCO_2$, a new equilibrium point, left shifted and located on a steeper portion of the isometabolic hyperbola, is established and thus the plant gain ($\Delta PaCO_2/\Delta VE$) is lower, protecting against instability (Fig. 3.2, panel b; see also Chaps. 4 and 5): in simple words, greater changes in ventilation are needed to determine smaller changes in $PaCO_2$. Therefore, other mechanisms should be involved. Indeed, an increased CO_2 response slope below eupnea during NREM sleep occurs at high altitude and causes a ventilatory overshoot following the rise in $PaCO_2$ during apnea, overcoming the stabilizing effect of reduced plant gain and leading to PB onset and mainteance (Fig. 3.2, panel b) [52]. While there is a general accordance about the key role of the increased chemosensitivity to hypercapnia in the PB genesis at high altitude, the role of the chemosensitivity to hypoxia is more debated. Indeed, in the classic study of Lahiri et al. the association between the hypoxic ventilatory response (HVR) and PB in lowlanders was mainly driven by the blunted HVR in the Sherpa group. The absence of a relationship between HVR and PB was further confirmed at 5050 m [52] as well as 6300 and 8050 m [53]. On the contrary, bilateral carotid body (CB) denervation prevents VA at high altitude, and cross-sectional studies in anesthetized cats also confirmed that several days of hypoxic exposure elicited increments in nerve firing from CB at any given PaO_2 during superimposed acute hypoxia. Furthermore, the carotid chemoreceptor glomus cells appear to thrive and multiply under conditions of sustained lack of oxygen [54].

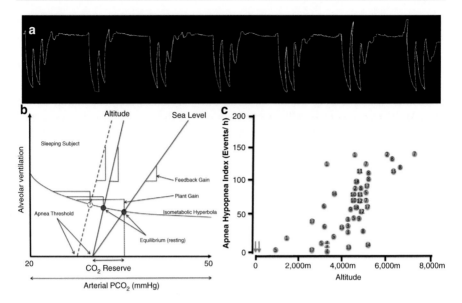

Fig. 3.2 Periodic breathing at high altitude

Panel a: Periodic breathing during sleep in the Regina Margherita Hut (4559 m) as described by Mosso in 1898 [51]

Panel b: Relationship between alveolar ventilation and alveolar PCO_2 at a fixed CO_2 production. High altitude increases the chemoreflex slope (*solid blue line*), but does not necessarily change the apnea threshold, and by doing so moves the equilibrium to an increased ventilation and lower PCO_2, thereby decreasing plant gain. If the apnea threshold is decreased with ventilatory acclimatization at altitude (*dotted blue line*), then ventilation further increases and PCO_2 decreases and plant gain is further decreased. Changing the slope of the ventilatory response to CO_2 above eupnea would alter susceptibility for transient ventilatory overshoots leading to periodic breathing. Other non-chemoreceptor factors (e.g., increased pulmonary pressures, behavioral drives, awake-to-sleep transitions, locomotion feedback) may favor ventilatory instability

Panel c: Relationship between altitude and apnea-hypopnea index. Each number refers to a different study; for further details please refer to Anslie PN et al [231]. Kind of concession of Anslie PN and colleagues.

However, after hypoxic acclimatization is completed in the intact animal, bilateral CB denervation reduces, but does not eliminate, continued hyperventilation on acute restoration of normoxia [55]. Recent evidence points to an interdependence of central medullary chemoreceptor activity on input from several sources, including CB (see also Chap. 5 for a detailed discussion) [56]. In summary, the central chemoreflex response to CO_2 is strongly influenced by the afferent discharge by CB during hypercapnia. Therefore, it is likely that hypoxia would cause an increased CB sensitivity, leading with time to an overall increase in the hypercapnic ventilatory response mediated by both peripheral and central chemoreceptors. The adrenergic overactivation observed at high altitude and presumably chemoreflex-mediated [57], together with neurohormonal activation, may also with time sustain the central chemoreflex increase independently from CB influences, thus justifying the sustained hyperventilation in VA, even after CB ablation [55]. Indeed, tonic hyperactivity of neurons at the level of the paraventricular nucleus and the rostral ventrolateral medulla was shown and correlated with the upregulation of the renin-angiotensin system and of angiotensin II type 1 receptors in the paraventricular nucleus [54].

Classically, it was believed that acute hypoxia stimulated CB, causing hyperventilation and systemic and cerebral spinal fluid (CSF) hypocapnia and respiratory alkalosis. After this initial phase, while arterial pH remained alkaline, CSF and, therefore, central chemoreceptors' pH would be quickly restored to normal via bicarbonate active transport across the blood–brain barrier, allowing the central chemoreceptors to sustain hyperventilation in VA and PB. However, CSF pH during acclimatization was shown to closely follow pH of arterial plasma, with CSF alkalinity increasing or remaining constant during hyperventilation. Therefore, CSF pH appeared to be primarily determined by, rather than a determinant of, VA and PB [54]. On the other hand, an important contributor that may change the chemoreflex response to CO_2 at high altitude is represented by the cerebral blood flow (CBF) reactivity. At sea level and in physiologic condition, an increase in the CBF, as obtained during hypercapnia, actually leads to CO_2 washout and to a blunted HCVR. CBF and CBF reactivity initially increase upon arrival at high altitude, but then CBF and its reactivity decline with VA and may thus contribute to the increase in HCVR and to breathing instability [52].

Other non-chemoreflex-mediated mechanisms that have been postulated are a direct influence of hypoxia on the brain, pulmonary J-receptors stimulation by pulmonary congestion/edema and pulmonary hypertension, leading to narrowed CO_2 reserve, as well as an increased rate of arousals [52].

While in normobaric hypoxia PB usually reduces over time, at high altitude there is instead an intensification of the phenomenon at least up to 15 days of exposure [58]. PB increases proportionally with altitude, while a small but progressive decrease in the average duration of the apnea–hypopnea events is described (Fig. 3.2, panel c) [52].

3.3.2.4 Treatment

Since there is a strong correlation between altitude and severity of PB (Fig. 3.2, panel c), the most rational treatment would be to descend. If this is not possible, there are several treatment options for PB, which can be broadly summarized in three different categories: medical gases, pharmacological interventions, and devices.

After the seminal paper of Lahiri, showing the positive effect of oxygen supplementation in a subject with sustained PB at 5300 m [59], the reduction in the number of apneas was also confirmed in a randomized controlled study (room air vs. 24 % O_2) performed in 18 lowlander volunteers sleeping at 3800 m, who also experienced improvement of sleep quality and showed reduced acute mountain sickness scores [60]. More recently, efficacy of oxygen supplementation ($FiO_2 = 0.25$) was also recently confirmed in Chilean miners at 4200 m, with PB reduction (PB%: 25 ± 18 in controls vs. 6.6 ± 5.6 in treated subjects, $p < 0.05$) and AHI reduction (34.9 ± 24.1 in controls vs. 8.5 ± 6.8 events/hour in treated subjects, $p < 0.05$) [61]. Small supplementation of CO_2 have a comparable stabilizing effect on breathing, probably due to the blunting of $PaCO_2$ fall during the hyperpneic phase of PB [62].

Among the pharmacological interventions, both acetazolamide and theophylline have been used to treat PB at high altitude. Acetazolamide, a carbonic anhydrase (CA) inhibitor, was found to improve oxygen saturation (from $72.0 \pm 2.1\%$ to $78.7 \pm 1.2\%$, $p < 0.001$) and to reduce the time spent in PB (from $80.4 \pm 3.5\%$ to $34.9 \pm 8.5\%$, $p < 0.001$), with no change observed in HVR [63]. The efficacy of carbonic anhydrase inhibitors is the result of ventilation and SaO_2 increase, driven by the metabolic acidosis and the slight CO_2 retention from vascular and red cell CA inhibition. CA inhibitors improve breathing stability by reducing the apneic CO_2 threshold and the chemosensitivity of peripheral chemoreceptors (see also Chap. 13) [64].

In a placebo-controlled trial, low-dose (300 mg/day) theophylline reduced symptoms of acute mountain sickness together with amelioration of PB and SaO_2 at 4559 m [65]. In a randomized, double-blind, placebo-controlled study the effects of theophylline (250 mg twice/day) on PB were compared to acetazolamide (250 mg twice/day) after fast ascent to high altitude (3454 m), with both drugs showing similar beneficial effect on PB; the only difference was that only acetazolamide (and not theophylline) improves basal SaO_2 during sleep [66].

Another respiratory stimulant, almitrine, was also studied, with no beneficial result (it rather increased PB) [67]. Similarly, benzodiazepines (temazepam) did not improve oxygen saturation compared to controls [68].

As for devices, some recent evidences have opened to the possibility of treating PB at high altitude with both CPAP, which actually halved PB in seven volunteers at 3800 m, and increased dead space (500 mL) through a fitted facemask, which improved PB, but only in subject with an AHI > 30 events/hour. The clinical application of both devices is obviously limited by compliance issues [52].

Considering that the increase in the chemoreflex gain is a key feature of PB at high altitude, regular yoga practice may be beneficial for healthy lowlanders in order to drive chemosensitivity back to the levels observed in highlanders, as Sherpa or Tibetan and to prevent or ameliorate PB [50].

3.3.3 Periodic Breathing in Neurological Diseases

3.3.3.1 Definition
Several neurological conditions may present with apneas/hypopneas along other symptoms, such as coma, stroke, Alzheimer's disease (AD), Multiple System Atrophy (MSA), Multiple Sclerosis (MS), Chiari Malformation (CM), epilepsy, amyotrophic lateral sclerosis (ALS), and neuromuscular disorders.

3.3.3.2 Epidemiology and Clinical Presentation

Sleep Disordered Breathing (SDB) in neurological disorders includes a range of conditions, including CSA, OSA, and sleep-related hypoventilation, or what may be called muscle-related sleep apnea (MRSA).

SDB prevalence widely varies from 10% to 70% depending on the underlying neurological condition [69]. Recent data report a very high prevalence of SDB in stroke patients, since most of them also have cardiovascular comorbidities predisposing to apneas, such as HF and AF [70]. A cross-sectional study of >6000 subjects in the general population from the Sleep Heart Health Study reported a modest but significant association of SDB with stroke [71]. On the other hand, SDB is frequent (44–72% of patients having an AHI $\geq$10) in acute ischemic stroke, with a prevalence ranging from 40% to 70%. A similar frequency of SDB in patients with transient ischemic attacks (TIAs), suggests that SDB may in some cases precede stroke. Further, after the acute phase of stroke, an improvement of SDB (around 40%) is observed in most patients within the first 3 months. Indeed, in a study performed in patients admitted for in-hospital rehabilitation after the acute phase of a stroke, the prevalence of OSA and CSA was 17% and 21% [72].

Apart from stroke, data on the prevalence and characteristics of SDB in other types of neurological disease are sparse. SDB are also detectable in 30–50% of AD patients [73]. In patients kept in residential institution the prevalence of OSA was reported to be 70% and 38% using an AHI cutoff of 5 and 20 events/hour, respectively. OSA has been associated with a significantly higher likelihood of developing cognitive impairment or dementia (see also Sect. 3.3.3.3), with the risk increasing with more sleep apnea events or a greater oxygen desaturations [74]. The prevalence of CSA is less known, but it is likely less common than OSA. Recent reports have also described a high prevalence of SDB, mainly OSA (up to 58%), and restless leg syndrome (up to 57%) in MS patients [75], with lower prevalence of CSA, unless the brainstem is involved. In MSA, the most typical sleep disorder is represented by REM sleep behavior disorder (violent dreams during nocturnal REM sleep and REM sleep without atonia), but central apneas, mainly during the night time, but also during the daytime, are frequently described in the later stage of the disease for MSA-related damage of central chemoceptive areas. Finally, 30–50% of patients with neuromuscular disorders also demonstrate SDB, as recently reviewed in [69, 76]. The most common SDB in neuromuscular disease is hypopneas/hypoventilation, with either prolonged period of hypoxia or a sawtooth pattern of desaturation dips, occurring during phasic REM sleep. This MRSA has also been named "pseudocentral" or "diaphragmatic" SDB. SDB and neuromuscular diseases are intimately linked and mainly related to the compromise of respiration mechanics. In amyotrophic lateral sclerosis (ALS), nocturnal breathing disturbance appears much earlier than daytime respiratory problems, due to the vulnerability of the respiratory system during sleep (especially during REM sleep), when accessory muscles do not lend support to the already weak diaphragm, leading to hypoventilation/MRSA. These events can be recognized by the timing of events corresponding to phasic REM sleep, by the SpO_2 profile and the greater reduction in chest wall relative to abdominal excursions. Nocturnal hypoventilation is usually accompanied by nocturnal hypercapnia with an arterial $PaCO_2 > 50$ mmHg for $> 5\%$ of monitoring time in adults or $> 2\%$ of monitoring time in children. Similar behaviors have been described in patients with myotonic dystrophy, in which also CSA has been described, in Duchenne muscular dystrophy, in which hypoventilation/MRSA may occur in all sleep stages and in Myasthenia Gravis, where OSA prevails on CSA, which is only rarely observed [69]. The higher prevalence of OSA in some subset of neuromuscular disease may be due to upper airway muscle hypotonia, whereas CSA may be due to concomitant cardiomyopathy potentially present in dystrophies [76].

Besides the different clinical presentation of each disease, the symptoms of apneas do not differ from the ones previously described in other conditions [69], although sometimes the clinical recognition of SDB may be more challenging due to the underlying clinical condition. However, it must be stressed that looking for SDB in neurological patients should be mandatory, not only for the very high prevalence, but also because SDB may lead to further neurologic damage and to a faster progression of the disease, especially in patients with background neurological frailty.

3.3.3.3 Pathophysiology

Patients with neurologic diseases are at risk for SDB development due to a combination of factors such as damage to areas of the brain that control respiration, muscular weakness, use of sedating medications and, in some cases, weight gain from limited physical activity. These mechanisms may sometimes coexist in the same patient. For the purpose of this essay, we will focus mainly on the affections of the central nervous system (CNS) and neuromuscular affections, usually leading to CSA and hypoventilation/MRSA, respectively. OSA usually coexists in neurologic patients, due to the very high prevalence of OSA and neurological disorders in the general population and especially in the elderly, making more difficult to establish a causal relationship between the two entities, also considering that OSA may frequently lead to neurological damage as outlined in the final part of this section.

Concerning CNS lesions, coma has always been the pivotal condition in which central apneas, in the form of Cheyne-Stokes respiration, is investigated. CSR, along with other cranial nerves testing, is indeed indicative of a higher lesion, generally diencephalic or encephalic, whereas disrupted and ataxic breathing usually manifests in more caudal lesions [77]. Coma is generally the result of a complex and extensive lesion (for the most part either ischemic/hemorrhagic or traumatic) and therefore, the presence of CSR in coma patients is only an expression of higher neurologic affections, but generally it gives no information about the key mechanisms leading to central events [77].

On the contrary, studies on selective brain lesions of ischemic nature (in patients with either stroke or macro- and microangiopathy) may help in clarifying which are the areas and the mechanisms responsible for CSA/CSR generation. The seminal paper of Plum and Brown in 1961 first described the association of CSR with stroke in 28 neurological patients. Although the neurological lesions of those patients were maybe too extensive to identify specific areas involved in the pathogenesis of CSR,

as the majority of patients presented with bilateral stroke and disturbed consciousness, this study opened to an extensive field of research.

Since then, several areas implicated in CSR pathophysiology have been identified also in patients with unilateral stroke and preserved vigilance, such as cingulate
cortex, supplementary motor cortex, insula, and thalamus (Fig. 3.3, panel a) [78].
Interestingly, these areas are involved in volitional control of respiration and autonomic balance, as reviewed by Macey et al. [79]. It is then reasonable to assume that
brain damage in those pivotal areas may cause either abolition or damping of the
neurological control from upper CNS centers on brainstem centers involved in
respiratory and cardiovascular stability [80]. Lesions in the internal capsule and the
pons due to lacunar strokes (diameter <20 mm) have also been associated with
Cheyne-Stokes respiration. A group of patients with lacunar strokes also experienced OSA, and authors speculated that this may be caused by either an increased
chemoreflex gain leading to OSA (see also Sect. 3.4.4) or to the damage of fibers in
the internal capsule controlling upper airway dilators [81].

The development of perilesional edema in stroke patients was also hypothesized
to play a role in the pathophysiology of central apneas, since the consequent rise in

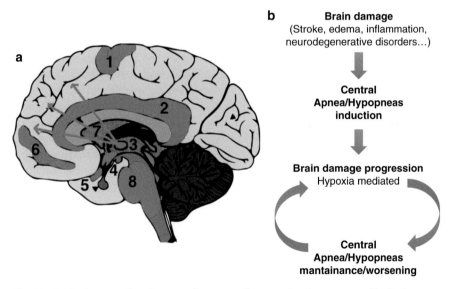

Fig. 3.3 Brain-damage-triggering central apneas and apnea-related sustenance of brain damage
Panel a: Brain areas that trigger sleep apnea when subjected to a stroke are shown. *1* motor cortex,
2 cingulate cortex, *3* thalamus, *4* hypothalamus, *5* Amygdala, *6* ventromedial prefrontal cortex, *7*
thalamocortical connections, *8* ponto-bulbar respiratory centers. These areas are involved in respiratory control and emotional and cognitive processing. Sleep apnea-derived chronic intermittent
hypoxia might perpetuate the damage. Multiple sclerosis plaques and Alzheimer plaques in the
brainstem respiratory centers might also trigger sleep apnea
Panel b: Brain damage (due to hypoxia/ischemia, stroke, inflammation, multiple sclerosis,
Alzheimer's disease, edema) can trigger sleep apnea due to loss of sovra and/or infratentorial control of respiration. Sleep apnea might further progress brain damage sustaining the anomaly. *AD*
Azheimer's disease, *MS* multiple sclerosis

intracranial pressure might activate brain autoregulatory metabolic mechanisms involving hypocapnic vasoconstriction to reduce cerebral blood volume; this mechanism may unmasking a pre-existing ventilatory instability imbalance [82].

The seminal study from Plum and Brown is also a unicum in demonstrating that stroke patients with CSR have an increased central response to carbon dioxide, since a 10% increase in CO_2 induced an 18 L/min increase in ventilation compared to 12 L/min increase of stroke patients without CSR and 5 L/min ventilatory increase observed in patients without CSR and in controls, respectively [80]. The pathological bases of this finding are currently unknown and would be of research interest. Finally, in the same paper, longer CSR cycles durations were found in stroke patients with occult cardiac dysfunction (LVEF < 40%) (66.6 ± 5.6 s vs. 46 ± 2.9 s, $p = 0.0006$) [83]. Therefore, measures of PB duration in CSR after a stroke might be a useful clinical tool for a complete and comprehensive assessment of the patient.

We have previously underlined how the loss of sovratentorial control of respiration might play a pivotal role in the genesis of CSA-CSR. It would be interesting to study how ischemic alterations of either brainstem respiratory centers or chemoreceptive areas might affect breathing stability. Unfortunately, strokes involving the brainstem are usually extremely critical and generally present with ataxic respiration [84]. However, the possibility that brainstem hypoperfusion might lead to CSA-CSR has been investigated in patients with macrovascular and, in particular, microvascular disorders.

In macrovascular disorders, CSA/CSR was described in patients with asymptomatic extracranial internal carotid (eICA) stenosis, with a prevalence up to 72% in case of severe stenosis ($\geq 70\%$) [85]. Reduced perfusion of the carotid body may induce ischemic changes in the CB that increase peripheral chemoreflex and decrease carotid baroreflex (for more details, see Chap. 5). These signals integrate in the nucleus of solitary tract and have an excitatory effect on medullary chemoreceptors, globally resulting in increased central and peripheral chemosensitivity and related autonomic deregulation. Detection of CSA-CSR in this clinical condition may help identify asymptomatic patients at risk for cerebrovascular and cardiovascular events [85].

As for microvascular disorders, a human model of microangiopathy (Fabry disease, FD) was used to study cortical and subcortical white matter alterations by means of Diffusion Tensor Imaging-MRI (DTI-MRI). Patients with FD that also had CSA-CSR showed a higher degree of white matter impairment (expressed as a higher DTI signal) in sovratentorial regions (subcortical white matter of the frontal lobe and internal capsule), and more pronounced brainstem DTI signal compared to healthy controls [86]. However, if these structural changes are the anatomical correlates of CSA-CSR is still undemonstrated.

Besides vascular patients, other CNS conditions are associated with respiratory instability; among them there are MSA, AD, MS, epilepsy, and Chiari I malformation.

The presence of central sleep apneas in MSA is related to a depressed response to hypercapnia [87] due to alterations of the Arcuate Nucleus (one of the central chemoreceptors) and marked gliosis and accumulation of the alpha sinuclein protein in the ventrolateral medulla [88]. This disruption results in a loss of function of those chemoreceptive areas with reduced response to carbon dioxide, in a fashion that resembles what happens in SIDS patients in whom apoptosis of the serotonergic chemoreceptors takes place (see Sect. 3.2.4).

Also AD patients show central apneas, especially in the latest phases of the disease; this is thought to depend on the disruption of brainstem respiratory regulation [89], together with neurotransmitter imbalance due to the loss of both neuroadrenergic neurons of the locus coeruleus (which is again a chemosensitive region) [90] and cholinergic neurons of the brainstem [91]. Moreover, neuronal damage due to CSA may in turn favor AD incidence and cognitive decline as in case of OSA, as we will further explain afterward.

MS patients show a high prevalence of SDB, but rarely manifest central apneas. Indeed, MS patients usually present with either obstructive or hypoventilation/MRSA events, probably because of muscular weakness. However, central apneic events have also been reported in MS in the presence of brainstem plaques [92]. Brainstem plaques are indeed associated with a higher central AHI compared to both controls and MS patients without brainstem involvement, underscoring again the key role of the brainstem in central apnea genesis. In addition to that, being olygodendrocytes the glial cells that are mostly affected by hypoxia [93], a possible association between MS onset and hypoxic insults on olygodendrocites may be hypothesized.

CSA has also been described in a case report of a patient with Chiari I malformation. This condition is associated with cerebellar tonsils herniation through the foramen magnum, with subsequent brainstem compression, which is in turn responsible for apnea generation; however, this finding has not been extensively investigated in more controlled studies and extensive populations [94].

Central apneas are also found in epilepsy, generally preceding the ictal phase, and have been related to sudden unexpected death in epilepsy (SUDEP); a possible role of amygdala involvement in the suppression of respiration was hypothesized [95, 96].

As mentioned at the beginning of the paragraph, besides CNS affections, neuromuscular disorders can also impact on the pathophysiology of sleep apnea.

From a general standpoint, both dystrophies and ALS are associated with muscle weakness and impaired diaphragmatic contraction; therefore, the elevated prevalence of SDB in these populations is likely to be related to a peripheral origin of the phenomenon, which is muscular weakness itself, with subsequent hypoventilation. However, in myotonic – or Steinert – dystrophy, apneas of central origin are more common (40–60 %) [97]; this phenomenon has been linked to autonomic imbalance and loss of medullary respiratory neurons (ventrolateral medullary neurons, dorsal central medullary neurons, and subtrigeminal nuclei) [98].

Up until now we have investigated the causes that can determine the onset of SDB in diverse neurological conditions; however, an increasing body of literature is available on the effects that apneas have on the brain. These studies have mainly been carried out in the setting of OSA, with only few studies focusing on CSA/CSR. Nonetheless, the same mechanisms of neuronal damage are likely to occur, since hypoxia/ischemia, sleep disruption, and cerebral inflammation are common features of both types of apneas.

Different neuropsychological studies have clarified that subjects with OSA have reduced cognitive and emotional abilities compared to healthy controls in different fields, from working memory, to attention, to higher executive and cognitive functions; they also have shown increased irritability and impulsive behaviors compared to controls, as well as increased depression and anxiety rates [99, 100]. These psychological findings set their biological bases in the damage of some key areas for the control of cognitive behavior and emotional processing.

Voxel-based and DTI-MRI studies in patients with OSA showed hypoxic damage in diverse brain regions: cingulate cortex, cerebellum, thalamo-cortical pathways, ventro-medial prefrontal cortex, insula, amygdala, hypothalamus, hippocampus, brainstem, and white matter are in fact all subjected to neuronal loss, gliosis, and atrophy (Fig. 3.3, panel a) [101–103]. Interestingly, postmortem studies on OSA subjects confirmed MRI results, demonstrating increased brainstem gliosis and increased rate of microinfarctions in apneic patients with reduced blood oxygen saturation [104]. It is noteworthy that the damaged areas identified by means of MRI techniques and autoptic studies are not only implied in cognitive and emotional processing, but they are also involved in sovratentorial control of autonomic balance [79]. Therefore, it is tempting to speculate that a vicious circle might take place in the setting of sleep apnea, where the primitive disruption of those core areas might induce apneas and vice versa (Fig. 3.3, panel b).

A possible role in the process leading to brain damage may be played by the inflammatory response. Both TNFa and IL-6 are indeed increased after sleep deprivation, but they are also elevated in stroke patients that subsequently develop OSA [70]. In addition, increased deposition of beta-amyloid and subsequent formation of amyloid plaques in the brain has been described, as well as increased formation of neurofibrillary tangles (NFT) of Tau protein [93]. The former association is relatively new and extremely interesting, as it represents a possible link between OSA and AD, in which the same anatomo-pathological alterations are found. As we have previously reported, AD is associated with SDB; in addition, patients that develop SDB earlier in life are at increased risk of mild cognitive impairment (MCI) and AD [105]. Finally, AD patients with SDB exhibit a more pronounced cognitive decline when compared to AD patients without SDB [106]. To strengthen this association, neuronal loss in the locus coeruleus (LC) in OSA patients has been reported, as well as in AD patients. LC is a neuroadrenergic brainstem nucleus that is implied in arousal, cardiovascular and respiratory balance, and chemosensitivity [90]; however, whether LC disruption is due to either apnea-induced hypoxia or to AD itself is not known, and further research is needed.

HF and AF are also associated with brain damage and increased AD prevalence. In fact, reduced brain perfusion due to HF is also responsible for the formation of amyloid plaques and NFT, while AF is notably an embolic source which is associated with a threefold increased risk for strokes (which, as we have reported, associated with SDB). Finally, it is interesting to notice that Donepezil, an anticholinesterase agent used in the treatment of AD, partially reverses the respiratory abnormalities, although the pathophysiological insights of the finding are not currently known.

Recent studies have also described an increased incidence of epilepsy in OSA patients, according to neuronal damage due to sleep fragmentation and hypoxia.

This insight is of particular interest, as new connections are likely to be found, but also because epilepsy and SUDEP could be in turn responsible for the negative outcomes observed in OSA patients.

3.3.3.4 Treatment

Currently, therapeutic strategies for CSA/CSR suppression in neurological patients have been rarely reported. More data are instead available regarding the treatment of OSA and hypoventilation/MRSA.

Considering that the presence of CSA/CSR after stroke is associated with poor outcome even in conscious patients [107], the treatment of central events may be of clinical interest. In a retrospective single-center analysis conducted in patients with stroke and no evidence of HF (>1 months from a stroke in the territory of the middle cerebral artery −7/15 patients, and the posterior cerebral artery −7/15 patients), the treatment with ASV significantly reduced AHI (46.7±24.3 vs. 8.5±12 event/hour, $p=0.001$) with a mean time use of ASV of 5.4±2.4 h at 3 months, a result that held at a 6-month follow-up. Notably, a previous ineffective attempt of treatment with either continuous (CPAP) or bi-level positive airway pressure (BIPAP) was described in the same population [108]. However, considering the paucity of data on treatment of CSA/CSR in stroke, and the negative finding observed in the large Adaptive Servoventilation trial performed in HF patients [109], larger randomized trials are needed also in this specific setting to further evaluate and establish the role of ASV with regard to survival, recurrent stroke, brain function, and cognitive impairment.

In stroke patients, CSR/CSA usually improve anyway in about half of the population within 1–3 months. In the interim, untreated OSA is associated with negative repercussion and worse outcome [110]. Treating moderate to severe OSA leads to longer survival (91, CI 76–106 months in the treated group vs. 52, CI 41–64 months in the untreated group, $p<0.001$) in a recent observational study performed in elderly patients with a 15 % prevalence of previous stroke [111]. In a randomized controlled study, early use of nasal CPAP seems to accelerate neurological recovery (evaluated by both Rankin and Canadian scales, all $p<0.05$), and to delay the appearance of cardiovascular events (14.9 vs. 7.9 months; $p=0.044$), although an improvement in patients' survival was not shown (0 % in the nasal CPAP group and 4.3 % in the control group, $p=0.161$).

CPAP was also effective in slowing cognitive decline in AD patients with OSA (at a 3-year follow-up, patients treated with CPAP showed a decline of −0.7 point by means of the Minimental State Evaluation, whereas non-CPAP patients showed a decline of −2.2 points, $p=0.013$) [112]. However, as pointed out by a long-term study by Bassett et al., long-term use of CPAP is difficult to achieve for the patients, as the majority of the patients drop out of the treatment [113]. Moreover, CPAP treatment did not affect survival in central sleep apnea, as pointed out by the CANPAP trial [114]. Therefore, since promising results were found for patients with SDB that undergo treatment, and since no treatment is available nowadays for the treatment of CSA, more research in this field should be pursued.

Pharmacological agents have also been investigated to treat sleep apnea in AD. Donepezil, an inhibitor of acetylcholinesterases, was able to improve total

REM time and total AHI (from 20.0 ± 15.9 to 9.9 ± 11.4, $p<0.035$). However, a subgroup analysis enlightened that only obstructive AHI and not central AHI was affected by the treatment, suggesting a role of the cholinergic system in OSA [115]. Nonetheless, treatment with Donepezil could represent a great choice of treatment, since it is commonly used in AD, and it is not associated with reduced sleep comfort as CPAP. Other pharmacological agents, such as theophylline and acetazolamide, have never been tried on these patients. A promising option may be theophylline, a respiratory stimulant, especially in patients who lost sovratentorial respiratory drive. Indeed, as we have previously described theophylline is effective in infants with underdeveloped central respiratory controllers, a condition similar to that sustaining SDB of different etiology in adult patients with neurological disorders (i.e., ischemia, infarction, neurodegenerative disorders). Finally, oxygen therapy was not evaluated in neurologic patients either, but it might be useful to reduce hypoxia-induced brain damage in patients with no other treatment option.

In neuromuscular disorders, non invasive ventilation reverses SDB events, with positive effects on MRA, OSA, and CSA. In some neuromuscular disorders, noninvasive ventilation (NIV) may improve sleep quality, often preventing or delaying invasive mechanical ventilation and also improving survival [116]. However, it should be reminded that NIV can be more difficult in this setting and sleep-disordered events related to NIV therapy may be observed in patients with neuromuscular disease. In fact, air leaks, ventilator–patient asynchrony, central events, and gloctic closure that contribute to desaturations, arousals, impaired sleep architecture and poor adherence have been described [76]. A potential alternative to NIV in patients with neuromuscular disorders might be exercise training and in particular respiratory muscle training, which has already shown some benefits in both patients with OSA and in HF patients with exertional ventilatory oscillations (see also Sect. 3.4.5).

3.3.4   Periodic Breathing and Kidney Failure

3.3.4.1 Definition
End-stage renal disease (ESRD) is a common clinical condition characterized by progressively reduced kidney function, with decreased glomerular filtration rate (GFR <30 mL/min/1.73 m^2). This condition is associated with metabolic acidosis and hypervolemia, and can lead to cardiovascular complications, including secondary heart failure, hypertension, pericarditis, and anemia.

3.3.4.2 Epidemiology
ESRD patients demonstrate 50–70 % of SDB, including insomnia, OSA, CSA, mixed apneas, nightmares, and restless leg syndrome, and up to 80 % of ESRD subjects also complain of subjective sleep disturbances [117]. OSA is the most prevalent disorder, with prevalence ranging between 16 % and 24 % [117]; obstructive AHI correlated with both urea and creatinine clearance in nondiabetic patients, while it only correlated with urea concentration in diabetics [118]. With regard to CSA, one

study demonstrated that patients with stage 3 chronic kidney disease (CKD, defined for a GFR < 60 ml/min/1.73 m^2) had a six times greater prevalence of central apneic events compared to patients with a GFR > 60 ml/min/1.73 m^2 (CAI: 5.9 ± 12.2 vs. 1.0 ± 2.1; $p = 0.01$). Therefore, it is reasonable to assume that there is a correlation between sleep apnea and kidney disease; however, due to the small cohorts of those studies, no definite statement can be made and further research is needed.

3.3.4.3 Clinical Implications and Complications

Symptoms of sleep disturbances in ESRD include snoring, increased diurnal sleepiness, arousals, and witnessed apnea [117], which reduces the quality of sleep and life in those patients. Patients with OSA and ESRD also refer nicturia, which is due to atrial natriuretic peptide (ANP) secretion in response to stretching of the cardiac walls related to the increment of intrathoracic pressure during the apneic event; nicturia is responsible for further destabilized breathing and arousals [119]. In addition, sleep disturbances are associated with increased sympathetic outflow and hemodynamic changes, as well as with increased incidence of adverse arrhythmias, leading to secondary cardiac disease, secondary pulmonary hypertension, and heart failure (see Chaps. 5 and 6). Increased plasma angiotensin II and aldosterone have also been described, which can in turn be responsible for sodium retention and sustained hypertension, overcoming the positive effect on natriuresis due to ANP. Furthermore, ESRD/OSA patients presented with increased vascular permeability due to CIH. Indeed, ERSD patients with SDB show peripheral edema more frequently than ERSD patients without SDB. Kidney biopsies of OSA patients also show glomerulosclerosis and glomerulomegaly (because of increased volume retention and blood flow), which can be responsible for massive proteinuria up until nephrotic syndrome. On the cognitive side, ESRD is itself associated with depression and cognitive and memory and executive impairment, which is worsened by overimposition of sleep apnea [73] (see Sect. 3.2.3.4).

SDB in patients with ESRD is associated with risk of fatal and nonfatal cardiovascular events. A 1 % decrease in average nocturnal saturation is associated with a 33 % increase in the incident risk. The risk of cardiovascular events is five times higher in patients with average nocturnal $SaO_2 < 95\%$ [120].

3.3.4.4 Pathophysiology

Before addressing deeply all the factors that contribute to the pathogenesis of SDB in ESRD, it is important to point out that most of the patients share metabolic and cardiovascular comorbidities, which per se are implied in the pathophysiology of sleep apnea. Therefore, separating the effects of CVD and kidney dysfunction is not always easy.

Since OSA is the most prevalent sleep abnormality in ESRD patients, its pathophysiology in this context has been studied the most. In OSA, as we will discuss more deeply in Sect. 3.4, craniofacial abnormalities as well as muscular weakness, together with obesity and metabolic abnormalities are of key importance. Increased volemia and interstitial edema can also contribute to mechanical obstruction of UA in ESRD patients [121].

In patients with ESRD, increased blood volume and interstitial edema may be particularly important, since peripheral edema, common in patients with ESRD and SDB, may be reabsorbed in lying conditions leading to rostral fluid shift during night and worsening of both OSA and CSA [122].

Furthermore, sleep apnea has been associated with ventilatory and blood gases abnormalities, and especially with impaired neuroreflexes in response to both pH and blood gases changes. There is evidence that ventilatory disturbances are also present in kidney patients. Rassaf et al. evaluated the hyperoxic cardiac chemoreflex sensitivity measured as the difference in the R–R intervals in the ECG before and after inhalation of pure oxygen (8 L O_2/min via a nose mask for 5 min), divided by the difference in the venous partial pressure of oxygen (normal values >3 ms/mmHg). CKD patients at stage 3 and 4 showed an impaired hyperoxic chemosensitivity compared to controls (2.1 ± 0.6 ms/mmHg vs. $6.7 \pm 0{,}9$ ms/mmHg, $p < 0.001$), with GFR being the only independent predictor for reduced hyperoxic chemosensitivity [123]. Beecroft et al. studied 58 ESRD patients receiving either conventional hemodialysis or peritoneal dialysis. They underwent overnight polysomnography and assessment of CO_2 chemosensitivity via modified Read's rebreathing technique, in both isoxic hypoxia (PO_2 6.65 kPa) and isoxic hyperoxia (PO_2 19.95 kPa) background. SDB was present in 66 % of the population, with the great majority of respiratory events being of OSA subtype. OSA in ESRD population is likely to be related to a high loop gain, considering that in the same study an increased chemosensitivity to hypercapnia was demonstrated, both in hypoxic and hyperoxic background conditions in ESRD patients with SDB compared with ESRD without SDB (in hypoxic conditions: 7.3 ± 3.5 vs. 3.5 ± 1.5 L/min/mmHg, $p < 0.001$; in hyperoxic conditions: 3.2 ± 1.3 vs. 1.7 ± 0.8 L/min/mmHg, $p < 0.001$) [117]. These data suggest that the sensitivity of both the central and peripheral chemoreceptors to CO_2 is increased in patients with sleep apnea and ESRD. Circadian differences in CO_2 sensitivity were also found, with higher values in the morning compared to the evening both in apneic and nonapneic patients; this fluctuation is thought to be due to hypothalamic circadian variation.

The mechanisms by which CKD causes cardiovascular autonomic resetting are not fully understood yet. Direct and indirect measures of sympathetic activity indicate that an adrenergic overdrive is common in CKD: several studies in animal models of renal failure suggest that excitation of renal afferent nerves results in increased efferent sympathetic nerve discharge [124, 125]. This may in turn lead to a brainstem modulation of input coming from peripheral chemoreceptors or directly influence central chemoreceptors, but currently this field of research is still to be defined.

Nakayama et al. demonstrated that in metabolic acidosis there is a left-ward shifting of CO_2 sensitivity curve, which can account for ventilatory instability [126]. However, Beecroft et al. did not find any pH alteration in ESRD patients with apneas versus those without, reducing the likelihood of the effects of metabolic acidosis on the central controllers of respiration in those patients [117].

Also uremia has been repeatedly taken into account in the pathogenesis of SDB; however, only one study investigated the potential effects of uremia on breathing control, showing that a transient fall in uremia concentration after hemodialysis was associated with increased CO_2 sensitivity, and that the fall could be prevented by adding urea to the dialysate. However, due to the reduced amount of studies available, no definite assumption can be made and further research is needed [127]. It is also possible to speculate on uremia-induced neuronal damage that can further impair breathing control and induce sleep apnea; however, this association has only been postulated and never fully demonstrated [128]. Interestingly, again Beecroft et al. did not find any difference in urea concentration in ESRD patients with or without SDB, at least in the first 24 h after dialysis; therefore, the real impact of uremia on sleep and respiration is still to be addressed [117].

Finally, the potential role of toxic protein has also been taken into account. Increased concentration of p-cresol and indoxyl sulfate was found in CKD patients compared to controls [129]. Those molecules (or other toxic proteins) are thought to be implied in atherosclerosis and cardiovascular disease progression and might play a role in SDB pathogenesis.

Another intriguing but still poorly characterized mechanism in patients with kidney disease and SDB is the role of inflammation. Increased levels of C-reactive protein (CRP), TNFa, and IL-6 were described in patients with kidney failure, and they are probably due to increased rate of infection, dialysis per se, and reduced renal clearance of pro-inflammatory cytokines [130]. Inflammation is an independent risk factor for atherosclerosis and cardiovascular dysfunction [131], which are themselves associated with sleep apnea. In addition, inflammation is tightly interconnected with OSA maintenance (see also Sect. 3.4.4).

Last but not least, an increased body of literature is available on the effects of kidney failure on brain damage. Several studies have demonstrated impaired cognitive performances in ESRD patients, as well as memory impairment, executive dysfunction, and psychiatric comorbidities [132–134]. On the other hand, as we have discussed in the Sect. 3.2.3.3, brain abnormalities might concur in the development of sleep disturbances. Several studies investigated both structural and functional abnormalities in the brain of CKD patients. DTI-MRI studies have demonstrated an increase in mean diffusivity and a reduction in fractional anisotropy in the white matter, especially in the corpus callosum, fornix, bilateral sagittal stratum, pons, cingulate cortex, radiate corona [133, 134]. These findings can both reflect brain damage and decreased myelinization or increased interstitial edema and water content [135]. As we have mentioned in Sect. 3.2.3.3, interstitial edema can have an impact on autoregulatory functions in the brain, thus inducing ventilatory instability [82]. Moreover, some of those regions (brainstem, cingulate cortex) show also a role in autonomic balance. Consequently, a sovratentorial pathogenetic role for SDB in ESRD patients is not unlikely.

3.3.4.5 Treatment

Among the various therapies that have been proposed to treat sleep disturbances in ESRD patients, only renal transplantation and nocturnal hemodialysis were found to be beneficial, supporting the theory of renal dysfunction as the initial trigger for SDB.

Nocturnal hemodialysis (NHD) was effective in reducing sleep disturbances in apneic responders. Fourteen patients who were undergoing conventional hemodialysis for 4 h on each of three days per week underwent overnight polysomnography, showing a prevalence of SDB of 57 % (AHI cutoff 15 events/hour: 7 patients with OSA, 1 patient with CSA/CSR). All patients were then switched to NHD for 8 h during each of six or seven nights a week. During NHD, serum creatinine concentration decreased compared to conventional hemodialysis. A similar behavior was observed for SDB, with a reduction of the AHI from 25 ± 25 to 8 ± 8 events/hour ($p = 0.03$), with the reduction occurring mainly in the seven patients with sleep apnea (AHI from 46 ± 19 to 9 ± 9 events/hour, $p = 0.006$), in whom also an increase in the minimal oxygen saturation (from 89.2 ± 1.8 to 94.1 ± 1.6 %, $p = 0.005$), transcutaneous partial pressure of carbon dioxide (from 38.5 ± 4.3 to 48.3 ± 4.9 mmHg, $p = 0.006$), and serum bicarbonate concentration (from 23.2 ± 1.8 to 27.8 ± 0.8 mmol per liter, $p < 0.001$) were observed [136].

In 1993, Langevin et al. reported two clinical cases of patients in which both OSA and CSA were markedly reduced after kidney transplantation (KT) [137]. A similar result was then found by Rodrigues et al. in 2010 in a more extensive population [138]. An AHI ≥ 5 was present in nine patients (26.5 %) prior to and seven (21 %) after transplantation (follow-up evaluation performed after 3–6 months), but no significant reduction in the mean AHI was found between the two study phases (5.3 ± 7.3 vs. 3.1 ± 4.5; $P > 0.05$). Possible explanations for partial failure of KT are the persistence of other sleep disturbances rather than OSA and CSA (such as restless leg syndrome) and the onset of secondary cardiovascular conditions such as CHF in kidney patients, which can further perpetuate the vicious circle leading to SDB, or the persistence of metabolic acidosis, uremic myopathy or neuropathy, anemia, hormonal imbalance, fluid overload, and inflammatory cytokines after transplantation [117]. Also a possible confounding effect of corticosteroid or immunosuppressive drugs given after transplantation cannot be excluded. Notably, KT was also associated with decreased mean diffusivity at DTI-MRI and improved cognitive performance in CKD patients [134].

Also CPAP was proposed for the treatment of OSA in CKD patients, and was found to be beneficial. Not only did it reduce the AHI (see Sect. 3.4), but it also increased renal plasma flow and reduced filtration fraction from 0.26 to 0.23 ($p < 0.001$), thus reducing hyperfiltration (which is associated to progressive kidney damage) [139].

3.3.5 Periodic Breathing and Pulmonary Hypertension

3.3.5.1 Definition
Pulmonary hypertension (PH) is defined as "an increase in mean pulmonary arterial pressure (PAPm) ≥ 25 mmHg at rest as assessed by right heart catheterization (RHC)," according to ESC/ERS Guidelines for the diagnosis and treatment of pulmonary hypertension [140].

The hemodynamic classification divides precapillary and postcapillary pulmonary hypertension. Precapillary pulmonary hypertension is defined as a resting mean pulmonary artery pressure (PAP) ≥ 25 mmHg with a pulmonary capillary wedge pressure (PWP) ≤ 15 mmHg; postcapillary pulmonary hypertension is defined by a PWP > 15 mmHg and it is further divided in isolated postcapillary PH (IPC-PH) with diastolic pressure gradient (DPG = diastolic PAP − mean PWP) < 7 mmHg and/or pulmonary vascular resistance PVR ≤ 3 Wood Unit (WU) and combined postcapillary and precapillary PH (CPC-PH) with DPG ≥ 7 mmHg and/or PVR > 3 WU [140].

3.3.5.2 Epidemiology and Risk Factors

According to the World Health Organization (WHO), PH is also classified in five groups. Group 1 includes PH of idiopathic, unknown, or heritable etiology (drug or toxin-induced PH, PH associated to connective tissue diseases, HIV infection, portal hypertension, congenital heart disease, chronic hemolytic anemia, and schistosomiasis). Group 2 includes PH due to left heart disease, group 3 PH due to pulmonary diseases (lung diseases and/or hypoxemia), and group 4 includes chronic thromboembolic pulmonary hypertension and other pulmonary artery obstructions. Finally, group 5 includes unusual hemodynamic PH with unclear and/or multifactorial mechanisms [141].

The prevalence and clinical severity of PH-related SDB remains uncertain and it is different according to the five different groups. The prevalence of SDB in group 2 and 3 of PH should be critically interpreted, as group 2 is mainly represented by heart failure, which is a very well-acknowledged determinant of CSA, and group 3, by definition, already includes OSA patients.

In group 1, a cross-sectional cohort study (52 patients from the Toronto pulmonary hypertension program) showed a prevalence of 71 % of SDB (AHI ≥ 5 events/hours), with 40 % having OSA and 31 % CSA. Using a higher AHI cutoff of 10 events/hour, the prevalence of SDB was 60 % [140].

The prevalence of sleep apnea has extensively been studied in patients with heart failure, but the number of reports simultaneously describing both pulmonary hemodynamics and apnea occurrence are rare. In a study performed by Solin et al. in 75 heart failure patients awaiting heart transplantation, SDB (AHI ≥ 5 events/hours) was observed in 71 % of the population, with 44 % presenting with CSA and 27 % with OSA. However, the presence of PH was not a prespecified entry criteria. Nonetheless, patients with CSA actually had average values of mean pulmonary pressure consistent with the PH definition (32.5 ± 1.6 mmHg), differently from OSA patients (20.4 ± 1.3 mmHg).

Soler et al. have recently found a high prevalence (52 %) of OSA (AHI ≥ 5 events/hours) also in patients with severe chronic obstructive pulmonary disease (COPD), the most prevalent disease included in group 3 PH [142]. Previous studies have reported OSA to be present in about 10–15 % of patients with COPD, similar to the general population [143].

To our knowledge, there is only one dedicated study that analyzed SDB in chronic thromboembolic pulmonary hypertension (CTEPH) or group 4: Jeremy et al. examined a population with CTEPH (notably with frequent right ventricular dysfunction) and observed that SDB (AHI $\geq$5 events/hour) was highly prevalent (57 %), with most apneas being again obstructive [144].

Recently, Dumistrascu et al. analyzed a population of 169 patients, enrolled at the Pulmonary Hypertension Unit of the University of Giessen Lung Center in Germany, with precapillary PH (exclusion criteria was a PWP >15 mmHg): 27 % of patients had SDB, using a higher AHI cutoff of 10 events/hours, with 16 % of OSA and 11 % of CSA. OSA mainly occurred in patients with CTEPH and COPD-associated PH, whereas most of cases with CSA were ascribable to pulmonary arterial hypertension (PAH) and "other" PH diagnoses [145].

3.3.5.3 Clinical Implications and Complications

Patients with PH usually present with dyspnea upon exertion, fatigue, lethargy, syncope with exertion and chest pain. PH is a serious condition that, if left untreated, may lead to right heart failure and cardiac output decrease, thus giving birth to SDB, which may in turn worsen PH, in a vicious circle self sustaining [140].

3.3.5.4 Pathophysiology

Different pathophysiological features characterize precapillary (PPH) and postcapillary PH (IPC-PH and CPC-PH) as well as the different clinical PH subgroups (Fig. 3.4).

Pulmonary arterial hypertension (PAH), including idiopathic and associated forms, and chronic thromboembolic pulmonary hypertension (CTEPH) represent the major groups of precapillary PH. These forms are characterized by an impaired ventilation-perfusion matching, whereby relatively small perturbations in ventilation can result in desaturation and hypoxic pulmonary vasoconstriction: hypoxia induces pulmonary vasoconstriction via its effects on pulmonary vascular smooth muscle and endothelial cells and therefore may lead to elevated pulmonary artery pressure [145].

Hildenbrand et al. analyzed a population of PPH (PAH and CTEPH) and observed that 77 % of the patients spent >10 % of the night with $SaO_2 < 90$ % (desaturators), and 52 % spent >50 % of the night with $SaO_2 < 90$ % (sustained desaturators), despite often normal daytime SaO_2. The only independent predictors of the mean nocturnal SaO_2 were the tricuspid pressure gradient and the daytime SaO_2 [146]. Nocturnal desaturators presented a higher prevalence of SDB (54 % vs. 38 % in nondesaturators). Sleep poses profound physiological alterations to the respiratory system even in healthy subjects, such as alterations in ventilation-perfusion, a reduced functional residual capacity due to a recumbent position and reduced respiratory drive with relative alveolar hypoventilation. In patients with PPH, these changes may lead to oxygen desaturation and may negatively interact, promoting sleep-related breathing disturbances. Indeed, hypoxia may favor SDB through hypoxia-mediated vasoconstriction, with consequent increased pulmonary hypertension and right ventricular pressure overload leading to reduced cardiac output. Moreover, hypoxia per se could stimulate peripheral chemoreceptors and lead to

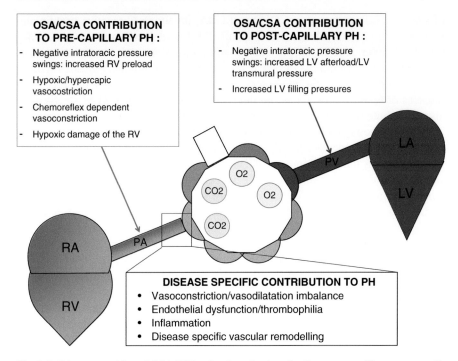

OSA/CSA CONTRIBUTION TO PRE-CAPILLARY PH :
- Negative intratoracic pressure swings: increased RV preload
- Hypoxic/hypercapic vasocostriction
- Chemoreflex dependent vasoconstriction
- Hypoxic damage of the RV

OSA/CSA CONTRIBUTION TO POST-CAPILLARY PH :
- Negative intratoracic pressure swings: increased LV afterload/LV transmural pressure
- Increased LV filling pressures

DISEASE SPECIFIC CONTRIBUTION TO PH
- Vasoconstriction/vasodilatation imbalance
- Endothelial dysfunction/thrombophilia
- Inflammation
- Disease specific vascular remodelling

Fig. 3.4 Disease-specific and OSA/CSA-related mechanisms leading to precapillary or postcapillary pulmonary hypertension. CO_2 carbon dioxide, *CSA* central sleep apnea, *PH* pulmonary hypertension, *LA* left atrium, *LV* left ventricle, O_2 oxygen, *OSA* obstructive sleep apnea, *PA* pulmonary artery, *PV* pulmonary veins, *RA* right atrium, *RV* right ventricle

CSA by shifting the $PaCO_2$ levels below the apneic threshold [147]. Unfortunately, neither the SaO_2 profile, nor the type of SDB (CSA/OSA) was reported in the study of Hildenbrand and thus it is difficult to infer whether part of the nocturnal desaturation is due to SDB or which pathophysiological mechanisms link PPH and SDB. In a recent study, Jeremy et al. confirmed the high prevalence of SDB in patients with CTEPH. In this population, a reduced cardiac index strongly predicted the presence and the severity of SDB, especially in the subgroup of patients with CSA [144].

In chronic obstructive pulmonary disease (COPD) (group III of WHO PH classification), a very high prevalence of OSA is commonly observed, so the term "overlap syndrome" (present in about 1 % of adults) has been created to define the coexistence of COPD and OSA. The coexistence of the two phenomena may be related to the high prevalence of the both COPD and OSA in the general population, but common risk factors such as body mass index and smoking may also influence the relationship. Cigarette smoking actually contributes to upper airway inflammation and edema, and certain medications used in COPD such as corticosteroids may foster central fat deposition. Furthermore, evidence of systemic inflammation in COPD and OSA, involving C-reactive protein and IL-6, in addition to nuclear factor-kappaB (NF-kB)-dependent pathways involving TNF-alpha and IL-8, provides insight into potential basic interactions between the two disorders [143]. The reduction of the pulmonary elastic recoil or the respiratory muscle fatigue associated with COPD (especially the accessory muscles of respiration such as the intercostal muscles during REM sleep), may also contribute to OSA development in group 3. Nocturnal oxygen desaturations, already common in COPD, are more severe in the overlap syndrome, thus predisposing to PH and accelerating right ventricular overload and failure. Among factors promoting the development of OSA, rostral fluid shift during sleep when supine should be remembered [122]: indeed fluid displacement from the legs during recumbency while in bed is known to narrow the upper airways cross-sectional area by increase in the mucosal water content, thus contributing to the pathogenesis of OSA.

OSA itself, without comorbid COPD, is considered a potential cause of PH and part of WHO group 3; in fact, PH is present in 12–34% of patients with OSA. However, the role of OSA in the development of PH and its mechanisms are not entirely clear [140].

Patients with OSA usually experience cyclical oxygen desaturations during sleep, with episodes lasting 10–40 s, followed by arousals and complete or partial re-oxygenation. Intermittent hypoxia can lead to polycythemia and PH [148]. Recent studies report the role of the involvement of numerous pathways involving ROS, perturbation of NO, angiogenic factors, and vasoactive agents, resulting in partially reversible vasoconstriction and increased pulmonary artery pressure. Wu et al. have shown that, although acute hypoxia (partial pressure of oxygen, 25–30 mmHg for 5–10 min) stimulates a reduction in reactive oxygen species (ROS), chronic hypoxia (48 h) actually increases ROS production in human pulmonary artery smooth muscle cells. This different pattern of response probably is a subcellular mechanism whose phenotypical expression is vasoconstriction in acute hypoxia and vascular remodeling in chronic hypoxia. In experiments in which mice were exposed to chronic intermittent hypoxia for 8 weeks, the induced PH was associated with increased lung levels of the NADPH oxidase subunits, an important source of superoxide production, that may contribute to the development of pulmonary vascular remodeling and hypertension [149]. Chronic intermittent hypoxia also causes suppression of endothelial nitric oxide synthase (eNOS) and impairment of endothelial-dependent nitric oxide (NO) vasodilation by an NF-kB-dependent mechanism [150]. Other potential pathways involved in OSA-related PH includes serotonin, angiopoietin-1, and endothelin-1. While some evidence about the role of these vascular peptides has been collected in heterogeneous animal models and clinical studies on PH, their specific role in patients with OSA is still to be demonstrated [140].

Most OSA patients present with normal oxygen saturation while awake, apart from those with underlying lung disease or obesity hypoventilation syndrome. The latter are at greater risk of having PH (59% higher than patients with OSA alone) due to the additional effect of hypercapnia [151].

Moreover, patients with OSA often develop systemic hypertension. As a result of the high frequency of diurnal hypertension and intermittent surges in arterial blood pressure due to respiratory events during sleep, patients with OSA often develop left ventricular hypertrophy and diastolic/systolic dysfunction (see also Sect. 3.4.3). Therefore, at least in a subset of patients, also a passive postcapillary component should be considered.

Finally, the effect of OSA on PH should be analyzed bearing in mind that especially during nighttime the ventilatory pattern is actually oscillatory and thus the hemodynamic consequences of OSA on the pulmonary vasculature are likely to be oscillatory as well. Indeed, the hemodynamic evaluation in patients with OSA showed very high PAP values at apnea or immediately after apnea, in particular during REM sleep [152, 153]. PWP was also studied and was found to increase progressively during apneas, confirming a postcapillary contribution on PAP increase during apneas [154].

In a few studies the transmural PAP was also evaluated, in order to estimate the distending pressure of the pulmonary artery, independently from any interference exerted by the intrathoracic pressure swings typical of OSA. Also after correcting for the intrathoracic pressure, a progressive increase of PAP from beginning to end of apnea was found [155–157].

Some of the mechanisms linking OSA to PH are likely to apply also to the CSR/CSA of patients with left-sided PH (group 2 of PH). A detailed focus on the background pathophysiology of heart failure and central apneas is beyond the aim of this chapter and will be discussed in depth in both Chaps. 4 and 5. PH due to left heart disease is surely composed by a passive component, associated with increased left atrial pressure possibly related to diastolic dysfunction and mitral regurgitation [158]. Beyond this passive component (which is the key feature of IPC-PH), a reactive component may occur and lead to the CPC-PH development. Vasoconstriction and "capillary stress failure" could be reversible or lead to muscularization of the small pulmonary arteries with medial hypertrophy and neointima formation [159]. A few investigations have analyzed the pathophysiology of PH in CSR/CSA of heart failure patients. Solin et al. [160] investigated the association between PAP and CSR in a population of unstable patients with advanced HF, screened for heart transplantation, with severe hemodynamic compromise. The authors hypothesized that higher PAP in patients with CSR could find a "passive" origin in the elevated pulmonary venous and end-diastolic LV pressure, also considering the finding of low pulmonary vascular resistances and transpulmonary gradient. A second study, by Christ et al. [161] was performed in a more stable population: only indirect signs of pulmonary hypertension, as expressed by pulmonary artery acceleration time, were found to be associated with both CSR and indexes of right ventricular dysfunction. In patients with heart failure is possible to assume that the effects of CSR on the pulmonary pressure are mainly linked to the direct effect of hypoxia on the pulmonary vasculature in the same way that occurs in patients with OSA. Nevertheless, it is possible that other mechanisms may take place. Interestingly, elevated sympathetic activity has been shown in a model of chronic intermittent hypoxia in healthy humans; in a similar fashion, patients with idiopathic pulmonary arterial hypertension had increased sympathetic nerve activity, which has yet to be characterized; however, a substantial component of increased sympathetic tone appears to be mediated by the arterial chemoreceptor reflex pathway [162]. In a study from our group, a population of chronic and stable HF patients and presumably low left ventricular filling pressures (no severe mitral regurgitation or diastolic dysfunction), the presence of CSR during the 24 h (AHI cutoff ≥15 events/hour) was associated with higher systolic PAP at echocardiography. Systolic PAP was indeed not only correlated with 24 h AHI, but also with chemosensitivity to hypoxia and hypercapnia, confirming a potential role of chemoreflex-mediated adrenergic discharge on pulmonary vasoconstriction [163].

3.3.5.5 Treatment

The vast majority of studies on SDB and PH have focused on the treatment of OSA in group 3 PH and are mainly based on CPAP administration. This is based on the clinical observation that patients with OSA and concomitant PH actually show increased mortality at 1-, 4-, and 8-year follow-up [164]. On the other hand, there are only a few trials that have explored the effect of treatment in other types of precapillary or postcapillary PH.

Alchanatis et al. examined the effect of CPAP therapy in six patients with OSA and PH; they were studied with pulsed-wave Doppler echocardiography for estimation of PAP before and after 6 months' effective treatment with CPAP: there was a significant reduction in mean PAP value from 25.6 ± 4.0 mmHg to 19.5 ± 1.6 mmHg ($P < 0.001$) [165]. In a prospective study involving 22 patients with OSA (mean AHI, 48.6 ± 5.2 events/h), five of whom had mean PAP ≥ 20 mmHg, 4 months of CPAP treatment decreased mean PAP from 17.0 ± 1.2 mmHg to 14.5 ± 0.8 mmHg in the entire group ($P < 0.05$), with the greatest reduction observed in patients with PH at baseline. The reduction in mean PAP was attributed to decreased pulmonary vascular resistance and decreased vasoconstrictive response to the hypoxic stimulus [166].

In a randomized, sham-controlled crossover study performed in ten patients with OSA and PH (right ventricular systolic pressure RVSP >30 mmHg estimated by Doppler echocardiograph) and no known cardiac or lung diseases, 12 weeks of CPAP therapy decreased RVSP from 28.8 ± 7.9 mmHg to 24.0 ± 5.8 mmHg ($P < 0.0001$), again with the greatest reduction in patients with either PH or left ventricular dysfunction at baseline [167]. The positive hemodynamic effects of CPAP treatment on PH in OSA patients are also supported by the reduction in endothelin-1, other markers of inflammation (namely CRP and IL-6) and platelet activation, as well as increase in NO metabolites observed after CPAP [168]. In patients with OSA and PH, a similar effect to CPAP on both PAP and systemic diastolic pressure at 3-, 6-, and 9-month follow-up was observed with uvulopalatopharyngoplasty [169].

Recently, in a randomized, placebo-controlled, double-blind, three period crossover trial, it was evaluated whether nocturnal oxygen therapy (NOT) or acetazolamide improved exercise performance and quality of life in patients with precapillary PH (16 with pulmonary arterial PH, 7 with chronic thromboembolic PH) and SDB. One week treatment with NOT improved nocturnal oxygenation and periodic breathing as well as exercise capacity, functional class and right ventricular function [170].

In postcapillary PH, some interesting information may be derived by the paper of Solin et al. [160]. In patients with severe heart failure with reduced ejection fraction, awaiting heart transplantation, in fact, not only the AHI was correlated with the PWP, but intensive medical therapy in seven patients with initially high PWP and central apneas (treated with increased diuretics and/or ACE inhibition, nitrates, carvedilol, or CPAP apart from the night of the respiratory recording in which CPAP was not applied) reduced both PWP (29.0 ± 2.6–22.0 ± 1.8 mmHg, $p < 0.001$) and AHI (38.5 ± 7.7–18.5 ± 5.3 events/hour, $p = 0.005$).

3.4 Obstructive Sleep Apnea

3.4.1 Definition

Obstructive sleep apnea (OSA) is defined by the adult obstructive sleep apnea task force of the American Academy of Sleep Medicine as "the occurrence of daytime sleepiness, loud snoring, witnessed breathing interruptions, or awakenings due to gasping or choking in the presence of at least five obstructive respiratory events" [171].

3.4.2 Epidemiology and Risk Factors

The exact prevalence of OSA is unknown and it is estimated to range between 10% and 17% of the US population, with the variation being in part due to the variable criteria used to define the disease (e.g., the number of apneic episodes per hour). Recently, the Wisconsin Sleep Cohort Study [171] estimated that 10% of men and 3% of women between 30 and 49 years and 17% of men and 9% of women between 50 and 70 years have moderate to severe OSA (AHI ≥ 15). The authors suggest that these prevalence rates are likely to increase due to the obesity pandemic, making OSA a global health issue. Besides obesity, also male gender, aging, alcohol consumption, smoking, drug addiction, enlarged neck circumference and nasal obstruction are risk factors independently correlated with AHI > 15 events/hour. Interestingly, in elderly subjects, the presence of OSA is poorly predicted by higher BMI and body habitus and snoring [172, 173].

3.4.3 Clinical Implications and Complications

OSA is characterized by recurrent collapse of the upper airways, resulting in substantially reduced (hypopnea) or complete cessation (apnoea) of airflow despite ongoing breathing efforts. The presentation of obstructive apneas is associated with snoring, reduced sleep quality, increased daytime sleepiness, and headaches; also witnessed apnea may be referred [171].

CIH is responsible for the development of negative cardiovascular and metabolic sequelae, as well as brain damage. CIH leads to increased sympathetic outflow by different mechanism. In particular, CIH could play a role in the increased activity of carotid chemosensitive cells and the inflammation of the carotid body, likely by the upregulation of angiotensinogen, AT receptors, and ACE expression in the carotid body [174, 175].

Hypercapnia occurring during apneas is itself a sympathetic stimulation factor, even if no significant increment in the responses to hypercapnia was found in apneic patients compared with control subjects (see below). Negative intrathoracic pressure, with the concomitant fluctuations in heart rate and systolic ejection volume, as well as arousals from sleep play secondary roles by potentiating the hypoxia-induced increase in sympathetic outflow [176], leading to chronic modifications in cardiovascular system, metabolic pathways, and nervous system.

Hypoxia and increased sympathetic activity predispose OSA patients to develop systemic hypertension (occurring in up to 60 % of patients with obstructive sleep apnea) [177] with left ventricular hypertrophy [178] and pulmonary hypertension (approximately in about 17–70 %: the variability of this range may be explained with the different cutoff used in different studies) [168]. Patients with severe OSA (defined by an AHI $\geq$30) are more frequently affected by atrial fibrillation (AF), complex ventricular ectopies and nonsustained ventricular tachycardia (NSVT) than patients with an AHI of <5 [179]. Furthermore, OSA is independently correlated to atherosclerosis, insulin resistance, hypercholesterolemia, and metabolic syndrome. Since OSA and metabolic syndrome share common features, the combination of the two has been labeled "Syndrome Z" [180]. Moreover, changes in cerebral blood flow and in oxygen availability, together with sleep fragmentation and sleep deprivation resulting from nocturnal episodes of complete or partial pharyngeal obstruction, may drive to progressive deterioration of brain function and cognitive dysfunction such as attention, executive functioning, motor efficiency, working memory, and long-term episodic memory [74, 181]. Finally, OSA is associated with reduced prognosis and quality of life (reduced work and scholar attention, excessive daytime sleepiness, increased road traffic accidents) [182].

3.4.4 Pathophysiology

The underlying pathophysiology of OSA is multifactorial and may considerably vary between individuals. Soft tissue morphology and bone abnormalities, together with decreased muscular tone of upper airway dilators, are long-established actors in the pathophysiology of OSA. Furthermore, the association between OSA and inflammation and metabolism has been recently studied, leading to new interesting insights in OSA pathophysiology (Fig. 3.5).

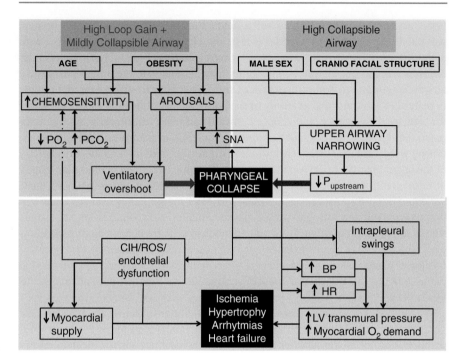

Fig. 3.5 Pathophysiological mechanisms leading to airway collapse in patients with OSA and consequent negative effects of OSA on the cardiovascular system. *BP* blood pressure, *CIH* chronic intermittent hypoxia, *ROS* reactive oxygen species, *HR* heart rate, *LV* left ventricular, *SNA* sympathetic nerve activity

During inspiration, the diaphragm acts as a pump creating intraluminal subatmospheric pressure, enabling air to get into the respiratory system. Airflow is directly related to the pressure gradient between the upstream pressure ($P_{upstream}$), which is equivalent to atmospheric pressure (P_{atm}) in free breathing, and the critical closing pressure (P_{crit}), defined as the negative pressure inside the airway at which the airway collapses. If P_{crit} is highly negative, the $P_{upstream}$ needed to ensure airway patency is small, and a great airflow may take place whenever a high negative intrapleural pressure is generated during inspiration. On the contrary, with P_{crit} approaching 0 cmH$_2$0 or P_{atm}, the $P_{upstream}$ required to maintain airway patency should be higher, and the range of airflow increase during inspiration is smaller, because the P_{crit} is easily overcome, leading to airway collapsibility. When P_{crit} equals P_{atm}, no pressure gradient is generated, no airflow takes place, and upper airways collapse [183]. Measurements in sleeping humans have shown that P_{crit} is < -10 cmH$_2$O in normal subjects with low airway resistance and minimal CO$_2$ retention during NREM sleep, while it is between -5 and 0 cmH$_2$O in snorers and even >0 cmH$_2$O in OSAS subjects [184].

Obesity is a major contributor to upper airway compression because of mechanical impediment to diaphragmatic contraction and increased adiposity in peripharyngeal regions [185], as well as under the mandible and within the tongue, soft palate, or uvula [186]. Gender is also associated with differences in P_{crit}, with males having less negative values than women (of about 2–3 cmH_2O). This gender difference in passive airway collapsibility may be related to the longer pharyngeal airway length and to a major content of soft tissue both in soft palate and tongue in males [187]. Abnormal anatomy of the upper airway regions is also responsible for increased resistance and reduced inward airflow. Nasal laryngoscopy, computed tomography and magnetic resonance imaging, or pharyngeal pressure monitoring were used in several studies to investigate the anatomy and the morphology of the upper airways in OSA patients, demonstrating a reduced mandibular length, inferior position of the hyoid bone, and retroposition of the maxilla in those patients [188, 189]. Moreover, by means of MRI imaging, Schwab et al. showed that retropalatal and retroglossal regions are smaller, soft palate is longer, tongue size is larger, and the quantity of subcutaneous fat is greater compared with normal subject. These characteristics encroach on airway diameter in the anterior–posterior plane, while the thickened pharyngeal walls encroach in the lateral plane, making the UA dilator muscle contraction mechanically disadvantageous [190, 191].

In addition, compromised activity of the UA dilator muscles (among them, the genioglossus muscle has been studied the most [192]) also plays a role in OSA pathophysiology. Upper airways are controlled by locally mediated mechanoreceptive reflex mechanisms that respond to negative pharyngeal pressure [193]; among those reflexes there is the genioglossus muscle (GG) negative pressure reflex, whereby the muscle is activated in response to rapid changes in negative intrapharyngeal pressure (subatmospheric or suction pressure) [194]. During wakefulness, patients with OSA appear to compensate for an anatomically compromised upper airway through protective reflexes that increase upper airways dilator muscles' activity to maintain airway patency. The genioglossus motor units in OSA patients are indeed recruited earlier and the motor units potentials show an increased temporal and spatial recruitment when compared with controls. It is likely that recurrent exposure to hypoxia, vibration due to snoring, abnormal movement, or compression of the pharyngeal musculature may lead to motor units' remodeling: fewer motor axons reinnervate the same number of muscle fibers to produce larger, longer, and often more complex motor units potentials [102].

On the contrary, during sleep, a diminished ability of the upper airway dilator muscles to maintain a patent airway during sleep was shown [195]. At the onset of sleeping, both in healthy individuals and in OSA, wake-related excitatory stimuli are lost and mechanoreceptor reflex responses may be significantly blunted. In particular, the GG negative pressure reflex is substantially diminished or lost completely. However, differently than in healthy controls, in OSA patients the loss of a protective reflex responsible for UA patency, coupled with anatomical abnormalities, is detrimental [194, 196]. Also the chemoreceptor activity has a substantial effect on upper airway muscle recruitment: a higher threshold for both inhibition (via hypocapnia) and activation (via hypercapnia) of the phrenic motor neurons was shown. In anesthetized rabbits, the GG muscle activity ceases before diaphragmatic activity during hypocapnia, whereas, during hypercapnia, increments of the activity from baseline are higher in the genioglossus than in the diaphragm [197].

Chemoreflex responses in OSA are affected by different factors such as age, gender, weight, and comorbidities such as diabetes, hypertension, and cardiovascular disease [198].

During hypoxia, OSA patients also exhibited a significantly greater increase in minute ventilation, heart rate, and mean arterial pressure, indicating greater peripheral chemoreceptor sensitivity in OSA, even after adjusting for all the aforementioned potential confounders; on the contrary, no significant change in the responses to hypercapnia was observed in OSA patients [199, 200]. However, obesity, a major risk factor in OSA, is an independent predictor of increased central chemoreflex sensitivity to CO_2 [199]. The mechanisms responsible for this phenomenon are not certain; however, authors speculated that it may be due to leptin, as leptin is raised in obesity and leptin-deficient mice show severe blunting of the HCVR [201]. Indeed, obese OSA patients actually exhibit an increased dynamic ventilatory response to hypercapnic hypoxia during sleep [202].

Recently, the correlations between OSA and the inflammatory status due to obesity have been studied. Fat depots are thought to be a rich source of humoral mediators and inflammatory cytokines, such as TNF-a and IL-6, which are elevated in OSA patients, but also ROS (produced by ANG –II-induced activation of NADPH oxidase), which induce carotid chemoreflex sensitization [203]. Moreover, OSA patients have a higher incidence of metabolic syndrome and diabetes than general population. OSA is in fact associated with greater values of insulin resistance as well as of plasma renin activity. It is possible that insulin resistance (through hyperinsulinemia) and plasma renin activity (through angiotensin II) stimulate sympathetic activity, leading to peripheral chemoreceptors overactivity but potentially also to central chemoreceptors overactivity [204].

The role of ventilatory control mechanisms in the pathogenesis of OSA is a matter of debate. Several studies indicate that the instability of respiratory control (see also Chaps. 4 and 5) can lead to periodic breathing and that complete or partial obstruction of upper airways can occur at the nadir of the ventilatory cycle (during central apneas/hypopneas) [205]. The hypothesis that basic instability of respiratory control is essential for the development of OSA is not new and was first postulated by Onal et al. in 1982, based on the observation that periodic breathing with repetitive central apnea was commonly observed in patients after tracheostomy for OSA treatment [206, 207]. After that, the relationship between loop gain and OSA has been further studied, and an increased loop gain in OSA patients was found [202, 208, 209], mainly due to increased controller gain rather than increased plant gain [210]. However, how elevated the chemoreceptor response must be is still debated, and the exact mechanism of chemoreflex influence in OSA pathophysiology is still unknown. There are two main potential mechanisms that are likely to be crucial. Firstly, elevated loop gain is expected to increase oscillations from the brainstem central pattern generator. While an increased chemoreflex stimulation not only increases ventilation, but also upper airway patency, pharyngeal obstruction does actually occur when chemoreflex stimulation and thus ventilatory and upper airway motor output are at their nadir. Furthermore, transient arousals, which are major determinants of the magnitude of the ventilatory overshoot at end-apnea, are likely to contribute to ventilatory instability together with overactive chemore-ceptors [180].

Overall, the extent to which ventilatory instability and neural reflexes impairment is pathophysiologically important in any given individual may relate to the anatomic properties of the airway, and vice versa. It is possible, in fact, that those factors that we have previously described, even if they all contribute to the genesis of obstructive apneas, play different relative roles in every single individual.

3.4.5   Treatment

The pathophysiology of OSA is characterized by a complex interaction among anatomical abnormalities of the upper airways, imbalanced neurochemical control of ventilation, airway muscle dilator recruitment and arousals.

Hence, when considering initiating any treatment, careful consideration on the patient's phenotype, along with his/her risk factors must be taken into account.

All patients should be counseled to adopt lifestyle modifications such as weight loss, avoidance of alcohol and other sedatives, smoking cessation, and good sleep hygiene that might reduce or eliminate known modifiable risk factors for OSA [211].

Noninvasive mechanical ventilation (NIV) still remains the most frequently used and the most efficient treatment in OSA. The American Academy of Sleep Medicine (formerly the American Sleep Disorders Association) guidelines for CPAP therapy recommend its use for patients with an apnea index ≥ 20 events/hour, and for symptomatic patients with an AHI or respiratory arousal index (mean number of arousals per hour of sleep) ≥ 10 events/hour [212]. NIV provides pneumatic splinting of the upper airways and is effective in reducing the AHI; NIV may be delivered in continuous (CPAP), bi-level (BPAP), or autotitrating (APAP or adaptive servo ventilation ASV) positive airway pressure modes. Partial pressure reduction during expiration (pressure relief) can also be added to these models. The mechanism of continuous positive airway pressure is debated, but probably it is related to an increased upstream pressure ($P_{upstream}$), so that the intraluminal pressure exceeds the surrounding pressure [213]. Continuous positive airway pressure also increases end-expiratory lung volume, which stabilizes the upper airway through caudal traction. Polysomnographic studies have demonstrated that treatment with CPAP is able to restore the patency of the airways throughout the respiratory cycle and to reverse apnea and hypopnea [213]. As explained above, CPAP therapy is not only associated with an increase in the upstream pressure given to the respiratory apparatus (which mechanically opens the airways), but it is also responsible for a reduction in the chemoceptive responses [214]. Spicuzza et al. found that in moderate to severe OSA, 1 month of nasal CPAP significantly decreased waking ventilatory response to normocapnic hypoxia (from 1.08 ± 0.07 L/min/%SaO$_2$ prior to treatment to 0.53 ± 0.02 L/min/%SaO$_2$ after treatment) but not to normoxic hypercapnia. In another study, Loewen et al. measured the dynamic ventilatory response to CO_2 in a group of severe OSA patients before and after 1 month of CPAP therapy and observed that ventilatory sensitivity to CO_2 was markedly diminished following CPAP therapy [215].

CPAP showed beneficial clinical effects in patients with OSA such as reduced daytime sleepiness and increased neurocognitive performance. Kribbs et al. reported the persistent improvement of the daytime sleepiness (measured by the Epworth Sleepiness Scale and Maintenance of Wakefulness Test) even after prolonged therapy, thus underlying the patient's compliance to the treatment [216].

Furthermore, prolonged CPAP significantly reduces diurnal sympathetic tone in patients with OSA [199]. In 2005 a prospective, long-term, observational study analyzed a population of 1651 subjects; these subjects, matched for age and BMI, were divided into four groups: healthy controls, snorers, mild to moderate OSA, and severe OSA. Patients with severe OSA showed an increased risk for fatal and non-fatal cardiovascular events; in this group treatment with CPAP significantly reduced cardiovascular outcomes [217].

Beyond weight loss, an alternative to CPAP action on $P_{up\ stream}$ is to decrease the critical collapse pressure (P_{crit}) reducing UA resistance, by either intervening on anatomical abnormalities or muscle strength [180].

Recently, a study of 570 subjects with severe OSA (apnea/hypopnea index (AHI) $\geq$ 30/h) and a control group of 269 subjects (AHI < 5/h) were followed up for a median of 79 months; initially, they all received CPAP, and mandibular advancing device (MAD) was subsequently offered to those who were nonadherent to CPAP. Both CPAP and MAD were equally effective in reducing the risk for fatal cardiovascular events in patients with severe OSA [218]. MADs represent the main noncontinuous positive airway pressure (non-CPAP) therapy for patients with obstructive sleep apnea (OSA); MADs reduce sleep apnea and daytime sleepiness and improve quality of life compared with placebo devices. CPAP and MADs usually had similar effects on daytime sleepiness, while CPAP seems more effective in reducing AHI (mean reduction from all studies of 83 %) when compared to MAD (mean reduction from all studies of 55 %). MADs are indicated in the treatment of patients with mild to moderate OSA (Recommendation Level A) and in patients who do not tolerate CPAP, according to European Respiratory Society Task Force [219].

Surgical approaches targeting different anatomical areas may have different outcomes; hence, it is crucial to precisely map the site of obstruction before surgery. The goal is to cure OSAS with the same efficacy as CPAP; however, a long-term follow-up is strongly recommended because of the high failure rates of the procedures; an objective pre- and postoperative measurement of OSAS severity is also crucial.

Among different surgical approaches, adenotonsillectomy is often performed in children and selected adults. Uvulopalatopharyngoplasty (UPPP) is recommended for obstruction confined to the velopharynx; however, the 95 % failure rate among patients with upper airway obstruction caudal to the velopharynx suggests recurrent obstruction at this level. Laser-assisted uvulopalatoplasty is a modified UPPP procedure that results in a less radical resection of palatal tissue. Tongue base surgery includes various procedures developed to remove excess of lingual tissue and increase the caliber of the retrolingual oropharynx in mild to moderate OSA [211].

More recently, other nonanatomical treatments were explored and tailored for patients with either high chemosensitivity or low arousal threshold; these treatments should reduce loop gain to stabilize central respiratory motor output, raise the arousal threshold, and recruit the airway dilator muscles [180]. The carbonic anhydrase inhibitor acetazolamide stimulates ventilation via a mild systemic metabolic acidosis and was shown to be partly effective in reducing central apneas of HF patients [220]. In a group of 13 patients with mild to severe OSA, 1 week of acetazolamide treatment reduced the loop gain by 41 % and AHI by 51 %. Interestingly, in one patient acetazolamide administration was associated with an increase in the loop gain, which was accompanied also by a significant increase in the AHI. Apart from reducing the loop gain, acetazolamide did not significantly alter pharyngeal anatomy/collapsibility, upper-airway gain, or arousal threshold [221]. Oxygen administration (via nasal cannula) has been proven to reduce chemosensitivity to CO_2, widen the CO_2 reserve between eupnea and the apneic threshold, and significantly reduce AHI in patients with HF and central apneas. Hyperoxia was also shown to reduce the AHI in a minority of patients with OSA, especially those with already elevated chemoreceptor gain [222].

Recent studies have focused on modifying the arousal threshold as a potential therapeutical option. The rationale around this type of treatment is dual: firstly, increasing the arousal threshold would per se have a positive effect on the loop gain, reducing the possibility of ventilatory overshoot usually associated with an arousal; secondly, the average increase in CO_2 levels depending on the maintenance of either the sleep state or a deeper sleep stage would warrant the chemoreflex stimulation of airway dilator muscles, restoring flow before the arousal. Several sedative agents are known to increase the arousal threshold, including ethanol, flurazepam, triazolam, pentobarbital, and trazodone. However, some of these drugs, such as alcohol and benzodiazepines may also impair the upper-airway dilator muscle responsiveness, paradoxically worsening apneas. Nonetheless, in a selected population of patients with OSA and particularly low arousal thresholds, eszopiclone (a non-benzodiazepine sedative) showed a promising reduction in the AHI by around 40–50 % [223].

Another emerging therapeutic option is to act on the neurochemical mechanisms of REM sleep–related hypotonia of upper airway muscles, as recently reviewed in [224]. In this respect, the withdrawal of the norepinephrine and serotonin-mediated excitatory inputs on upper airway muscles seems to play a critical role [225]. Unfortunately, the results of trials testing drugs with an action on this neurobiological pathway are conflicting. One crossover trial performed in 20 OSA patients compared paroxetine (specific serotonin reuptake inhibitor, antidepressant) versus placebo and showed a significant difference in AHI with average reduction of 6.1 events/hour (95 % CI −11.00 to −1.20) in the paroxetine arm. Three placebo control studies have compared the effect of mirtazapine (mixed antagonist and agonist acting on serotonin receptors) on OSA. While Carley et al. in 2007 reported a significant reduction in mean AHI (15 mg and 4.5 mg of mirtazapine, AHI reduction 52% and 46%, respectively) [226], Marshall et al. in 2008 found a significant increase in AHI in the mirtazapine arm (both with 15 mg and 30 mg dosages) [227]. The lack of any preenrollment evaluation of LG state may possibly account for the controversial results of these studies.

As also suggested in patients with neuromuscular disorders, inspiratory muscle training seems to show some benefit in patients with OSA, who are intolerant to CPAP, with positive reductions in systolic and diastolic blood pressures (-12.3 ± 1.6 and -5.0 ± 1.3 mmHg, respectively; $p<0.01$) and plasma norepinephrine levels (536.3 ± 56.6 vs. 380.6 ± 41.2 pg/mL, $p=0.01$), nighttime arousals and amelioration of sleep (Pittsburgh Sleep Quality Index scores: 9.1 ± 0.9 vs. 5.1 ± 0.7; $p=0.001$). These favorable results were achieved without any effect on the AHI and may be mediated by a reduced stimulation of the ergoreflex by respiratory muscles [228]. The same positive finding was also replicated in HF patients and this time accompanied by both improvement of functional capacity and reduction in exertional ventilatory oscillations [229].

Anatomic substrate, ventilatory instability, and neurochemical reflexes represent the main actors in the OSA pathophysiology, as well as the main therapeutic targets. The management of the single patient, thus, should not disregard the individual pathophysiological background and should aim at identifying the specific features of the single patient and treating them in a tailored approach.

Conclusions

Central and obstructive sleep apneas are complex disorders that may be present in different clinical scenarios, from cardiac to neurologic and pulmonary conditions. The identification of sleep disturbances is crucial for the comprehensive treatment of the underlying condition, since apneas are associated with increased sympathetic outflow and neural damage, worsened cardiovascular outcomes and overall reduced quality of life. On the other hand, the most appropriate treatment for sleep disturbances is strongly dependent on a deeper understanding of the pathophysiological mechanisms underlying respiratory instability in that specific disease background. In this respect, a global and wide vision of the apnea phenomenon, rather than a narrow and deeply redundant approach, related to the peculiar researcher point of view, may warrant a faster advancement even in remote fields of interest.

References

1. Rigatto H, Brady UP. Periodic breathing and apnea in preterm infants: 2. Hypoxia as a primary event. Pediatrics. 1972;50:219–28.
2. Brooks JG. Apparent lifethreatening events and apnea of infancy. Clin Perinatol. 1992;4:80938.
3. Henderson DJ. The effect of gestational age on the incidence and duration of recurrent apnoea in newborn babies. Aust Paediatr J. 1981;4:2736.

4. Razi PP, Razi NM, DeLauter M, Pandit PB. Periodic breathing and oxygen saturation in preterm infants at discharge. J Perinatol. 2002;22:442–4.
5. Wilkinson MH, Cranage S, Berger PJ, Blanch N, Adamson TM. Changes in the temporal structure of periodic breathing with postnatal development in preterm infants. Pediatr. 1995;38:533–8.
6. NIH Consens Statement Online. Infantile Apnea and Home Monitoring. 1986;6(6):1–10.
7. Abu-Shaweesh J, Baird TM, Martin RJ. Apnea and bradycardia of prematurity. Neonatal Respiratory Disorders. 2nd ed. London: Arnold; 2003. pp. 424–36.
8. Kiechl Kohlendorfer U, Hof D, Peglow UP, Traweger Ravanelli B, Kiechl S. Epidemiology of apparent life threatening events. Arch Dis Child. 2005;90(3):297300.
9. Wigfield RE, Fleming PJ, Berry PJ. Can the fall in Avon's sudden infant death rate be explained by the observed sleeping position changes? BMJ. 1993;304:282–3.
10. Blair PS, Sidebotham P, Berry PJ. Major changes in the epidemiology of sudden infant death syndrome: a 20-year population based study of all unexpected deaths in infancy. Lancet. 2006;367:314–9.
11. Oliveira AJ, Nunes ML, Fojo-Olmos A, Reis FM, da Costa JC. Clinical correlates of periodic breathing in neonatal polysomnography. Clin Neurophysiol. 2004;115:2247–51.
12. Sale SM. Neonatal apnoea. Best Pract Res Clin Anaesthesiol. 2012;323–36:24.
13. Fleming PJ, Blair PS, Pease A. Sudden unexpected death in infancy: aetiology, pathophysiology, epidemiology and prevention in 2015. Arch Dis Child. 2015;100:984–8.
14. Fenner A, Schalk U, Hoenicke H, Wendenburg A, Roehling T. Periodic breathing in premature and neonatal babies: incidence, breathing pattern, respiratory gas tensions, response to changes in the composition of ambient air. Pediatr Res. 1973;7:174–8.
15. Marcus C, Carroll JM, Donnelly D. Sleep and breathing in children, Second Edition: Developmental changes in breathing during sleep. New York: Medical; 2008. pp. 185–91.
16. Raynes-Greenow CH, Hadfield RM, Cistulli PA, Bowen J, Allen H, Roberts CL. Sleep apnea in early childhood associated with preterm birth but not small for gestational age: a population-based record linkage study. Sleep. 2012;35(11):1475–80.
17. Marcus CL, Brook LJ, Draper KA, Gozal D, Halbower AC, Jones J, et al. Diagnosis and management of childhood obstructive sleep apnea syndrome. Pediatrics. 2012;130(3): 576–84.
18. Clinical practice guideline: diagnosis and management of childhood obstructive sleep apnea syndrome. Pediatrics. 2002;109(4):704–12.
19. Martin RJ, DiFiore JM, Jana L, Davis RL, Miller MJ, Coles SK, et al. Persistence of the biphasic ventilator response to hypoxia in preterm infants. J Pediatr. 1998;132:960–4.
20. Krauss A, Klain D, Waldman S, Auld P. Ventilatory response to carbon dioxide in newborn infants. Pediatr Res. 1975;9:46–50.
21. Khan A, Qurashi M, Kwiatkowski K, Cates D, Rigatto H. Measurement of the CO_2 apneic threshold in newborn infants: possible relevance for periodic breathing and apnea. J Appl Physiol. 2005;98:1171–6.
22. Pickens D, Schefft G, Thach B. Prolonged apnea associated with upper airway protective reflexes in apnea of prematurity. Am Rev Respir Dis. 1988;137(1):113–8.
23. Lee J, Stoll B, Downing S. Properties of the laryngeal chemoreflex in neonatal piglets. Am J Physiol. 1977;233:R30–6.
24. Abu-Shaweesh J, Dreshaj I, Haxhiu M, Martin R. GABAergic mechanisms are involved in superior laryngeal nerve stimulation-induced apnea. J App Physiol. 2001;90:1570–6.
25. Runold M, Lagercrantz H, Fredholm B. Ventilatory effect of an adenosine analogue in unanaesthetized rabbits during development. J App Physiol. 1986;61:255–9.
26. Wilson C, Martin R, Jaber J, Abu-Shaweesh J, Jafri A, Haxhiu M, et al. Adenosine A2A receptors interact with GABAergic pathways to modulate respiration in neonatal piglets. Respir Physiol Neurobiol. 2004;141:201–6.
27. Abu-Shaweesh J, Martin R. Neonatal apnea: what's new? Pediatr Pulmonol. 2008;937(944):43.
28. Kinney H, Richerson G, Dymecki S, Darnall R, Nattie E. The brainstem and serotonin in the sudden infant death syndrome. Annu Rev Pathol. 2009;4:517–50.

29. Kinney H. Abnormalities of the brainstem serotonergic system in the sudden infant death syndrome: a review. Pediatr Dev Pathol. 2005;8:507–24.
30. Gerhardt T, McCarthey J, Bancalari E. Effect of aminophylline on respiratory center activity and metabolic rate in premature infants with idiopathic apnea. Pediatrics. 1979;63:537–42.
31. Abu-Shaweesh J. Activation of central adenosine A(2A) receptors enhances superior laryngeal nerve stimulation-induced apnea in piglets via a GABAergic pathway. J Appl Physiol. 2007;103(4):1205–11.
32. Al-Matary S, Kutbi I, Quaiashi M, Khalil M, Alvaro R, Kwiatkowski K, et al. Increased peripheral chemoreceptor activity may be critical in destabilizing breathing in neonates. Semin Perinatol. 2000;28:264–72.
33. Gauda E, Shirahata M, Mason A, Pichard L, Kostuk E, Chavez-Valdez R, Gauda EB. Shirahata M, Mason A, Pichard LE, Kostuk EW, Chavez-Valdez R. Inflammation in the carotid body during development and its contribution to apnea of prematurity. Respir Physiol Neurobiol. 2013;185:120–31.
34. Pawar A, Peng YJ, Jacono F, Prabhakar N. Comparative analysis of neonatal and adult rat carotid body responses to chronic intermittent hypoxia. J Appl Physiol. 2008;104:1287–94.
35. Bhattacharjee R, Kim J, Kheirandish-gozal L, Gozal D. State of the art obesity and obstructive sleep apnea syndrome in children: a tale of inflammatory cascades. Ped. Pulm. 2011;323:313–23.
36. Mitchell R, Kelly J. Adenotonsillectomy for obstructive sleep apnea in obese children. Otolaryngol Head Neck Surg. 2004;131:104–8.
37. Arens N, Sin S, Wylie-Rosett J, Wootton D, McDonough J, Shifteh K. Upper airway structure and body fat composition in obese children with obstructive sleep apnea syndrome. Am J Respir Crit Care Med. 2011;183(6):782–7.
38. Punjabi N, Beamer B. Alterations in glucose disposal in sleep-disordered breathing. Am J Respir Crit Care Med. 2009;179:235–40.
39. Koren D, Sullivan K, Mokhlesi B. Metabolic and glycemic sequelae of sleep disturbances in children and adults. Curr Diab Rep. 2015;15(1):562.
40. Tapia IE, Bandla P, Traylor J, Karamessinis L, Huang J, Marcus CL. Upper airway sensory function in children with obstructive sleep apnea syndrome. Sleep. 2010;33(7):968–72.
41. Arens R, Muzumdar H. Pulmonary physiology and pathophysiology in obesity childhood obesity and obstructive sleep apnea syndrome. J App Physiol. 2010;108(2):436–44.
42. Marcus CL, Lutz J, Carroll JL, Bamford O. Arousal and ventilatory responses during sleep in children with obstructive sleep apnea. J App Physiol. 1998;84(6):1926–36.
43. Baird T. Clinical correlates, natural history and outcome of neonatal apnoea. Sem Neonatol. 2004;9(3):205–11.
44. Aubier M, DeTroyer A, Sampson M. Aminophylline improves diaphragmatic contractility. New Eng J Med. 1981;305:249–52.
45. Xie A, Wong B, Phillipson E, Slutsky A, Bradley T. Interaction of hyperventilation and arousal in the pathogenesis of idiopathic central sleep apnea. Am J Respir Crit Care Med. 1994;150:489–95.
46. Solin P, Roebuck T, Johns D, Walters E, Naughton M. Peripheral and central ventilatory responses in central sleep apnea with and without congestive heart failure. Am J Respir Crit Care Med. 2000;162:2194–200.
47. Xie A, Rutherford R, Rankin F, Wong B, Bradley T. Hypocapnia and Increased ventilatory responsiveness in patients with idiopathic central sleep apnea. Am J Respir Crit Care Med. 1955;152:1950.
48. Xie A, Rankin F, Rutherford R, Bradley T. Effects of inhaled CO_2 and added dead space on idiopathic central sleep apnea. J App Physiol. 1997;82(3):918–26.
49. Quadri S, Drake C, Hudgel D. Improvement of idiopathic central sleep apnea with zolpidem. J Clin Sleep Med. 2009;5(2):122–9.
50. Spicuzza L, Gabutti A, Porta C, Montano N, Bernardi L. Yoga and chemoreflex response to hypoxia and hypercapnia. Lancet. 2000;356(9240):1495–6.
51. Mosso A. A life of man on the high Alps. London: T Fisher Unwin; 1898.

52. Ainslie PN, Lucas SJ, Burgess KR. Breathing and sleep at high altitude. Respir Physiol Neurobiol. 2013;188(3):233–56.
53. West J, Peters JR, Aksnes G, Maret K, Milledge J, Schoene R. Nocturnal periodic breathing at altitudes of 6,300 and 8,050 m. J App Physiol. 1986;61:280–8.
54. Dempsey J, Powell F, Bisgard G, Blain G, Poulin M, Smith C. Role of chemoreception in cardiorespiratory acclimatization to, and deacclimatization from, hypoxia. J Appl Physiol. 2014/1985;116:858–66.
55. Barnard P, Andronikou S, Pokorski M, Smatresk N, Mokashi A. Time-dependent effect of hypoxia on carotid body chemosensory function. J Appl Physiol. 1987;63:685–91.
56. Dempsey J, Smith C, Blain G, Xie A, Gong Y, Teodorescu M. Role of central/peripheral chemoreceptors and their interdependence in the pathophysiology of sleep apnea. Adv Exp Med Biol. 2012;758:343–9.
57. Hansen J, Sander M. Sympathetic neural overactivity in healthy humans after prolonged exposure to hypobaric hypoxia. J Physiol. 2003;546(Pt 3):921–9.
58. Burgess K, Lucas S, Shepherd K, Dawson A, Swart M, Thomas K, et al. Worsening of central sleep apnea at high altitude – a role for cerebrovascular function. J App Physiol. 2013;114:1021–8.
59. Lahiri S, Maret K, Sherpa M. Dependence of high altitude sleep apnea on ventilatory sensitivity to hypoxia. Resp Physiol. 1983;52:281–301.
60. Luks A, van Melick H, Batarse R, Powell F, Grant I, West J. Room oxygen enrichment improves sleep and subsequent day-time performance at high altitude. Respir Physiol. 1998;113:247–58.
61. Moraga F, Jiménez D, Richalet J, Vargas M, Osorio J. Periodic breathing and oxygen supplementation in Chilean miners at high altitude (4200 m). Respir Physiol Neurobiol. 2014;203:109–15.
62. Berssenbrugge A, Dempsey J, Iber C, Skatrud J, Wilson P. Mechanisms of hypoxia-induced periodic breathing during sleep in humans. J Physiol. 1983;343:507–24.
63. Sutton J, Houston C, Mansell A, McFadden M, Hackett P, Rigg J. Effect of acetazolamide on hypoxemia during sleep at high altitude. N Engl J Med. 1979;301(24):1329–31.
64. Teppema L, Rochette F, Demedts M. Ventilatory effects of acetazolamide in cats during hypoxemia. J App Physiol. 1992;72:717–23.
65. Kupper T, Strohl K, Hoefer M, Gieseler U, Netzer C, Netzer N. Low-dose theophylline reduces symptoms of acute mountain sickness. J Trav Med. 2008;15:307–14.
66. Fischer R, Lang S, Leitl M, Thiere M, Steiner U, Huber R. Theophylline and acetazolamide reduce sleep-disordered breathing at high altitude. Eur Resp J. 2004;23:47–52.
67. Hackett P, Roach R, Harrison G, Schoene R. Respiratory stimulants and sleep periodic breathing at high altitude: almitrine versus acetazolamide. Am Rev Respir Dis. 1987;135:896–8.
68. Dubowitz G. Effect of temazepam on oxygen saturation and sleep quality at high altitude: randomised placebo controlled crossover trial. BMJ. 1998;316(7131):587–9.
69. Deak M, Kirsch D. Sleep-disordered breathing in neurologic conditions. Clin Chest Med. 2014;35(3):547–56.
70. Ifergane G, Ovanyan A, Toledano R, Goldbart A, Abu-Salame I, Tal A, et al. Obstructive sleep apnea in acute stroke: a role for systemic inflammation. Stroke. 2016;47:1–7.
71. Shahar E, Whitney C, Redline S, Lee E, Newman A, Javier Nieto F, et al. Sleep-disordered breathing and cardiovascular disease: cross-sectional results of the sleep heart healthy study. Am J Resp Crit Care Med. 2001;163:19–25.
72. Somers V, White D, Amin R, Abraham W, Costa F, Culebras A, Daniels S, Floras J, Hunt C, Olson L, Pickering T, Russell R, Woo M, Young T. Sleep apnea and cardiovascular disease: an American Heart Association/American College of Cardiology Foundation Scientific Statement from the American Heart Association Council for High Blood Pressure Research Professional Education Committee, Council on Clinical Cardiology, Stroke Council, and Council on Cardiovascular Nursing. J Am Coll Cardiol. 2008;52:686–717.
73. Chokrovery S. Sleep disorder – Italian edition. Milan: Time Science; 2000. pp. 555–8.

74. Yaffe K, Laffan A, Harrison S. Sleep-disordered breathing, hypoxia, and risk of mild cognitive impairment and dementia in older women. JAMA. 2011;306(6):613–9.
75. Marrie R, Reider N, Cohen J, Trojano M, Sorensen P, Cutter G, et al. A systematic review of the incidence and prevalence of sleep disorders and seizure disorders in multiple sclerosis. Mult Scler. 2015;21(3):342–9.
76. Aboussouan L. Sleep-disordered breathing in neuromuscular disease. Am J Respir Crit Care Med. 2015;191:979–89.
77. Victor A. Adams and Victor's, principles of neurology. Milano: The McGraw-Hill Companies, Publishing Group Italia; 2002. pp. 363–5.
78. Hermann D, Siccoli M, Kirov P, Gugger M, Bassetti C. Central periodic breathing during sleep in acute ischemic stroke. Stroke. 2007;38:1082–4.
79. Macey P, Ogren J, Kumar R, Harper R. Functional imaging of autonomic regulation: methods and key findings. Front Neurosci. 2016;9(513):1–23.
80. Plum F, Brown H. Neurogenic factors in periodic breathing. Trans Am Neurol Assoc. 1961;86:39–42.
81. Bonnin-Vilaplana M, Arboix A, Parra O, Garcìa-Eroles L, Montserrat J, Massons J. Sleep-related breathing disorders in acute lacunar stroke. J Neurol. 2009;256:2036–42.
82. De Paolis F, Colizzi E, Milioli G, Grassi A, Riccardi S, Parrino L, et al. Acute shift of a case of moderate obstructive sleep apnea syndrome towards one of severe central sleep apnea syndrome after an ischemic stroke. Sleep Med. 2012;13:763–6.
83. Nopmaneejumruslers C, Kaneko Y, Hajek V, Zivanovic V, Bradley D. Cheyne-Stokes respiration in stroke. Am J Respir Crit Care Med. 2005;171:1048–52.
84. Howard R, Rudd A, Wolfe C, Williams A. Pathophysiological and clinical aspects of breathing after stroke. Postgrad Med J. 2001;77:700–2.
85. Rupprecht S, Hoyer D, Hagemann G, Witte O, Schwab M. Central sleep apnea indicates autonomic dysfunction in asymptomatic carotid stenosis: a potential marker of cerebrovascular and cardiovascular risk. Sleep. 2010;33(3):327–33.
86. Duning T, Deppe M, Brand E, Stypmann J, Becht C, Heidbreder A, et al. Brainstem involvement as a cause of central sleep apnea: pattern of microstructural cerebral damage in patients with cerebral microangiopathy. PLoS One. 2013;8(4), e60304.
87. McNicholas W, Rutherford R, Grossman R, Moldofsky H, Zamel N. Abnormal respiratory pattern generation during sleep in patients with autonomic dysfunction. Am Rev Respir Dis. 1981;128:429–33.
88. Benarroch E, Schmeichel A, Low P, Parisi J. Depletion of putative chemosensitive respiratory neurons in the ventral medullary surface in multiple system atrophy. Brain. 2007;130:469–75.
89. Boeve B. Update on the diagnosis and management of sleep disturbances in dementia. Sleep Med Clin. 2008;33:247–360.
90. Gargaglioni L, Hartzler L, Putnam R. The locus coeruleus and central chemosensitivity. Respir Physiol Neurobiol. 2010;173(3):264–73.
91. Tomlinson B, Irving D. Cell loss in the locus coeruleus in senile dementia of Alzheimer type. J Neurol Sci. 1981;49(3):419–28.
92. Braley T, Segal B, Chervin R. Sleep-disordered breathing in multiple sclerosis. Neurology. 2012;79:929–36.
93. Daulatzai M. Death by a thousand cuts in alzheimer's disease: hypoxia – the prodrome. Neurotox Res. 2013;24:216–43.
94. St Louis E, Jinnur P, McCarter S, Duwell E, Bennaroch E, Kentarci K, et al. Chiari 1 malformation presenting as central sleep apnea during pregnancy: a case report, treatment considerations, and review of the literature. Frontier Neurol. 2014;5(195):1–8.
95. Schuele S, Afshari M, Afshari Z, Macken M, Asconape J, Wolfe L, et al. Ictal central apnea as a predictor for sudden unexpected death in epilepsy. Epilepsy Behav. 2011;22:401–3.
96. Dlouhy BJ, Gehlbach BK, Kreple CJ, Kawasaki H, Granner MA, Welsh MJ, Howard MA, Wemmie JA, Richerson GB. Breathing inhibited when seizures spread to the amygdala and upon amygdala stimulation. J Neurosci. 2015;35(28):10281–10289.

97. Bianchi M, Di Blasi LAC, Santoro M, Masciullo M, Conte G, Valenza V, et al. Prevalence and clinical correlates of sleep disordered breathing in myotonic dystrophy types 1 and 2. Sleep Breath. 2014;18:579–89.
98. Ono S, Kanda F, Takahashi K. Neuronal loss in the medullary reticular formation in myotonic dystrophy: a clinicopathological study. Neurology. 1996;46(1):228–31.
99. Rosenzweig I, Glasser M, Polsek D, Leschziner G, Williams S, Morrell M. Sleep apnoea and the brain: a complex relationship. Lancet Respir Med. 2015;15:1–11.
100. Beebe D, Gozal D. Obstructive sleep apnea and the prefrontal cortex: towards a comprehensive model linking nocturnal upper airway obstruction to daytime cognitive and behavioral deficits. J Sleep Res. 2002;11:1–16.
101. Tahmasian M, Rosenzweigc I, Eickhoffd S, Sepehryf A, Lairdg A, Morrell M, et al. Structural and functional neural adaptations in obstructive sleep apnea: an activation likelihood estimation meta-analysis. Neurosci Behav Rev. 2016;65:142–56.
102. Rosenzweig I, Glasser M, Polsek D, Leschziner G, Williams S, Morrell M. Sleep apnoea and the brain: a complex relationship. Lancet Respir Med. 2015;3:404–14.
103. Morrell M, Jackson M, Twigg G, Ghiassi R, McRobbie D, Quest R, et al. Changes in brain morphology in patients with obstructive sleep apnoea. Thorax. 2010;65:908–14.
104. Gelber R, Redline S, Ross G, Petrovitch H, Sonnen J, Zarow C, et al. Associations of brain lesions at autopsy with polysomnography features before death. Neurology. 2015;84(3):296–303.
105. Guarnieri B, Adorni F, Musicco M, Appollonio I, Bonanni E, Caffarra P, et al. Prevalence of sleep disturbances in mild cognitive impairment and dementing disorders: a multicenter italian clinical cross-sectional study on 431 patients. Dement Geriatr Cogn Disord. 2012;33:50–8.
106. Osorio R, Gumb T, Pirraglia E, Varga A, Lu S, Lim J, et al. Sleep-disordered breathing advances cognitive decline in the elderly. Neurology. 2015;84:1964–71.
107. Rowat A, Dennis M, Wardlaw J. Central periodic breathing observed on hospital admission is associated with an adverse prognosis in conscious acute stroke patients. Cerebrovasc Dis. 2006;21:340–7.
108. Brill A, Rösti R, Hefti J, Bassetti C, Gugger M, Ott S. Adaptive servo-ventilation as treatment of persistent central sleep apnea in post-acute ischemic stroke patients. Sleep Med. 2014;15:1309–13.
109. Cowie M, Woehrle H, Wegscheider K, Angermann C, d'Ortho M, Erdmann E, et al. Adaptive servo-ventilation for central sleep apnea in systolic heart failure. N Engl J Med. 2015;373:1095–105.
110. Sahlin C, Sandberg O, Gustafson Y, Bucht G, Carlberg B, Stenlund H, et al. Obstructive sleep apnea is a risk factor for death in patients with stroke: a 10-year follow-up. Arch Intern Med. 2008;168:297–301.
111. López-Padilla D, Alonso-Moralejo R, Martínez-García M, De la Torre Carazo S, Díaz de Atauri M. Continuous positive airway pressure and survival of very elderly persons with moderate to severe obstructive sleep apnea. Sleep Med. 2016;19:23–9.
112. Troussière AC, Monaca Charley C, Salleron J. Treatment of sleep apnoea syndrome decreases cognitive decline in patients with Alzheimer's disease. J Neurol Neurosurg Psychiatry. 2014;85:1405–8.
113. Bassetti C, Milanova M, Gugger M. Sleep-disordered breathing and acute ischemic stroke diagnosis, risk factors, treatment, evolution, and long-term clinical outcome. Stroke. 2006;37:967–72.
114. Bradley T, Logan A, Kimoff J, Sériès F, Morrison D, Ferguson K, et al. Continuous positive airway pressure for central sleep apnea and heart failure. New Eng J Med. 2005;353:2025–33.
115. Moraes W, Poyares D, Sukys-Claudino L, Guilleminault C, Tufik S. Donepezil improves obstructive sleep apnea in Alzheimer disease: a double-blind, placebo-controlled study. Chest. 2008;133(3):677–83.

116. Irfan M, Selim B, Rabinstein A, St Louis E. Neuromuscular disorders and sleep in critically ill patients. Crit Care Clin. 2015;31:533–50.
117. Beecroft J, Duffin J, Pierratos A, Chan C, McFarlane P, Hanly P. Enhanced chemo-responsiveness in patients with sleep apnoea and end-stage renal disease. Eur Respir J. 2006;28:151–8.
118. Unruh M, Sanders M, Redline S. Sleep apnea in patients on conventional thrice-weekly hemodialysis: comparison with matched controls from the Sleep Heart Health Study. J Am Soc Nephrol. 2006;17:3503–9.
119. Chakravorty I, Manu Shastry M, Farrington K. Sleep apnoea in end-stage renal disease: a short review of mechanisms and potential benefit from its treatment. Nephrol Dial Transplant. 2007;22:28–31.
120. Zoccali C. Sleep apnoea and nocturnal hypoxaemia in dialysis patients: mere risk-indicators or causal factors for cardiovascular disease? Nephrol Dial Transplant. 2000;15:1919–21.
121. Anastassov G, Trieger N. Edema in the upper airway in patients with obstructive sleep apnea syndrome. Oral Surg Oral Med Oral Pathol Oral Radiol Endod. 1998;86:644–7.
122. White L, Bradley T. Role of nocturnal rostral fluid shift in the pathogenesis of obstructive and central sleep apnoea. J Physiol. 2013;591:1179–93.
123. Rassaf T, Schueller P, Westenfeld R, Floege J, Eickholt C, Hennersdorf M, et al. Peripheral chemosensor function is blunted in moderate to severe chronic kidney disease. Int J Cardiol. 2012;155:201–5.
124. Ye S, Ozgur B, Campese V. Renal afferent impulses, the posterior hypothalamus, and hypertension in rats with chronic renal failure. Kidney Int. 1997;51:722–7.
125. Ye S, Zhong H, Yanamadala V, Campese V. Renal injury caused by intrarenal injection of phenol increases afferent and efferent renal sympathetic nerve activity. Am J Hypertens. 2002;15:717–24.
126. Nakayama H, Smith C, Rodman J, Skatrud J, Dempsey J. Effect of ventilatory drive on carbon dioxide sensitivity below eupnea during sleep. Am J Respir Crit Care Med. 2002;165(9):1251–60.
127. Hamilton R, Epstein P, Henderson L, Edelman N, Fishman A. Control of breathing in uremia: ventilatory response to CO_2 after hemodialysis. J Appl Physiol. 1976;41:216–22.
128. Benz R, Pressman M, Masood I. Sleep disorders associated with chronic kidney disease. In: Gööz M, editor. Chronic kidney disease. Rijeka, Croatia: InTech 2012. pp. 383–400.
129. Huang S, Shu K, Cheng C, Wu M, Yu T, Chuang Y, et al. Serum total p-cresol and indoxyl sulfate correlated with stage of chronic kidney disease in renal transplant recipients. Transplant Proc. 2012;44(3):621–4.
130. Carrero J, Stenvinkel P. Inflammation in end-stage renal disease-what have we learned in 10 years? Semin Dial. 2010;23(5):498–509.
131. Stenvinkel P, Alvestrand A. Inflammation in end-stage Renal disease: sources, consequences, and therapy. Semin Dial. 2002;15(5):329–37.
132. Qiu Y, Lv X, Su H, Jiang G, Li C. Structural and functional brain alterations in end stage renal disease patients on routine hemodialysis: a voxel-based morphometry and resting state functional connectivity study. Plos one. 2014;9(5), e98346.
133. Chou M, Hsieh T, Lin Y, Hsieh Y, Li W, Chang J, et al. Widespread white matter alterations in patients with end-stage renal disease: a voxelwise diffusion tensor imaging study. Am J Neuroradiol. 2013;34:1945–51.
134. Gupta A, Leppingc R, Yua A, Pereac R, Honeac R, Johnsonc D, et al. Cognitive function and white matter changes associated with renal transplantation. Am J Nephrol. 2016;43:50–7.
135. Kong X, Wen J, Qi R, Luo S, Zhong J, Chen H, et al. Diffuse interstitial brain edema in patients with end-stage renal disease undergoing hemodialysis: a tract-based spatial statistics study. Medicine. 2014;93(28):1–9.
136. Hanly P, Pierratos A. Improvement of sleep apnea in patients with chronic renal failure who undergo nocturnal hemodialysis. N Engl J Med. 2001;344(2):102–7.
137. Langevin B, Fouque D, Leger P, Robert D. Sleep apnea syndrome and end-stage renal disease. Cure after renal transplantation. Chest. 1993;103:1330–5.

138. Rodrigues C, Marson O, Togeiro S, Tufik S, Ribeiro A, Tavares A. Sleep-disordered breathing changes after kidney transplantation: a polysomnographic study. Nephrol Dial Transplant. 2010;25(6):2011–5.
139. Adeseun G, Rosas S. The impact of obstructive sleep apnea on chronic kidney disease. Curr Hypertens Rep. 2010;12(5):378–83.
140. Kholdani C, Fares W, Mohsenin V. Pulmonary hypertension in obstructive sleep apnea: is it clinically significant? A critical analysis of the association and pathophysiology. Pulm Circ. 2015;5(2):220–7.
141. Galiè N, Humbert M, Vachiery J, Gibbs S, Lang I, Torbicki A, Simonneau G, Peacock A, Vonk Noordegraaf A, Beghetti M, Ghofrani A, Sanchez M, Hansmann G, Klepetko W, Lancellotti P, Matucci M, McDonagh T, Pierard L, Trindade P. 2015 ESC/ERS Guidelines for the diagnosis and treatment of pulmonary hypertension. Rev Esp Cardiol (Engl Ed). 2016;69(2):177.
142. Soler X, Gaio E, Powell F. High prevalence of obstructive sleep apnea in patients with moderate to severe chronic obstructive pulmonary disease. Ann Am Thorac Soc. 2015;12:1219–25.
143. McNicholas W. Chronic obstructive pulmonary disease and obstructive sleep apnea: overlaps in pathophysiology, systemic inflammation, and cardiovascular disease. AM J Resp Crit Med. 2009;180:692–700.
144. Jeremy E, William R, DeYoung P, Kim N, Malhotra A, Owens R. Usefulness of low cardiac index to predict sleep-disordered breathing in chronic thromboembolic pulmonary hypertension. Am J Cardiol. 2016;117:1001–5.
145. Dumitrascu R, Tiede H, Eckermann J, Mayer K, Reichenberger F, Ghofrani H, et al. Sleep apnea in pre- capillary pulmonary hypertension. Sleep Med. 2013;14:247–51.
146. Florian F, Blocha E, Speichc R, Ulricha S. Daytime measurements underestimate nocturnal oxygen desaturations in pulmonary arterial and chronic thromboembolic pulmonary hypertension. Respiration. 2012;84:477–84.
147. Schulz R, Baseler G, Ghofrani H, Grimminger F, Olschewski H, Seeger W. Hypocapnia in PH is mainly due to reactive hyperventilation in response to hypoxemia. Eur Respir J. 2002;19:658–63.
148. Marrone O, Bonsignore M. Pulmonary haemodynamics in obstructive sleep apnoea. Seep Med Rev. 2002;6(3):175–93.
149. Nisbet R, Graves A, Kleinhenz D, Rupnow H, Reed A, Fan T. The role of NADPH oxidase in chronic intermittent hypoxia- induced pulmonary hypertension in mice. Am J Resp Cell Mol Biol. 2009;40:601–9.
150. Foresi A, Leone C, Olivieri D, Cremona G. Alveolar-derived exhaled nitric oxide is reduced in obstructive sleep apnea syndrome. Chest. 2007;132:860–7.
151. Kauppert C, Dvorak I, Kollert F, Heinemann F, Jorres R, Pfeifer M. Pulmonary hypertension in obesity-hypoventilation syndrome. Respir Med. 2013;107:2061–70.
152. Coccagna G, Mantovani M, Brignani F, Parchi C, Lugaresi E. Continuous recording of the pulmonary and systemic arterial pressure during sleep in syndromes of hypersomnia with periodic breathing. Bull Physiopathol Respir. 1972;8(5):1159–72.
153. Tilkian A, Guilleminault C, Schroeder J, Lehrman K, Simmons F, Dement W. Hemodynamics in sleep-induced apneas. Ann Intern Med. 1976;85:714–9.
154. Buda A, Schroeder J, Guilleminault C. Abnormalities of pulmonary artery wedge pressures in sleep-induced apnea. Int J Cardiol. 1981;1:67–74.
155. Marrone O, Bellia V, Ferrara G, Milone F, Romano L, Salvaggio A, et al. Transmural pressure measurements. Importance in the assessment of pulmonary hypertension in obstructive sleep apneas. Chest. 1989;95(2):338–42.
156. Schafer H, Hasper E, Ewig S, Koehler U, Latzelsberger J, Tasci S, et al. Pulmonary haemodynamics in obstructive sleep apnoea: time course and associated factors. Eur Respir J. 1998;12:679–84.
157. Scharf S. Cardiovascular effects of airways obstruction. Lung. 1991;169:1–23.

158. Enriquez-Sarano M, Rossi A, Seward J, Bailey K, Tajik A. Determinants of pulmonary hypertension in left ventricular dysfunction. J Am Coll Cardiol. 1997;29(1):153–9.
159. Haddad F, Kudelko K, Mercier O, Vrtovec B, Zamanian R, de Jesus PV. Pulmonary hypertension associated with left heart disease: characteristics, emerging concepts, and treatment strategies. Prog Cardiovasc Dis. 2011;54(2):154–67.
160. Solin P, Bergin P, Richardson M, Kaye D, Walters E, Naughton M. Influence of pulmonary capillary wedge pressure on central apnea in heart failure. Circulation. 1999;99:1574–9.
161. Christ M, Grimm C, Rostig SEA. Association of right ventricular dysfunction and Cheyne–Stokes respiration in patients with chronic heart failure. J Sleep Resp. 2003;12:161–7.
162. Velez-Roa S, Ciarka A, Najem B, Vachiery J, Naeije R, van de Borne P. Increased sympathetic nerve activity in pulmonary artery hypertension. Circulation. 2004;110:1308–12.
163. Giannoni A, Raglianti V, Mirizzi G, Taddei C, Del Franco A, Iudice G, et al. Influence of central apneas and chemoreflex activation on pulmonary artery pressure in chronic heart failure. Int J Cardiol. 2016;202:200–6.
164. Minai O, Ricaurte B, Kaw R, Hammel J, Mansour M, McCarthy K, et al. Frequency and impact of pulmonary hypertension in patients with obstructive sleep apnea syndrome. Am J Cardiol. 2009;104(9):1300–6.
165. Alchanatis M, Tourkohoriti G, Kakouros S, Kosmas E, Podaras S, Jordanoglou J. Daytime pulmonary hypertension in patients with obstructive sleep apnea: the effect of continuous positive airway pressure on pulmonary hemodynamics. Respiration. 2001;68:566–72.
166. Sajkov D, Wang T, Saunders N, Bune A, McEvoy R. Continuous positive airway pressure treatment improves pulmonary hemodynamics in patients with obstructive sleep apnea. Am J Respir Crit Care Med. 2002;165:152–8.
167. Arias M, Garcia-Rio F, Alonso-Fernandez A, Martinez I, Villamor J. Pulmonary hypertension in obstructive sleep apnoea: effects of con- tinuous positive airway pressure: a randomized, controlled cross-over study. Eur Heart J. 2006;27:1106–13.
168. Ismail K, Roberts K, Manning P, Manley C, Hill N. OSA and pulmonary hypertension: time for a new look. Chest. 2015;147(3):847–61.
169. Marvisi M, Vento M, Balzarini L, Mancini C, Marvisi C. Continuous positive airways pressure and uvulopalatopharyngoplasty improves pulmonary hypertension in patients with obstructive sleep apnoea. Lung. 2015;193:269–74.
170. Ulrich S, Keusch S, Hildenbrand F, Lo Cascio C, Huber L, Tanner F, et al. Effect of nocturnal oxygen and acetazolamide on exercise performance in patients with pre-capillary pulmonary hypertension and sleep-disturbed breathing: randomized, double-blind, cross-over trial. Eur Heart J. 2015;36:615–22.
171. Epstein L, Kristo D, Strollo P, Friedman N, Malhotra A, Patil S, et al. Clinical guideline for the evaluation, management and long-term care of obstructive sleep apnea in adults. J Clin Sleep Med. 2009;5(3):263–76.
172. Peppard P, Young T, Barnet J, Palta M, Hagen E, Hla K. Increased prevalence of sleep-disordered breathing in adults. Am J Epidemiol. 2013;177:1006–14.
173. Young T, Shahar E, Nieto F, Redline S, Newman A, Gottlieb D, et al. Predictors of sleep-disordered breathing in community-dwelling adults: the Sleep Heart Health Study. Arch Intern Med. 2002;162(8):893–900.
174. Lam S, Liu Y, Ng K, Liong E, Tipoe G, Leung P. Up-regulation of a local renin-angiotensin system in the carotid body during chronic intermittent hypoxia. Exp Physiol. 2014;99:220–31.
175. Lam SY, Tipoe GL, Liong EC, Fung ML. Chronic hypoxia upregulates the expression and function of proinflammatory cytokines in the rat carotid body. Histochem Cell Biol. 2008;130:549–59.
176. Baguet JP. Hypertension and obstructive sleep apnoea syndrome: current perspectives. J Hum Hypert. 2009;23:432–43.
177. Boysen P, Block A, Wynne J, Hunt L, Flick M. Nocturnal pulmonary hypertension in patients with chronic obstructive pulmonary disease. Chest. 1979;76:536–42.

178. Hedner J, Ejnell H, Caidahl K. Left ventricular hypertrophy independent of hypertension in patients with obstructive sleep apnoea. J Hypertens. 1990;8:941–6.
179. Hersi AS. Obstructive sleep apnea and cardiac arrhythmias. Ann Thorac Med. 2010;5(1):10–7.
180. Dempsey J, Veasey S, Morgan B, O'Donnell C. Pathophysiology of sleep apnea. Physiol Rev. 2010;90(1):47–112.
181. Onen F, Onen H. Obstructive sleep apnea and cognitive impairment in the elderly. Psychol Neuropsychiatr Vieil. 2010;8(3):163–9.
182. George C. Sleep ? 5: driving and automobile crashes in patients with obstructive sleep apnoea/hypopnoea syndrome. Thorax. 2004;59:804–80.
183. Chwartz A, Smith P, Wise R, Gold A, Permutt S. Induction of upper airway occlusion in sleeping individuals with subatmospheric nasal pressure. J Appl Physiol. 1988;64:535–42.
184. Isono S, Morrison D, Launois S, Feroah T, Whitelaw W, Remmers J. Static mechanics of the velopharynx of patients with obstructive sleep apnea. J Appl Physiol. 1993;75:148–54.
185. Shelton K, Woodson H, Gay S, Suratt P. Pharyngeal fat in obstructive sleep apnea. Am Rev Respir Dis. 1993;148:462–6.
186. Stauffer J, Buick M, Bixler E, Sharkey F, Abt A, Manders E, et al. Morphology of the uvula in obstructive sleep apnea. Am Rev Respir Dis. 1989;140:724–8.
187. Jordan A, Wellman A, Edwards J, Schory K, Dover L, MacDonald M, et al. Respiratory control stability and upper airway collapsibility in men and women with obstructive sleep apnea. J Appl Physiol. 2005;99:2020–7.
188. Riley R, Guilleminault C, Herran J, Powell N. Cephalometric analyses and flow-volume loops in obstructive sleep apnea patients. Sleep. 1983;6:303–11.
189. Rivlin J, Hoffstein V, Kalbfleisch J, McNicholas W, Zamel N, Bryan A. Upper airway morphology in patients with idiopathic obstructive sleep apnea. Am Rev Resp Dis. 1984;129:355–60.
190. Schwab R, Gefter W, Pack A, Hoffman E. Dynamic imaging of the upper airway during respiration in normal subjects. J Appl Physiol. 1993;74:1504–14.
191. Leiter J. Upper airway shape: it is important in the pathogenesis of obstructive sleep apnea? Am J Resp Crit Care Med. 1996;153:894–8.
192. Van Lunteren E. Muscle of the pharynx: structural and contractile properties. Ear NoseThroat J. 1993;72:27–33.
193. Pillar G, Fogel R, Malhotra A, Beauregard J, Edwards J, Shea S, et al. Genioglossal inspiratory activation: central respiratory vs mechanoreceptive influences. Respir Physiol. 2001;127:23–38.
194. Horner R, Innes J, Morrell M, Shea S, Guz A. The effect of sleep on reflex genioglossus muscle activation by stimuli of negative airway pressure in humans. J Physiol. 1994;476:141–51.
195. Mezzanotte W, Tangel D, White D. Waking genioglossal electromyogram in sleep apnea patients versus normal controls (a neuromuscular compensatory mechanism). J Clin Invest. 1992;89:1571–9.
196. Wheatley J, Mezzanotte W, Tangel D, White D. Influence of sleep on genioglossus muscle activation by negative pressure in normal men. Am Rev Respir Dis. 1993;148:597–605.
197. Haxhiu M, Mitra J, van Lunteren E, Prabhakar N, Bruce E, Cherniack N. Responses of hypoglossal and phrenic nerves to decreased respiratory drive in cats. Respiration. 1986;50:130e8
198. Deacon N. The role of high loop gain induced by intermittent hypoxia in the pathophysiology of obstructive sleep apnoea. Sleep Med Rev. 2015;22:3–14.
199. Narkiewicz K, Kato M, Pesek C, Somers V. Human obesity is charac- terized by a selective potentiation of central chemoreflex sensitivity. Hypertension. 1999;33:1153–8.
200. Sin D, Jones R, Man G. Hypercapnic ventilator response in patients with and without obstructive sleep apnea: do age, gender, obesity, and daytime $PaCO_2$ matter? Chest. 2000;117:454e9.
201. O'Donnell C, Tankersley C, Polotsky V, Schwartz A, Smith P. Leptin, obesity, and respiratory function. Respir Physiol. 2000;119:163–70.
202. Younes M, Ostrowski M, Thompson W, Leslie C, Shewchuk W. Chemical control stability in patients with obstructive sleep apnea. Am J Respir Crit Care Med. 2001;163:1181–90.

203. Peng Y, Raghuraman G, Khan S, Kumar G, Prabhakar N. Angiotensin II evokes sensory long-term facilitation of the carotid body via NADPH oxidase. J Appl Physiol. 2011;111:964–70.
204. Trombetta I, Maki-Nunes C, Toschi-Dias E, Alves M, Rondon M, Cepeda F, et al. Obstructive sleep apnea is associated with increased chemoreflex sensitivity in patients with metabolic syndrome. Sleep. 2013;36(1):41–9.
205. Hudgel D, Chapman K, Faulks C, Hendricks C. Changes in inspiratory muscle electrical activity and upper airway resistance during periodic breathing induced by hypoxia during sleep. Am Rev Respir Dis. 1987;135:899–906.
206. Weitzman E, Kahn E, Ollack C. Quantitative analysis of sleep and sleep apnea before and after tracheostomy in patients with the hypersomnia sleep apnea syndrome. Sleep. 1980;3:407–23.
207. Onal E, Lopata M. Periodic breathing and the pathogenesis of occlusive sleep apnea. Am Rev Respir Dis. 1982;126:676–80.
208. Hudgel D, Gordon E, Thanakitcharu S, Bruce E. Instability of ventilatory control in patients with obstructive sleep apnea. Am J Respir Crit Care Med. 1998;158(4):1142–9.
209. Meza S, Younes M. Ventilatory stability during sleep studied with proportional assist ventilation (PAV). Sleep. 1996;19(10 Suppl):S164–6.
210. Gederi E, Nemati S, Edwards B, Clifford G, Malhotra A, Wellman A. Model-based estimation of loop gain using spontaneous breathing: a validation study. Respir Physiol Neurobiol. 2014;15(201):84–9.
211. Ryan C. Sleep 9: an approach to treatment of obstructive sleep apnoea/hypopnoea syndrome including upper airway surgery. Thorax. 2005;60:595–604.
212. The Report of an American Academy of Sleep Medicine Task Force. Sleep related breathing disorders in adults: recommendations for syndrome definition and measurement techniques in clinical research. Sleep. 1999;22(5):667–89.
213. Sullivan C, Issa F, Berthon-Jones M, Eves L. Reversal of obstructive sleep apnoea by continuous positive airway pressure applied through the nares. Lancet. 1981;1:862–5.
214. Loewen A, Ostrowski M, Laprairie J, Atkar R, Gnitecki J, Hanly P, et al. Determinants of ventilator instability in obstructive sleep apnea: inherent or acquired? Sleep. 2009;32:1355e65.
215. Spicuzza L, Bernardi L, Balsamo R, Ciancio N, Polosa R, DiMaria G. Effect of treatment with nasal continuous positive airway pressure on ventilator response to hypoxia and hypercapnia in patients with sleep apnea syndrome. Chest. 2006;130:774e9.
216. Kribbs N, Pack A, Kline L. Effects of one night without nasal CPAP treatment on sleep and sleepiness in patients with obstructive sleep apnea. Am Rev Respir Dis. 1993;147:1162–8.
217. Marin J, Carrizo S, Vicente E, Agusti A. Long-term cardiovascular outcomes in men with obstructive sleep apnoea-hypopnoea with or without treatment with continuous positive airway pressure: an observational study. Lancet. 2005;365(9464):1046.
218. Anandam A, Patil M, Akinnusi M, Jaoude P, El-Solh A. Cardiovascular mortality in obstructive sleep apnoea treated with continuous positive airway pressure or oral appliance: an observational study. Respirology. 2013;18(8):1184–90.
219. Marklund M, Verbraecken J, Randerath W. Non-CPAP therapies in obstructive sleep apnoea: mandibular advancement device therapy. Eur Respir J. 2012;39(5):1241–7.
220. Javaheri S. Acetazolamide improves central sleep apnea in heart failure: a double-blind, prospective study. Am J Respir Crit Care Med. 2006;173:234–7.
221. Edwards BA, Sands SA, Eckert DJ, White DP, Butler JP, Owens RL, et al. Acetazolamide improves loop gain but not the other physiological traits causing obstructive sleep apnoea. J Physiol. 2012;590(5):1199–211.
222. Wellman A, Jordan A, Malhotra A, Fogel R, Katz E, Schory K, et al. Ventilatory control and airway anatomy in obstructive sleep apnea. Am J Respir Crit Care Med. 2004;170(11):1225–32.
223. Eckert D, Owens R, Kehlmann G, Wellman A, Rahangdale S, Yim-Yeh S, et al. Eszopiclone increases the respiratory arousal threshold and lowers the apnoea/hypopnea index in obstructive sleep apnoea with a low arousal threshold. Cli Sci (Lond). 2011;120:505–14.
224. Mason M, Welsh E, Smith I. Drug therapy for obstructive sleep apnoea in adults. Cochrane Database Syst Rev. 2013;31(5):CD003002.

225. Fenik V, Davies R, Kubin L. REM sleep-like atonia of hypoglossal (XII) motoneurons is caused by loss of noradrenergic and serotonergic inputs. Am J Respir Crit Care Med. 2005;172:1322–30.
226. Carley D, Olopade C, Ruigt G, Radulovacki M. Efficacy of mirtazapine in obstructive sleep apnea syndrome. Sleep. 2007;30(1):35–41.
227. Marshall N, Yee B, Desai A, Buchanan P, Wong K, Crompton R. Two randomized placebo-controlled trials to evaluate the efficacy and tolerability of mirtazapine for the treatment of obstructive sleep apnea. Sleep. 2008;31(6):824–31.
228. Vranish JR, Bailey EF. Inspiratory muscle training improves sleep and mitigates cardiovascular sysfunction in obstructive sleep apnea. Sleep. 2016. [Epub ahead of print].
229. Dall'Ago P, Chiappa GR, Guths H, Stein R, Ribeiro JP. Inspiratory muscle training in patients with heart failure and inspiratory muscle weakness: a randomized trial. J Am Coll Cardiol. 2006;47:757–63.
230. Thach, BT. Reflux associated apnea in infants. Evidence for a laryngeal chemoreflex, Am J Med. 1997;103(5A):120S–124S.
231. Anslie PN. Breathing and sleep at high altitude. Respiratory Physiology & Neurobiology. 2013:188;233–256.

Pathophysiology of Central Apneas in Heart Failure

4

Mathematical Models, Animal and Clinical Studies

Alberto Giannoni, Maria Sole Morelli, and Darrel Francis

Abbreviations

β	CO_2 solubility in blood
$P_{a_{CO_2}}$	Arterial concentration of CO_2
$C^*_{A_{CO_2}}$	Steady-state alveolar CO_2 fraction
$C_{A_{CO_2}}$	Displacement of alveolar CO_2 fraction
$C_{aB_{CO_2}}$	Arterial concentration of CO_2 in the brain
$C_{aT_{CO_2}}$	Arterial concentration of CO_2 in tissues
CBF	Cerebral blood flow
$C_{M_{CO_2}}$	Concentration of CO_2 in the muscle
$C_{O_{CO_2}}$	Concentration of CO_2 in other tissues
$C_{v_{CO_2}}$	Venous concentration of CO_2
$C\overline{v}_{CO_2}$	The mixed venous CO_2 concentrations
$C_{vB_{CO_2}}$	Venous concentration of CO_2 in the brain
$C_{vM_{CO_2}}$	Venous concentration of CO_2 in the muscle
$C_{vO_{CO_2}}$	Venous concentration of CO_2 in tissues (except muscles)
$C_{vT_{CO_2}}$	Venous concentration of CO_2 in tissues

A. Giannoni (✉)
Division of Cardiology and Cardiovascular Medicine, Fondazione Toscana Gabriele Monasterio, Pisa, Italy
e-mail: alberto.giannoni@ftgm.it

M.S. Morelli
Scuola Superiore Sant'Anna, Pisa, Italy

Centro di Ricerca "E. Piaggio", University of Pisa, Pisa, Italy
e-mail: msole.morelli@gmail.com

D. Francis
International Centre for Circulatory Health, National Heart and Lung Institute, Imperial College London, London, UK
e-mail: darrel@DrFrancis.org

© Springer International Publishing Switzerland 2017
M. Emdin et al. (eds.), *The Breathless Heart*,
DOI 10.1007/978-3-319-26354-0_4

CSF	Cerebrospinal fluid
FRC	Functional residual capacity
CO_2	Carbon dioxide
CSR	Cheyne-Stokes respiration
D_{CO_2}	Transport coefficient across the blood-brain barrier
$\dot{F}_{ACO_2}$	Alveolar volume fraction in the lung
F_{ICO_2}	Inspired CO_2 volume fraction
GP	Central gain
GC	The peripheral gain
IC	Threshold value for the activation of central chemoreceptor
IP	Threshold value for the activation of peripheral chemoreceptor
K_{CO_2}	Slope of dissociation curve of CO_2
LG	Loop gain
mlv	Effective lung volume of CO_2
MR	Metabolic rate of CO_2 production
MRB	The metabolic production rates of CO_2 in the brain
MRT	The metabolic production rates of CO_2 in tissues
MRM	Metabolic rate of CO_2 production in the muscle
MRO	Metabolic rate of CO_2 production in tissues (except muscles)
O_2	Oxygen
PB	Periodic breathing
P_{ICO_2}	CO_2 partial pressure of inspired CO_2
$P_{a_{CO_2}}$	Arterial pressure of CO_2
$Pa_{CO_2}^P$	Arterial blood gas tensions at peripheral chemoreceptors
$P^*a_{CO_2}^C$	Arterial CO_2 gas tension at central chemoreceptors at steady state
$P_{A_{CO_2}}$	Alveolar pressure of CO_2
$P_{a_{O_2}}$	Arterial pressure of O_2
$P^*a_{O_2}$	Arterial O_2 tension at steady state
PB	Barometric pressure
P_{BCO_2}	Partial pressure of CO_2 in the brain
$PCR(t)$	P_{CO_2} at chemoreceptor site
P_{CSFCO_2}	Partial pressure of CO_2 in CSF
P_{CO_2}	Partial pressure of CO_2
P_{O_2}	Partial pressure of O_2
$Pa_{O_2}^P$	O_2 tensions at peripheral chemoreceptors
$P_{v_{CO_2}}$	Venous CO_2 pressure
PW	Water vapour pressure at body temperature
$\dot{Q}$	Cardiac output
$\dot{Q}_B$	Brain-blood flow
$\dot{Q}_M$	Blood flow to muscle compartment
$\dot{Q}_O$	Blood flow to other tissue compartments
τ_1	Mixing time constant in the heart
τ_2	Mixing time constant in the lungs
τaB	Arterial transport delay from the brain to the lungs
τa_0	Lung to carotid body delay

$\tau a T$	Arterial transport delay from tissues to the lungs
T_{CO_2}	Lung washout time constant for CO_2
T_{O_2}	Lung washout time constant for O_2
τP	Absolute delays from the lungs to the carotid body
$\tau v B$	Venous transport delay from the brain to the lung
$\tau v T$	Venous transport delay from tissues to the lung
TF	Transfer function
va	Arterial blood volume (l)
$\dot{V}_A$	Alveolar ventilation
$\dot{V}_A^*$	Alveolar ventilation at steady state
$\bar{V}_A$	Displacement of alveolar ventilation
vB	The volume of brain compartment
VC	Centrally controlled ventilation
VP	Peripherally controlled ventilation
v_{CO_2}	The lung storage volume of CO_2
v_{CSF}	CSF volume
VE	Expiratory ventilation
VI	Inspiratory ventilation
vL	The volume of lung compartment
vM	Volume of the muscles
vO	Volume of the other tissues
vs	Equivalent storage volume of CO_2
vT	The volume of brain compartment
v_{TCO_2}	Volume of CO_2 in the tissue compartment

4.1   Introduction

The pathophysiology of central apneas in heart failure (HF) is incredibly complex and multifactorial. Although numerous theoretical and experimental works on periodic breathing (PB) and Cheyne-Stokes respiration (CSR) have been published so far, a thorough understanding of the mechanisms involved and their interactions has not been achieved yet.

Only 56 years after the description of Cheyne in 1874, the first noteworthy pathophysiological theory of CSR was given by Traube. He described two types of CSR, namely, that with an intracranial lesion in the presence of an intact heart and that with cardiac disease but no alteration in the brain. He believed that a diminished arterial blood supply to the brain caused a diminished respiratory centre activity, being the pathogenic factor common to both types of CSR [1].

Since then, a plethora of studies have progressively increased our awareness of the pathophysiology underlying central apneas, showing that the idea of Traube of diminished respiratory centre activity, at least in heart failure, was completely wrong. In this scientific asymptotic motion towards the real pathophysiological background of CSR, a great acceleration was given by the use of mathematical modelling. Based on a priori information derived by both animal and human studies, more and more accurate models have been elaborated, not only to disentangle the complexity hidden behind CSR but also to design rational therapeutic approaches.

4.2   Introduction to Mathematical Modelling

Biological models are useful tools to describe the behaviour of biological systems without any experimental tests. In particular, mathematical models are characterized by mathematical relations, which describe a system and quantitatively represent reality using a certain degree of approximation. The principal aims of the first models in medicine and biology were to describe organ and tissue physiology. Later models were used to unveil the pathophysiology of specific diseases, to define diagnostic and therapeutic algorithms or recently to exploit medical instrumentations and devices [2]. Several classifications are available to describe different kinds of model:

- Deterministic models (all relations between input and output signals are known without uncertainty) and stochastic models (some degree of uncertainty is present and constitutive relation could include probability values; output values are aleatory values)
- Static models (output signals depend only on current values) and dynamic models (output signals depend on all the temporal evolution of the system)
- Continuous time models (relations between signals consider the whole time window) and discrete time models (signals are defined in a particular instant)
- Lumped parameter models (consider only temporal variations) and distributed parameter models (also spatial variations are considered)

Usually to build a model, different approaches are available, specifically "black box" and "grey box" model or "white box":

- A "black box" model (Fig. 4.1a) is a model where it is possible only to observe the reaction of the output to a particular input, with no information about the internal workings of the system. This kind of model is a universal model applicable to whichever system with predictive capacity. However, the mathematical representation may be complex, and it may be difficult to establish the exact number of necessary elements, leading either to the loss of predictive capacity (if too much parameters are used) or to the bad representation of the signal (if not enough parameters are used). Further, the physiological and clinical interpretation of the mathematical structure may be problematic.
- A "grey box" model is a model where some knowledge about the nature of the system or of the process that generates signals is known. The equations of the model are not universal, but they focus to reproduce a particular physiological/pathophysiological process, and the parameters that describe the model can be

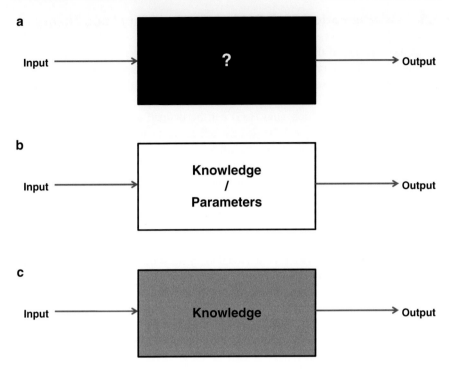

Fig. 4.1 Schematic representation of different model approaches: (**a**) black box model, (**b**) white box model, (**c**) grey box model

given a precise a priori significance. The number of parameters can be defined: (i) considering the physiological and/or clinical knowledge or (ii) considering the fitting relationship between the output of the model and the measured data. "If some variables are not known and a fitting between output and measured data is necessary, the model becomes an instrument to explain all the variance of the signal; we then have a grey box (Fig. 4.1c). Not all parameters are found using fitting method, but only the parameters in which the variability between subjects can explain the major part of variability of measured data. In this way, the complexity of the model is only due to the number of parameters found with fitting method. This number may be based on physiological and/or clinical knowledge, giving also a real significance to the parameters, thus providing predictive capacities that can be used to anticipate the results of different kind of manoeuvres in patients. Some drawbacks have to be highlighted: the numerical algorithm to find parameters is not universal, and there is no certainty that it converges to acceptable results; long computing time is necessary and, moreover, some limitative assumptions must be made [3].

- In a "white box" model, all parameters are known from the a priori knowledge (Fig. 4.1c), and thus the model becomes only a simulation instrument for improving the knowledge of the system or for simple didactical aims.

4.3   Mathematical Basis Behind the Instability Loop Theory

In the past decades, different mathematical models have been proposed to describe PB and CSR. The overall accepted hypothesis is that the respiratory control system could be seen as a closed-loop system, with a determinate transit time in the feed-back loop.

Mathematically, the loop gain (LG) can be defined as the ratio between the response to a disturbance and the disturbance itself. Generally, if LG is high, the system reacts quickly to a perturbation, while if it is low, there is a slower effect [4]. The principal elements influencing a loop gain are called controller gain and plant gain. In the respiratory system, the controller gain is represented by the sensitivity of the chemoreceptors, which is their response as the change in ventilation per unit change in partial pressure of carbon dioxide and oxygen (PCO_2, PO_2), while the plant gain is represented by the lungs, and it can be expressed as the change in PCO_2 or PO_2 per unit change in ventilation. The connection between the controller and the plant in the ventilatory system is represented by the blood circulating between the lung and the chemoreceptors (Fig. 4.2). In the ventilatory system, if LG < 1 every respiratory disturbance produces a small and proportionate response in the system, with ventilation more or less slowly returning to stability. On the other hand, if LG ≥ 1, every respiratory disturbance produces a large and disproportionate response in the system, with ventilation waxing and waning, and the system beco-meing unstable (Fig. 4.3).

In mathematical modelling, increases in controller and plant gains may result in endless cycling. However, the conditions for "mathematical" instability are rarely met in humans, so that periodic breathing (PB) is much more likely to be transient.

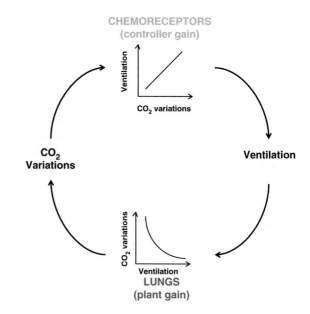

Fig. 4.2 Loop gain applied to the ventilatory system. From the lungs to chemoreflex (*left*): any change in CO_2 (independent variable) is sensed by chemoreceptors (controller gain), which drive a change in ventilation (dependent variable). From chemoreflex to the lungs (*right*): the change in ventilation (independent variable) leads to a change in CO_2 (dependent variable) at the lung level (plant gain)

The mechanical constraints on ventilation, as well as mechanical and neural linkages to other systems that modulate the respiratory control system activity, prevent instability in the engineering sense from occurring and limit the duration and magnitude of ventilatory oscillations. As a result, periodic breathing and instability in biological systems are much less precise terms than they are in engineering and most often occur in states of low damping rather than frank instability [5].

In an oversimplified view, increased chemoreflex gain, increased plant gain and increased circulatory time are commonly considered the key elements responsible for the increase in the global LG and for the PB/CSR onset and maintenance [6–14].

Alteration in the gain of the chemoreceptors in heart failure patients has been well documented in the experimental and the clinical setting and will be examined into detail in Chap. 5. In summary, an increased sensitivity to hypoxia and/or to hypercapnia due to overactive peripheral/central chemoreceptors is responsible for an exaggerated ventilatory response, whenever a change in the respiratory gases occurs [7–9]. The delay in transfer information between the plant and the controller gain (lung and chemoreceptor, respectively), due to prolonged circulation time, causes the temporal extension of any stimulus on the chemoreflex system, because

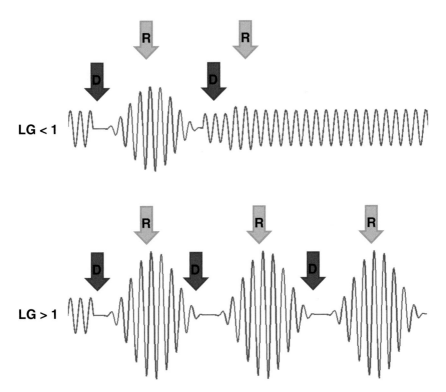

Fig. 4.3 Ventilatory response for different values of LG: if LG <1 (*up*), after an apnoea (first disturbance represented in *red arrow*), the ventilation quickly returns to the regular pattern (response in *green arrow*). On the other hand, if LG > 1 (*bottom*) after a disturbance, an oscillation occurs

chemoreceptors feel the gas changes with a certain delay [15]. The consequent ventilatory overshoot, depending on delayed and increased chemoreceptive response, drives the arterial CO_2 below the apnoeic threshold with the onset of central apnoea. During apnoea, CO_2 rises again above the chemoreflex threshold, and thus another cycle of the PB pattern materializes [6–8].

Although included in all mathematical models of ventilatory instability, the plant gain is less well understood and has been less commonly studied in the clinical setting, as compared to the controller gain. Reductions in lung volume are thought to increase plant gain since smaller lung volumes are less effective at damping changes in CO_2 and O_2, thus favouring instability. Furthermore, a reduction in the lung diffusion capacity and in the gas stores in the lung may also cause a higher variation in the blood gases once the chemoreflex is stimulated, further amplifying ventilatory instability and favouring/maintaining PB/CSR [16].

4.4 History of Mathematical Modelling and Periodic Breathing

Although recognition of the basic closed-loop nature of the respiratory control system was implicit in the work of Haldane and Priestley in 1905 [17], the first explicit quantitative formulation was given by Gray in 1945 [18], with algebraic model restricted to the steady-state response to CO_2 inhalation, anoxaemia and acid-base metabolic disturbances. However, the first dynamic analysis of the respiratory system appeared in 1954 by Grodins and colleagues, who tried to simulate the dynamic effect of CO_2 inhalation, using a proportional controller and reproducing the on and off transients in blood gases and ventilation that were observed when humans inhaled a CO_2-enriched gas mixture [19, 20]. With the development of large computing facilities and as more was learned about the respiratory control from animal and human studies, several workers using both analogic and digital simulations have progressively refined and extended subsequent models. This has allowed the simulation of different physiological and pathophysiological scenarios, better resembling the complexity of the human body. Greater success in simulating PB/CSR was obtained with mathematical models that included oxygen sensors and oxygen stores, multiple body compartments in addition to the brain and the effects on ventilation of simultaneous changes in PCO_2 and PO_2. The more complex models include oxygen and carbon dioxide chemoreceptors, the effects of brain hypoxia, the effects of hypoxia and hypercapnia on cerebral blood flow (CBF) in the controller and a compartmentalized version of the body tissues connected to the controller by motor and sensory nerves and the circulation.

4.4.1 Horgan and Lange Model (1962) [21]

One of the first mathematical models specifically designed to reproduce PB was originally made by Horgan and Lange. They developed an analogue model that reproduced the classic experiment of Douglas and Haldane [17] in which, in normal subjects, periodic breathing was induced after forced hyperventilation. The first model assumption was that only CO_2 variations represented the input element influencing the controller. In the closed-loop control system that they considered, every input and output of the system, such as ventilation and CO_2 concentration, could be identified.

A time delay of 10–15 s was considered, derived from in vivo observation. Considering that the model aimed at reproducing PB experimentally induced in healthy subjects, the short time delay used in the model was obviously taken from healthy subjects.

To reproduce periodic breathing in the analogue model, a revised form of chemoreceptor characteristics of Gray was used [22], as for the controller gain. In fact, referring to the Gray algorithm, a linear relationship between CO_2 and alveolar ventilation starting from no ventilation and progressively rising to normal ventilation as CO_2 increase was employed. However, using this equation and increasing ventilation, it was not possible to reproduce experimental PB, but only a smoother fluctuation of ventilation. Therefore, Horgan and Lange introduced a CO_2 threshold (39 mmHg) below which the linear relationship between ventilation and CO_2 was interrupted and alveolar ventilation falls straight to 0 from a fixed predetermined value (3 l/min), somehow anticipating the apnoea threshold concept:

$$\dot{V}_A = \begin{cases} 0 & \text{if} \quad P_{a_{CO_2}} < 39 \text{ mmHg} \\ 2P_{a_{CO_2}} - 75 & \text{if} \quad P_{a_{CO_2}} > 39 \text{ mmHg} \end{cases} \tag{4.1}$$

where $\dot{V}_A$ is the alveolar ventilation (l/min) and $P_{a_{CO_2}}$ is the arterial partial pressure (mmHg). Using this modified controller gain equation, they were able to reproduce the ventilatory changes of experimental PB.

They first introduce mathematical equations also for the lung and the circulatory compartments. In the lung compartment, they estimated the CO_2 balance as the net rate of CO_2 being delivered by blood equal to the rate of CO_2 expired plus the time rate of increase of CO_2 in lung volume:

$$\frac{\dot{Q}\left(C_{v_{CO_2}} - C_{a_{CO_2}}\right)}{100} = \left[\dot{V}_A P_{a_{CO_2}} + \frac{d}{dt}(\text{FRC})P_{a_{CO_2}}\right]\frac{1}{(P_B - P_W)} \tag{4.2}$$

where $\dot{Q}$ was the cardiac output (l/min), $C_{v_{CO_2}}$ was the venous concentration of CO_2 (%), $C_{a_{CO_2}}$ was the arterial concentration of CO_2 (%), FRC was the functional residual capacity (l), PB is the barometric pressure (mmHg) PW is the water vapour pressure at body temperature (mmHg). $P_{a_{CO_2}}$ (arterial) was considered equivalent to $P_{A_{CO_2}}$ (alveolar), because they assumed that the partial pressure of CO_2 at both sides of the alveolar membrane was the same, considering the large surface area and small membrane thickness of the lung membrane.

In the circulatory compartment, they aimed to evaluate the venous CO_2 concentration, and they were able to estimate it adding to the CO_2 arterial concentration, the CO_2 produced by peripheral tissues, which depends on the metabolic rate.

Furthermore, they also considered that the body is capable to store a large amount of CO_2, which is able to smooth out CO_2 variation, and they also included it in the following equation:

$$Q\frac{C_{v_{CO_2}}}{100} = Q\frac{C_{a_{CO_2}}}{100} + MR - \frac{d}{dt}\left(v_s \frac{P_{v_{CO_2}}}{P_B - P_W}\right) \qquad (4.3)$$

where MR is the metabolic rate of CO_2 production (l/min), v_s is the equivalent storage volume of CO_2 (l) and $P_{v_{CO_2}}$ is the venous CO_2 pressure (mmHg).

Combining the lung and the circulatory compartment equation and providing a circulatory delay of 10–15 s, it was possible to closely reproduce the arterial and venous CO_2 fluctuation obtained by Haldane after inducing experimental PB.

In summary this model dynamically reproduced the respiratory system introducing the following characteristics: (1) a nonlinear chemoreceptor system; (2) damping components, mainly based on the lung volume; and (3) a time delay.

Using this model, it was already possible to employ spontaneous PB/CSR simply decreasing pH and lung volume or increasing time delay. With normal chemosensitivity value and without increased feedback time, very large variations of other parameters were necessary to cause ventilatory instability.

4.4.2   Longobardo Model (1966) [10]

The last concepts introduced in the Horgan and Lange model put the basis for the birth of Longobardo et al. digital model. In fact, the principal idea proposed by the authors was that PB and central apneas might not occur only after hyperventilation in healthy subjects but also at high altitudes and in patients with metabolic alkalosis, neurological disorders and congestive heart failure [17, 23, 24]. The aim of this model was then to reproduce PB/CSR under circumstances comparable to those in which ventilatory instability spontaneously occurs. Authors confirmed the validity of their model using both experimental data on human subjects found in other works and data acquired during CSR experimentally induced in dogs [25].

The model was divided in two principal parts: a regulated system and a controller (Fig. 4.4). The regulated system included CO_2 and O_2 stored in the lungs and body tissues, as described in [26, 27]. CO_2 was stored in three different compartments, the arterial CO_2 stores, the venous CO_2 store in the muscle and the venous CO_2 store in other tissues.

- The arterial CO_2 compartment was represented by arterial blood and functional residual capacity of the lung. In this compartment, the difference between the net rate at which CO_2 is brought into the arterial CO_2 store by the blood and the rate at which CO_2 leaves the arterial stores in the expired air was considered equal to the rate of change in the CO_2 arterial store. The equation can be written as

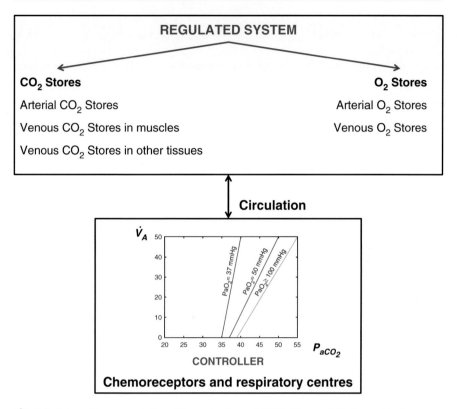

Fig. 4.4 Schematic representation of Longobardo model [10]. The model is formed by two compartments: the regulated system and the controller. The first compartment is the regulated system, divided in CO_2 and O_2 stored in the lung and other body tissues. The controller included chemoreceptors and other respiratory centres, and it is described using data by Nielsen and Smith [28]

$$\dot{Q}\left(C_{v_{CO_2}} - C_{a_{CO_2}}\right) - \frac{\dot{V}_A P_{a_{CO_2}}}{P_B - P_W} = \frac{d}{dt}\left(\frac{FRC}{P_B - P_W}\right)P_{a_{CO_2}} + v_a C_{a_{CO_2}} \qquad (4.4)$$

where $\dot{Q}$ is the cardiac output (l/min), $C_{v_{CO_2}}$ is the venous concentration of CO_2 (%), $C_{a_{CO_2}}$ is the arterial concentration of CO_2 (%), $\dot{V}_A$ is the alveolar ventilation (l/min), $P_{a_{CO_2}}$ is the arterial pressure of CO_2 (mmHg), PB is the barometric pressure (mmHg), PW is the water vapour pressure at body temperature (mmHg), FRC is the functional residual capacity (l) and va is the arterial blood volume (l).

- The venous CO_2 compartments had two different equations for muscles and the remaining other tissues. Generally, the rate at which CO_2 left the muscles/other tissues and the metabolic production of CO_2 by the muscles/other tissues were equal to the rate of change of CO_2 in the muscle/other tissues. For the muscles, this could be expressed as

$$\dot{Q}_M \left(C_{a_{CO_2}} - C_{vM_{CO_2}} \right) + MR_M = \frac{d}{dt} \left(v_m C_{M_{CO_2}} \right) \tag{4.5}$$

where $\dot{Q}_M$ is the blood flow to muscle compartment (l/min), $C_{vM_{CO_2}}$ is the venous concentration of CO_2 in the muscle (%), MRM is the metabolic rate of CO_2 production in the muscle (l/min), vM is the volume of the muscles (l) and $C_{M_{CO_2}}$ is the concentration of CO_2 in the muscle (%). For other tissues, the equation became

$$\dot{Q}_O \left(C_{a_{CO_2}} - C_{vO_{CO_2}} \right) + MR_O = \frac{d}{dt} \left(v_O C_{O_{CO_2}} \right) \tag{4.6}$$

where $\dot{Q}_O$ is the blood flow to other tissue compartments (l/min), $C_{vO_{CO_2}}$ is the venous concentration of CO_2 in other tissues (%), MRO is the metabolic rate of CO_2 production in other tissues (l/min), vO is the volume of the other tissues (l) and $C_{O_{CO_2}}$ is the concentration of CO_2 in other tissues (%).

Also, O_2 is stored in the arterial and venous compartments, but differently from CO_2, in tissue a small quantity of O_2 is stored, and so no equation for this part was considered in the model. The other two equations were similar to the two introduced for CO_2, and they are not reported in this chapter.

The controller part included chemoreceptor and respiratory centres, sensitive both to CO_2 and O_2 variations and to changes in afferent neurological stimuli. For the controller, a model based on the work of Nielsen and Smith was used [28]. Briefly, they studied the effects of CO_2 variations on ventilation in condition of different regimen of hypoxia in two subjects. They demonstrated that after a certain threshold of $P_{a_{CO_2}}$, $\dot{V}_A$ increased in a linear fashion with $P_{a_{CO_2}}$, in a fashion which depends on the background level of hypoxia, so that the lowest was the hypoxic condition, the steepest the chemoreflex sensitivity to hypercapnia was. Below that threshold $\dot{V}_A$ randomly varied independently from the CO_2 values, thus identifying the chemoreflex threshold. Comparison between normal conditions (green line in Fig. 4.4) and hypoxic stimulation (red and blue lines in Fig. 4.4) was considered demonstrating that in hypoxia, the variation of $P_{a_{CO_2}}$ required to induce apnoea decreased (or the apneic threshold increased). The equation describing this behaviour of the controller was

$$\dot{V}_A = 1.81 \left(P_{a_{CO_2}} - 31 \right) + \frac{23.53 \left(P_{a_{CO_2}} - 31 \right)}{P_{a_{O_2}} - 32.44} - 15 \tag{4.7}$$

where $P_{a_{O_2}}$ is the arterial pressure of O_2. The two compartments were considered connected through the circulation, and a 6 s latency between the changes in the lung and the sensing of the controller was used.

Using the model it was possible to reproduce the appearance of PB/CSR in five different physiological and pathological conditions:

Case (I): CSR in normal individuals after prolonged hyperventilation as in the Douglas and Haldane experiment [17]. Driving down $P_{a_{CO_2}}$ to 14 mm led to apnoea lasting 105 s and to CSR with 30 s cycles, while a lesser degree of hyperventilation, with $P_{a_{CO_2}} > 14$ mm, did not produce apnoea and CSR but only PB.

Case (II): CSR in patients with heart failure and prolonged circulation time [24]. Less marked hyperventilation driving $P_{a_{CO_2}}$ to 25 mm was followed by apnoea and CSR despite initially higher levels of oxygen saturation, with CSR cycle time varying directly with lung-to-brain circulation time.

Case (III): CSR in patients with metabolic alkalosis. A $P_{a_{CO_2}}$ driven to 18 mm was this time sufficient to reproduce apnoea and CSR.

Case (IV): CSR in patients with neurological disorders [23]. The slope of the controller curve was increased by 1.5 times, and the apnoeic threshold was increased, with similar findings as in Case III, but with shorter cycle time due to the steepened slope. Further trials with the models showed that PB/CSR was possible even though there was no arterial hypoxaemia, consistently with the findings of Brown and Plum of CSR not abolished in some neurologic patients after oxygen administration [23].

Case (V): CSR in normal individuals at high altitude [29]. Again as in Case III, a $P_{a_{CO_2}}$ driven to 18 mm was this time sufficient to reproduce apnoea and CSR, with the same cycle time seen at sea level but larger ventilatory fluctuations.

The model was also applied and fitted with the experimental data obtained by the same group in dogs, where again CSR was induced by mechanical hyperventilation [25].

4.4.3 Grodins Model (1967) [20]

In 1967, Grodins et al. developed a compartment model where O_2, CO_2 and nitrogen concentration were in two different compartments: the controller characterized by central and peripheral chemoreceptors and the plant constituted by the lung, brain, cerebrospinal fluid (CSF) and tissues interconnected through the circulating blood. Nitrogen was passive in the model and so it was possible to consider only two subsystems for CO_2 and O_2. Blood flowed with four different delays in arterial and venous systems from the lung to the brain and tissues and from the brain and tissue to the lung, respectively.

Differently from the Horgan and Lange model, where only the lung and circulatory systems were provided, with the aim to reproduce the CO_2 variation in the venous and arterial system obtained by experimental PB [17], in the Grodins model, also the brain and the tissues were included, increasing the complexity and the usability of the model. Considering only the CO_2 part of the model (as an O_2 part was also employed), the equations of CO_2 concentrations in the brain, lungs and tissues were

$$\text{Brain}: \quad \dot{C}_{BCO_2} = \frac{1}{v_B}\left[MR_B + Q_B\left(C_{aBCO_2} - C_{vBCO_2}\right) - D_{CO_2}\left(P_{BCO_2} - P_{CSFCO_2}\right)\right]$$

$$\text{Lungs}: \quad \dot{F}_{ACO_2} = \frac{1}{v_L}\left[V_I F_{ICO_2} - V_E F_{ACO_2} + \beta Q\left(C_{vCO_2} - C_{aCO_2}\right)\right]$$

$$\text{Tissues}: \quad \dot{C}_{TCO_2} = \frac{1}{v_T}\left[MR_T + \left(Q - Q_B\right)\left(C_{aTCO_2} - C_{vTCO_2}\right)\right]$$

$$(4.8)$$

where vB, vL and vT are the volumes of the brain, lung and tissue, respectively(l); MRB and MRT are the metabolic production rates of CO_2 in the brain and tissues, respectively (l/min); $\dot{Q}$ is the cardiac output, while $\dot{Q}_B$ is the brain-blood flow (l/min); and C_{aBCO_2}, C_{aCO_2} and C_{aTCO_2} are the arterial concentration of CO_2, while C_{vBCO_2}, C_{vCO_2} and C_{vTCO_2} are the venous concentration of CO_2 in the brain, lungs and tissues, respectively. D_{CO_2} is a transport coefficient across the blood-brain barrier (l/min mmHg), P_{BCO_2} is the partial pressure of CO_2 in the brain and P_{CSFCO_2} is the partial pressure of CO_2 in cerebrospinal fluid (CSF) (mmHg). Finally, $\dot{F}_{ACO_2}$ is the alveolar volume fraction in the lung, F_{ICO_2} is the inspired CO_2 volume fraction and VI and VE are the inspiratory and expiratory ventilation, respectively (l/min). The β-value is a numerical factor to convert gas volume usually expressed in the blood in standard temperature and pressure and dry (STPD) to BTPS which specifically applies to the lung environment (body temperature and pressure, saturated) and represents the CO_2 solubility. Specifically, β is the CO_2 solubility in blood and is equal to $863 / \left(P_B - P_W\right)$ where PB is the barometric pressure and PW is the water vapour pressure at body temperature.

Based on the assumption that, usually, F_{ICO_2} is equal to zero, a CO_2 equilibrium is expected between the venous level and the brain/tissues; the arterial CO_2 in the brain/tissue corresponds to arterial CO_2 values in the lung after a certain delay (τ):

$$
\begin{aligned}
C_{vBCO_2} &= C_{BCO_2} \\
C_{vTCO_2} &= C_{TCO_2} \\
C_{aBCO_2} &= C_{aCO_2}\left(t - \tau_{aB}\right) \\
C_{aTCO_2} &= C_{aCO_2}\left(t - \tau_{aT}\right)
\end{aligned}
\qquad (4.9)
$$

The model defined the venous CO_2 as a function of brain and tissue CO_2 (C_{BCO_2} and C_{TCO_2}, respectively) and venous transport delay from the brain to the lung (τvB) and tissue to the lung (τvT):

$$C_{vCO_2} = \frac{1}{Q}\left[Q_B C_{BCO_2}\left(t - \tau_{vB}\right) + \left(Q - Q_B\right)C_{TCO_2}\left(t - \tau_{vT}\right)\right] \qquad (4.10)$$

It was then possible to write Eq. 4.8 in terms of partial pressure translating both volume fraction and concentration in terms of partial pressure. The volume fraction value is related to the partial pressure through the Dalton law:

$$F_{ACO_2} = \frac{P_{ACO_2}}{P_B - P_W} \tag{4.11}$$

considering that P_{ACO_2} and P_{aCO_2} are equal. Concentrations are related to partial pressure considering the dissociation curves:

$$
\begin{aligned}
C_{aCO_2} &= K_1 + K_{CO_2} P_{aCO_2}, \\
C_{vCO_2} &= K_1 + K_{CO_2} P_{vCO_2}, \\
C_{aBCO_2} &= K_1 + K_{CO_2} P_{aBCO_2}, \\
C_{vBCO_2} &= K_1 + K_{CO_2} P_{vBCO_2}.
\end{aligned}
\tag{4.12}
$$

where K_1 and K_{CO_2} are constant values. Combining the previous equations, it is possible to write the Grodins model as

$$\text{Brain}: \quad \dot{P}_{BCO_2} = \frac{1}{v_B K_{CO_2}} \begin{bmatrix} MR_B + K_{CO_2} Q_B \left(P_{aCO_2} \left(t - t_{aB} \right) - P_{BCO_2} \right) \\ -D_{CO_2} \left(P_{BCO_2} - P_{CSFCO_2} \right) \end{bmatrix}$$

$$\text{Lungs}: \quad \dot{P}_{ACO_2} = \frac{1}{v_L} \left[-V_E P_{ACO_2} + 863 K_{CO_2} Q \left(P_{vCO_2} - P_{aCO_2} \right) \right]$$

$$\text{Tissues}: \quad \dot{P}_{TCO_2} = \frac{1}{v_T K_{CO_2}} \left[MR_T + \left(Q - Q_B \right) K_{CO_2} \left(P_{aCO_2} \left(t - t_{aT} \right) - P_{TCO_2} \right) \right]$$

$$\tag{4.13}$$

And Eq. 4.10 can be rewritten as

$$P_{vCO_2} = \frac{1}{Q} \left[Q_B P_{BCO_2} \left(t - \tau_{vB} \right) + \left(Q - Q_B \right) P_{TCO_2} \left(t - \tau_{vT} \right) \right] \tag{4.14}$$

In addition, the CSF CO_2 partial pressure can be written as

$$\text{CSF}: \quad \dot{P}_{CSFCO_2} = \frac{1}{v_{CSF} k \alpha_{CO_2}} \left[D_{CO_2} \left(P_{BCO_2} - P_{CSFCO_2} \right) \right] \tag{4.15}$$

where v_{CSF} is the CSF volume (l), k is a conversion factor from atmospheric pressure to mmHg ($k = 1/760$) and α_{CO_2} is a solubility coefficient for CO_2 in CSF.

At last, from the Grodins model, it was possible to have an estimate of the variation in the arterial pressure of CO_2 (P_{aCO_2}), which reflects the alveolar pressure of CO_2, and the the variation in the venous pressure of CO_2 (P_{vCO_2}), which may be derived from the variation in the brain and tissue values of CO_2 (P_{BCO_2} and P_{TCO_2}, respectively).

The transport delays are not constant but in each part of the system they change following variation in cardiac output, as exemplified by the lung to the carotid body delay (τa_0) that is also used in the controller function (see below):

$$\tau_{a0} = \frac{1.062}{\dfrac{1}{\tau_{a0} - \tau_{a0}(1)} \displaystyle\int_{t-\tau_{a0}}^{t-\tau_{a0(1)}} Q\,dt} + \frac{0.008}{\dfrac{1}{\tau_{a0}(1)} \displaystyle\int_{t-\tau_{a0}(1)}^{t} Q_B\,dt}$$

(4.16)

In each equation used to define the time delay, including that used for chemoreflex delay, the numerator represents the volume of the vascular segment through which blood flows at the appropriate "past-average rate" defined by the denominator.

The Grodins model was an evolution as compared with Horgan and Lange model, also because the controller was not only represented by a single chemoreflex sensitive to CO_2, but rather by two chemosensory areas, namely, peripheral and central chemoreceptors. Grodins considered the global ventilation as given by the contribution of both peripherally controlled ventilation (*VP*) and centrally controlled ventilation (*VC*).

The peripheral ventilation (or ventilatory response to peripheral chemoreceptor) was influenced by both PCO_2 and O_2 according to the following equation:

$$V_P = G_P e^{-0.05 P_{aO_2}(t-\tau_{a0})}\left(P_{aCO_2}(t-\tau_{a0}) - I_P\right)$$

(4.17)

where *GP* is the peripheral gain, *IP* is a threshold value for the activation of peripheral chemoreceptor, P_{aO_2} is the arterial partial pressure of O_2 and τ_{a0} is the transport delay between the lungs and carotid body (as defined in Eq. 4.16).

On the other hand, the central ventilation (or ventilatory response to central chemoreceptors) was influenced only to PCO_2 linearly, as in steady state, and in particular there was a dependence on H^+ through acid-base relation that is directly related to P_{CSFCO2}:

$$V_C = G_C\left(P_{CSFCO_2}(t) - I_C\right)$$

(4.18)

where *GC* is the central gain and *IC* is a threshold value for the activation of central chemoreceptor.

The inclusion of a second group of chemoreceptors (as expressed by central ventilation) was related to the cornerstone discovery made by Mitchell in 1963 [30] of a chemosensory area on the ventrolateral medullary (VLM) surface discovered after increasing H^+ concentration in the cerebrospinal fluids of anaesthetized cats. That also explained the inclusion of a cerebrospinal compartment in the model (originally not provided).

All the equations of the model were used to study different conditions: hypercapnia (1 %, 3 % and 5 % of CO_2) and recovery, hypoxia at sea level (10 %, 8 % and 6 % of O_2) and recovery and altitude hypoxia (15,000, 18,000 and 20,000 ft). Using the model it was possible to reproduce the steady-state ventilatory responses to gas variations observed in real studies. In particular, it was possible to mathematically obtain a fast ventilatory response to CO_2 administration in the first minute (30 % of the global ventilatory response) similar to that experimentally obtained in animals by Lambertsen and Dejours [31, 32], in which a fast (peripheral) and slow (central) component in the CO_2 response were observed. It was also possible to reproduce the ventilatory effects related to changes in blood pH. Moreover, after a prolonged period of hypoxia, a short period of PB was obtained by mathematical simulation. The same periodic breathing pattern also emerged at 20,000 ft (6096 m). The main limitation of this model was its overall complexity, making it hardly clinically applicable, and the need for extreme variations in the input parameters to reproduce PB.

4.4.4 The Mackey-Glass Model (1977) [33]

While the main aim of the first mathematical models was to describe in general the ventilatory system and the chemical control of ventilation, in the Mackey and Glass model, the main aim was to describe oscillatory instabilities, using PB/CSR as one example of dynamic perturbation of physiological variables. Therefore, differently from the growing complexity of algorithms previously described, this model was oversimplified to a specific scenario, which was the PB/CSR pattern observed in neurological and cardiovascular diseases.

Hence, the respiratory changes were described using a closed-loop control system with a single compartment and a single time delay. The compartment in the model was represented by the peripheral tissues; the blood flows through tissues, where metabolic activity occurs, and then in the lungs, where gas exchange occurs; and finally the blood flows from lungs to the brain with a certain delay due to the transport time (Fig. 4.5).

In steady state, the CO_2 concentration is increased by metabolic production with a constant speed and reduced through ventilation. The model was described using partial pressure of CO_2 instead of concentration and was expressed as

$$\frac{dP_{aCO_2}}{dt} = MR - \alpha P_{aCO_2} V \tag{4.19}$$

where P_{aCO_2} is the arterial partial pressure of CO_2 (mmHg), MR is the metabolic production rate (l/min), α is a constant value and V is the ventilation (l/min). The ventilation is a function of the time delay between the lungs and the brain (τ) and depends on P_{aCO_2} through a sigmoidal Hill function (where Vm is the maximum ventilation and n and Θ are coefficients adjusted to fit the experimental observation) [34].

$$V = V_m \frac{P_{aCO_2}^n}{\Theta^n + P_{aCO_2}^n} \tag{4.20}$$

Specifically, typical values incorporated in the model were $V_m = 80$ l/min, $\alpha = 0.0214$, $\tau = 0.15$ min and $MR = 6$ mmHg/min.

Fig. 4.5 Diagram of
Mackey-Glass model [33].
A single compartment
representing the peripheral
tissue was considered. The
blood flows through tissue
and then in the lungs
where gas exchanges
occurs. After the lungs, the
blood goes to the brain
with a certain transport
time delay (τ)

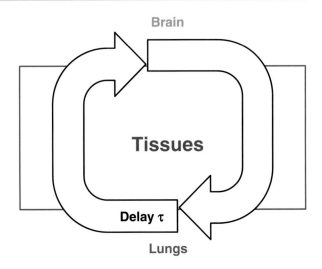

Combining Eqs. 4.19 and 4.20, we obtain the final equation of the model as follows:

$$\frac{dP_{aCO_2}}{dt} = MR - \alpha P_{aCO_2} V_m \frac{P^n_{aCO_2}}{\Theta^n + P^n_{aCO_2}} \tag{4.21}$$

It is possible to study the stability of Eq. 4.21 near to the steady state where $P^*_{aCO_2}$ is the partial pressure of CO_2 (40 mmHg), the ventilation is V^* (7 l/min) and the slope of CO_2 curve is S^* (i.e. chemoreflex sensitivity). In this particular condition, $n = P^*_{aCO_2} S^* V_m / V^* \left(V_m - V^*\right)$ and $\Theta^n = P^*_{aCO_2} \left(V_m - V^*\right)/V^*$ and the system became unstable if

$$S^* > S_{cr} = \frac{\pi V^*}{2MR\tau} \tag{4.22}$$

Considering a minute ventilation of 7 l/min and a metabolic rate of 6 mmHg/min, the critical chemosensitivity or S_{cr} was found to be 7.44 l/(min mmHg), which was above the chemosensitivity range (2–6 l/min/mmHg) in healthy subjects evaluated by steady-state CO_2 tests. Furthermore, in condition of instability, the period of oscillation calculated was 4τ (around 36 s), similar to the cycle length evaluated in a clinical study published in 1961 by Brown and Plum in CSR subjects mainly with neurological disorders and thus with a short circulatory time [23]. The model shows that for S=10 l/(min mmHg), the envelope of ventilation is similar to ventilation in PB (Fig 4.6).

In a more recent modified version of Mackey-Glass model [35], also the rhythm of the central generator was considered. The instantaneous ventilation V_I, for constant value of CO_2, was

$$V_I = V\left(1 + \cos 2\pi ft\right) \tag{4.23}$$

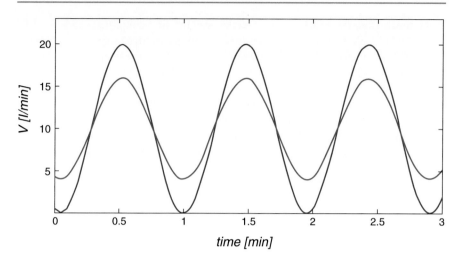

Fig. 4.6 Ventilation in Mackey-Glass model. A low amplitude in ventilation is found including a value of S near to the S_{cr} (in *red line* S=7.7 l/(min mmHg)). A larger amplitude result is found when S = 10 l/(min mmHg) is used (*blue line*). This results is similar to ventilation in PB

where f is the frequency of separate breath. Equation 4.21 became

$$\frac{dP_{aCO_2}}{dt} = MR - \alpha P_{aCO_2} V_m \frac{P^n_{aCO_2}}{\Theta^n + P^n_{aCO_2}} \left(1 + \cos 2\pi ft\right) \qquad (4.24)$$

To study the frequency of the control feedback loop, the authors supposed that the frequency of the generator had a weak dependence on CO_2 level at the previous time, and this control was necessary to maintain constant the level of CO_2 in gas. This dependence was represented using a small modulation of the frequency near to the steady state as

$$f = f_0 + \upsilon \left(P_{aCO_2} - P^*_{aCO_2}\right) \qquad (4.25)$$

where $\upsilon \ll 1$ is the modulator parameter and f_o is the frequency of normal respiration (one breath in 4 s). Studying the parameters variations, authors demonstrated that:

- If $\tau < \tau_{cr}$ and $0 < \upsilon < 0.005$, normal breathing occurs.
- If $\tau > \tau_{cr}$ and $\upsilon = 0$ (no frequency modulation of the generator), an almost periodic result is obtained with the same respiration frequency of healthy subjects.
- If $\tau > \tau_{cr}$ and $\upsilon > 0$, the typical PB trend is observed with higher-frequency oscillation.

The increase in frequency (which was observed also in experimental data during periodic breathing) seems to be caused not only by modulation but also by nonlinearity and time delay.

In conclusion, the Mackey-Glass model was the first simplified model of PB/CSR with the great advantage of describing ventilatory dynamics with a limited number of parameters. This was achieved by employing a nonlinear analysis based on the sigmoidal Hill function and by assuming a single controller, a single compartment and a single time delay. Whether mathematically appealing for its simplicity, as also stated by the authors, the crudeness of the mathematical model makes comparison with experimental data difficult to realize. Furthermore, while specifically designed for the study of PB/CSR, the changes in the key parameters (i.e. chemoreflex gain or time delay) needed to make the system oscillate were quite extreme and far from those observed in both animal and human studies.

4.4.5 The Khoo Model (1982) [12]

Periodic breathing occurs not only in pathological conditions as heart failure and brainstem lesions, but also in physiological condition as during sleep and at high altitude [36–38]. Differently from Mackey and Glass, Khoo et al. developed a model that was able to simulate PB not only in pathological but also in physiological conditions. This time the controller was not limited to a single chemoreflex system, but both peripheral (carotid) and central (medullary) controllers were used in the model. Furthermore, three body compartments (brain, lung and tissue) were again incorporated in the system. Finally, two different time delays from the lung to peripheral chemoreceptors and from the lung to the brain were included, and dead space was also considered a part of the ventilatory algorithm. To solve the equations of this nonlinear system, a restricted analysis to a sufficient small regime of $PaCO_2$ and PaO_2 was considered, making a linearization of the equations of the system. In this way, the stability properties of the linearized system can be described in terms of analytic expression and examined using a frequency response method.

In the model, some assumptions were considered to describe the different parts of the model, namely, the lung, the body tissue and the peripheral/central controllers.

Lung compartment was represented as a single alveolar compartment perfused by the entire blood flow. The CO_2 capacity storage was considered greater than O_2 capacity storage. Moreover, the alveolar gas tensions were assumed in equilibrium with arterial gas tension. The equation describing this compartment was

$$\frac{dPa_{CO_2}}{dt} = \frac{863\dot{Q}}{v_{CO_2}}\left(C\bar{v}_{CO_2} - Ca_{CO_2}\right) + \frac{P_{ICO_2} - Pa_{CO_2}}{v_{CO_2}}\dot{V}_A \qquad (4.26)$$

where Pa_{CO_2} is the arterial CO_2 partial pressure (mmHg), $\dot{Q}$ is the cardiac output (l/min), v_{CO_2} is the lung storage volume of CO_2 (l), $C\bar{v}_{CO_2}$ is the mixed venous CO_2 concentrations (%), Ca_{CO_2} is the arterial CO_2 concentrations (%), P_{ICO_2} is the CO_2 partial pressure of inspired CO_2 (mmHg) and $\dot{V}_A$ is the alveolar ventilation (l/min). This equation was very similar to the one used by Grodins (Eq. 4.9), apart from the inclusion of P_{ICO_2} and the substitution of lung volume with CO_2 volume in the lung.

In the body tissue compartment, the quantity of CO_2 returning from the tissues to the lungs is equilibrated with the corresponding gas tension found in the compartment. Moreover, the metabolic production of CO_2 is constant in resting condition:

$$\frac{dC\overline{v}_{CO_2}}{dt} = \frac{\dot{Q}}{v_{TCO_2}}\left(Ca_{CO_2} - C\overline{v}_{CO_2}\right) + \frac{MR_{CO_2}}{vt_{CO_2}} \tag{4.27}$$

where v_{TCO_2} is the volume of CO_2 in the tissue compartment and MR is the metabolic production rate of CO_2 (l/min). It was possible to change CO_2 concentration in CO_2 partial pressure using the dissociation curve function:

$$Ca_{CO_2} = K_{CO_2} \cdot Pa_{CO_2} + 0.244 \tag{4.28}$$

The same relation expressed for arterial blood was assumed to be also valid for venous blood, body tissue and brain tissue.

The $P_{a_{CO_2}}$ and $P_{a_{O_2}}$ leaving the lungs arrive to chemoreceptors with a typical time delay (τ_c for transport from lungs to central chemoreceptor and τ_p for transport from lungs to peripheral chemoreceptor) Moreover, P_aCO_2 and P_aO_2 are distorted by the mixing in the heart and in arterial vascular system: this was derived from the lung-tochemoreceptor transfer function proposed by Lange et al. [39].

The steady-state ventilatory response ($\dot{V}_E^*$) to $P_{a_{CO_2}}$ and $P_{a_{O_2}}$ is

$$\dot{V}_E^* = \dot{V}_P + \dot{V}_C^* = G_P e^{-0.05 Pa^P_{O_2}}\left(Pa^P_{CO_2} - I_P\right) + G_C\left(P^*a^C_{CO_2} - I_C\right) \tag{4.29}$$

The first component ($\dot{V}_P$) is assumed to be related to peripheral response, while the second ($\dot{V}_C^*$) is the steady-state central response. Moreover, GP and GC are the peripheral and central gain, respectively; IP and IC are the peripheral and central chemoreflex threshold, respectively; $Pa^P_{O_2}$ and $Pa^P_{CO_2}$ are the arterial blood gas tensions at peripheral chemoreceptors; and $P^*a^C_{CO_2}$ is the arterial CO_2 gas tension at central chemoreceptors at steady state. Assuming that the central controller responds only to the tissue Pa_{CO2} of the brain (P_{BCO_2}), the instantaneous response to the central controller becomes

$$\dot{V}_C = G_C\left(P_{BCO_2} - \frac{MR_B}{\dot{Q}_B \cdot K_{CO_2}} - I_C\right) \tag{4.30}$$

where MRB is the metabolic production rates of CO_2 in the brain (l/min) and $\dot{Q}_B$ is the brain-blood flow (l/min). To study the stability of the system is sufficient to observe the transfer function (TF) of the system itself. Generally, a perturbation to a system (input) that operates in steady-state condition provokes a response (output), and the TF represents the ratio between the perturbation applied and the response to the system itself. TF is simply a complex quantity that has a magnitude (LG) and a phase shift (φ) that are functions of frequency. The stability can be studied using the Nyquist criterion [40]. Briefly, if there exists a frequency f_c where $\varphi = 180°$, the value of LG determines the condition of stability: if $LG(f_c) \geq 1$, the system is unstable and the oscillation produced by the perturbation is maintained or amplified; otherwise, the system is stable and after the perturbation the system returns to its original state. In the Khoo model, a perturbation with a specific cycle time (T) is applied to $\dot{V}_A$, and a corresponding variation in $\dot{V}_E$ is produced. To obtain the expression of LG and φ, the three components that form the overall loop transfer function are considered, namely, the peripheral CO_2 and O_2 TF and the central CO_2 TF.

The peripheral CO_2 loop gain $LG_{P_{CO_2}}$ and phase $\varphi_{P_{CO_2}}$ were expressed in the model by the equation:

$$LG_{P_{CO_2}} \approx \frac{G_P e^{-0.05 P a_{O_2}} \left(P^* a_{CO_2} - PI_{CO_2} \right)}{v_{CO2}} \Bigg/ \sqrt{\left[1+\left(\omega T_{CO_2}\right)^2\right]\left[1+\left(\omega t_1\right)^2\right]\left[1+\left(\omega t_2\right)^2\right]} \cdot T_{CO_2}^2$$

(4.31)

$$\varphi_{P_{CO_2}} \approx \omega\tau_P + \tan^{-1}\left(\omega\tau_1\right) + \tan^{-1}\left(\omega\tau_2\right) + \tan^{-1}\left(\omega T_{CO_2}\right)$$

(4.32)

where T_{CO_2} is the lung washout time constant for CO_2 (min), τ_1 is the mixing time constant in the heart, τ_2 is the mixing time constant in the lungs, τP is the absolute delays from the lungs to the carotid body and $\omega = 2\pi/T$.

The peripheral O_2 loop gain $LG_{P_{O_2}}$ and phase $\varphi_{P_{O_2}}$ were expressed as

$$LG_{P_{O_2}} \approx \frac{0.05 G_P e^{-0.05 P a_{O_2}} \left(P^* a_{CO_2} - I_P \right)\left(PI_{O_2} - P^* a_{O_2} \right)}{v_{O_2}} \Bigg/ \sqrt{\left[1+\left(\omega T_E\right)^2\right]\left[1+\left(\omega t_1\right)^2\right]\left[1+\left(\omega t_2\right)^2\right]} \cdot T_E^2$$

(4.33)

$$\varphi_{P_{O_2}} \approx \omega\tau_P + \tan^{-1}\left(\omega\tau_1\right) + \tan^{-1}\left(\omega\tau_2\right) + \tan^{-1}\left(\omega T_E\right)$$

(4.34)

where $P^* a_{O_2}$ is the arterial O_2 tension and at steady state and $T_E \approx 1/\left(\dot{V}_A^*/v_{O_2} + 1/T_{O_2}\right)$ (where T_{O_2} is the lung washout time constant for O_2 (min)).

The central loop gain LGC and the phase φC were instead defined by the algorithm:

$$LG_C \approx \frac{G_P\left(P^* a_{CO_2} - PI_{CO_2} \right)}{v_{CO_2}} \Bigg/ \sqrt{\left[1+\left(\omega T_b\right)^2\right]\left[\frac{1+\left(\omega T_{CO_2}\right)^2}{1+\left(\omega t_1\right)^2}\right]\left[1+\left(\omega t_2\right)^2\right]} \cdot T_{CO_2}^2$$

(4.35)

$$\varphi_C \approx \omega\tau_P + \tan^{-1}\left(\omega\tau_1\right) + \tan^{-1}\left(\omega\tau_2\right) + \tan^{-1}\left(\omega T_{CO_2}\right) + \tan^{-1}\left(\omega T_b\right)$$

(4.36)

Table 4.1 Loop gain at sea level in subjects during wakefulness and sleep and at high altitude in awake subjects

	Sea level (awake)			Sea level (sleep)					High altitude (awake)			
									8000 ft		**14,000 ft**	
	A1	**A2**	**A3**	**S1**	**S2**	**S3**	**S4**	**S5**	**M1**	**M2**	**H1**	**H2**
LG	0.17	1.35	0.28	0.85	0.93	~1	~>1	1.5	0.9	0.89	1.6	1.44

A1 = sea level, awake, normal condition; A2 = sea level, awake, normal condition, hyperventilation of 2 min; A3 = sea level, awake, drop in cardiac output of 15 %, smaller lung volume, lower saturation level, slightly higher controller gain. S1 = sea level, sleep; S2 = S1 + drop in cardiac output of 15 %; S3 = S2 + smaller lung volume; S4 = S3 + lower saturation level; S5 = S4 + slightly higher controller gain; M1 = high altitude, supine position, 8000 ft; M2 = high altitude, upright position, 8000 ft; H1 = high altitude, supine position, 14,000 ft; H2 = high altitude, upright position, 14,000 ft

where $T_b = v_b / \dot{Q}_b$.

Looking at the equations, we can notice that LG and φ are independent to the effects due to body tissue compartment. On the contrary, LG and φ are indirectly influenced by the cardiac output, which act on transport lags (τ_1, τ_2, τP) and lung washout time (T_{CO_2} and T_{O_2}), as well as on the operating of the system (as characterized by PaCO$_2$).

Using the mathematical model, Khoo reproduced different physiological and pathophysiological conditions, as summarized in Table 4.1. At sea level, in awake state, in normal condition (A1), the LG was relatively low and the system was stable. After 2 min of hyperventilation (A2), 2 other minutes of apnoea occurs, with CO$_2$ quickly restored to normal levels, but O$_2$ remains low for the long washout time of O$_2$ at sea level. This increases the LG (>1) and leads to PB resembling the Douglas and Haldane experiment [17]. In sleep conditions (S1–S5), if compared with the awake condition (A1–A3), small physiological variations had greater effects on LG. In fact, in normal state (S1) higher LG was already observed compared to awake state (A1), due to the 2 % drop in O$_2$ and the rise in PCO$_2$, despite the expected reduction during night of the central chemosensitivity [36]. Modifying the system by a drop (15 %) in cardiac output (S2), as happens in patients with heart failure (HF), increased the LG and produced a cycle length of about 60 s as in HF. Starting from the same condition of S2 and reducing also the lung volume (S3) and the O$_2$ saturation levels (S4), i.e. assuming the supine position, the LG became > 1 leading to ventilatory instability. Whether also a small increase in the chemoreflex sensitivity (S5) occurred, LG became > 1 determining ventilatory instability and PB/CSR.

In summary in the Khoo model, small physiological variation led to a wide range of LG only during sleep and not in awake conditions (A3). Furthermore, apart from the case of cardiac output decrease, the cycle length was rather stable and approximates 30 s, concordantly with experimental findings in subjects with normal cardiac output [41, 42].

At high altitude the hypoxic conditions progressively increased the loop gain (in the table, M stands for 8000 ft and H for 14,000 ft). The effect of postural changes form supine (M1 and H1) to standing position (H2 and M2) seemed to decrease the LG of about 10 % at each altitude level. The inhalation of CO$_2$ led to a reduction of

LG (as occurs in periodic breathing, where CO_2 can eliminate the phenomenon), and also inhalation of O_2 at high altitude decreased LG reducing the PB likelihood [17]. On the other hand, the same effect was not observed at sea level [43]. The authors also found that the instability of respiratory system was prevalently due to peripheral control in case of normal central controller sensitivity and normal circulatory delay, and so they suggested that PB was mediated by peripheral chemoreceptors. The model also demonstrated that LG was independent from CO_2 and O_2 in peripheral tissues suggesting that storage of the gases in the lungs is the first source of oscillation in respiration.

4.4.6   The Carley and Shannon Model (1988) [44]

The model proposed by Carley and Shannon was a "minimal" model of PB/CSR. In fact, the previous models simulated PB/CSR using a number of parameters > 15. Although allowing the models a wide range of applicability, the large number of parameters introduces two disadvantages. Since some of these parameters exhibit a wide range of values in a population, such simulations can hardly test the model's ability to account for PB of individuals. Furthermore, the validation of the model in the experimental setting would require the estimation of each of the 15 or more parameters for each subject. In the Mackey-Glass model, only six parameters were incorporated in nonlinear differential equation. However, unusually high changes in those parameters were necessary to induce PB/CSR, and the model did not allow the study of the mechanisms governing the frequency of ventilatory oscillations, as the only dynamic element considered was circulation delay. Hence, Carley and Shannon designed a model to specifically describe PB, without incorporating elements considered unimportant for the genesis of ventilatory oscillations. Further, authors restricted the model to a specific limited range around an equilibrium to linearize the nonlinear equations, as previously made by Khoo [12].

The model was a single-loop control system, where a single controller, a single compartment (controlled system) and a single time delay were considered. In this case, the transfer function (TF) was a dimensional system parameter that has a magnitude LG and a phase φ shift that are functions of frequency and was expressed as

$$TF(f) = A(f)B(f)D(f) \qquad (4.37)$$

where $A(f)$, $B(f)$ and $D(f)$ represent the TF of the controller gain, the controlled system and the pure delay, respectively. The controller was represented by chemoreceptors and in the model it was considered as a linear instantaneous controller.

Starting from the input/output relationship of the controller,

$$\dot{V}_A(t) = \left(P_{CR}(t) - S\right) \otimes A(t) \qquad (4.38)$$

where $\dot{V}_A$ is the alveolar ventilation, $PCR(t)$ is the PCO_2 at chemoreceptor site, S is the controller set point and the $\otimes$ symbol represents the convolution operator. Using the following predetermined assumptions:

- At every variation of $P_{a_{CO_2}}$, the respiratory controller acts immediately and linearly to adjust ventilation.
- The sole effect of changes in $P_{a_{O_2}}$ is to alter the controller sensitivity to disturbances in $P_{a_{CO_2}}$.
- Variation of $P_{a_{CO_2}}$ in the lungs is detected in carotid bodies and the brainstem with the same circulatory time delay.

It was possible to obtain the equations describing magnitude ($LGA(f)$) and phase ($\varphi A(f)$) of controller, which were expressed as follows:

$$LG_A(f) = \sqrt{\begin{array}{c}\left[LG_{A_C}(f)\cos\left(j_{A_C}(f)\right)+LG_{A_P}(f)\cos\left(j_{A_P}(f)\right)\right]^2 \\ +\left[LG_{A_C}(f)\sin\left(j_{A_C}(f)\right)+LG_{A_P}\sin\left(j_{A_P}(f)\right)\right]\end{array}}^{-2} \tag{4.39}$$

$$\varphi_A(f) = \tan^{-1}\left(\frac{LG_{A_C}(f)\sin\left(\varphi_{A_C}(f)\right)+LG_{A_P}(f)\sin\left(\varphi_{A_P}(f)\right)}{LG_{A_C}(f)\cos\left(\varphi_{A_C}(f)\right)+LG_{A_P}\cos\left(\varphi_{A_P}(f)\right)}\right) \tag{4.40}$$

where the pedex AC and AP stand for the central and peripheral chemoreceptors, respectively.

In the controlled system, all the process concerning gas exchanges were described. Again starting from input/output relationship of the controlled system for incremental changes in equilibrium,

$$B = \frac{dPa_{CO_2}}{d\dot{V}_A} \tag{4.41}$$

where B is the equilibrium value of the magnitude of $B(f)$ (mmHg/l min), considering the lung equilibration time constant TL (min) as

$$T_L = \frac{mlv}{\dot{Q}(P_B - P_W)K_{CO_2} + \dot{V}_A} \tag{4.42}$$

where mlv is the effective lung volume of CO_2 (l), PB is the barometric pressure (mmHg), PW is the water vapour pressure at body temperature (mmHg) and K_{CO_2} is the slope of dissociation curve of CO_2, using the following predetermined assumptions:

- In the lung, a diffusion process for gas exchanges between the alveolar and the blood occurs, with an equilibrium between the two compartments.
- There is no intracardiac shunting of blood.
- Mixed venous PCO_2, cardiac output, circulation delay and mean lung volume are constant.
- The same linear dissociation curve is applied to both the arterial and the venous blood.

The magnitude ($LGB(f)$) and phase ($\varphi B(f)$) of controlled system were elaborated in the following equations:

$$LG_B(f) = \frac{B}{\left[\left(2\pi fT_L\right)^2 + 1\right]^{0.5}} \quad (4.43)$$

$$\varphi_B(f) = -\left[\pi + \tan^{-1}\left(2\pi fT_L\right)\right] \quad (4.44)$$

The time delay compartment has no effect on the amplitude, but a phase shift is introduced:

$$LG_D(f) = 1 \quad (4.45)$$

$$\varphi_D(f) = -2\pi fD \quad (4.46)$$

where D is the pure delay. Combining all equations of magnitude and phase, the global magnitude ($LG(f)$) and phase ($\phi(f)$) can be simply expressed as

$$LG(f) = \frac{AB}{\left[\left(2\pi fT_L\right)^2 + 1\right]^{0.5}} \quad (4.47)$$

$$\varphi(f) = -2\pi fD - \tan^{-1}\left(2\pi fT_L\right) - \varphi_A(fc) \quad (4.48)$$

where $A = LG_A(0)$ and fc are the critical frequency value where the phase is 180°. For this value of frequency, the stability of the model is ensured if the magnitude of the LG is <1. Specifically, the stability depends on AB (the incremental equilibrium of LG) and f_cT_L (terms that govern the attenuation of LG at the critical frequency) that can be represented as

$$AB = \frac{AP\overline{v}_{CO_2}\dot{Q}K_{CO_2}\left(P_B - 47\right)}{\left[\dot{V}_A + \dot{Q}K_{CO_2}\left(P_B - 47\right)\right]^2} \quad (4.49)$$

$$f_cT_L = \frac{f_c mlv}{\dot{V}_A + \dot{Q}K_{CO_2}\left(P_B - 47\right)} \quad (4.50)$$

where $P\overline{v}_{CO_2}$ is the mixed venous P_{CO_2}.

In conclusion in the Carley and Shannon model, beyond ventilation, only five parameters resulted to be essential to study the model and were

- A (magnitude of A(f) at f=0)
- $\dot{Q}K_{CO_2}$ (cardiac output x slope of CO_2 dissociation curve)
- $P\overline{v}_{CO_2}$ (mixed venous PCO_2)

- mlv (effective lung volume of CO_2)
- TL (lung equilibration time constant)

Using the model it was possible to build a curve relating the LG values and relative stability of the system (R), so that the higher the R value was, the higher the instability of the system and its tendency to produce oscillatory breathing patterns. This relationship was sigmoidal and exhibited a break point near to LG = 0.5. When LG was lower than 0.5, the system was defined overdamped, since variations in the fundamental parameters were unable to produce instability. On the contrary, when LG was between 0.5 and 1, the system was defined underdamped, and even minor variations in key parameters were able to make the system unstable and oscillatory.

Differently from previous models, the system was simple to use and easily allow evaluation of model performance. The average values for the parameters of interest were derived from healthy subjects and the validity of the model tested in that population. PB oscillations were easily obtained in underdamped condition, only with minor changes in the fundamental parameters (around 25 % changes on the average values). However, the system constraints due to the many a priori assumptions may have led to over- or underestimation of the LG. Indeed, neither changes in heart rate, blood pressure, cardiac output and time delay, nor fluctuations in lung volumes were considered in the model (all these parameters were a priori defined constant). Moreover, the ability to predict the behaviour of the controller may be imprecise, since only a single chemoreceptor group was provided, and the known CO_2 signal smoothing due to heart and vasculature mixing [39] was not integrated in the model.

4.4.7 The Francis Model (2000) [14]

Francis and colleagues developed an analytic approach to describe the dynamics of cardiorespiratory stability/instability in patients with chronic heart failure to predict the onset of PB/CSR. The model was developed to solve analytically the dynamics of respiratory control in PB/CSR avoiding the complexity of iterative models, in line with the approaches of Mackey/Glass and Carley/Shannon. A unified general theory was elaborated in order to provide clinicians a rigorous but comprehensible mathematical tool to understand the pathophysiology and to help in designing rational treatments of PB/CSR in heart failure. Indeed, the model wants both to predict stability starting from preliminary clinical data and to understand the effects of parameter changes on stability.

Again as in Khoo [12], the analysis was limited around the steady state, thus applying linear mathematics. CO_2 and O_2 oscillate in antiphase during PB and the state of blood gases was represented as a single variable. Furthermore a single time delay and a single chemoreflex compartment were considered, using CO_2 chemosensitivity as the main driving force influencing ventilation.

In the model the rate of increase of lung CO_2 stores ($v_L \dfrac{dC_{ACO_2}}{dt}$) was expressed as

$$v_L \frac{dC_{ACO_2}}{dt} = \dot{V}_A^* C_{ACO_2}^* - \left[\left(\dot{V}_A + \overline{V}_A \right)\left(C_{ACO_2}^* + C_{ACO_2} \right) \right] - b\dot{Q}C_{ACO_2} \qquad (4.51)$$

where $C_{ACO_2}^*$ is the steady-state alveolar CO_2 fraction, while C_{ACO_2} is the displacement of alveolar CO_2 fraction; vL is the lung volume; $\dot{V}_A^*$ is the alveolar ventilation at steady state, while $\overline{V}_A$ is the displacement of alveolar ventilation; β is the CO_2 solubility in blood; and $\dot{Q}$ is the cardiac output. In particular, $\dot{V}_A^* C_{ACO_2}^*$ is the metabolic production of CO_2, $\left(\dot{V}_A + \overline{V}_A \right)\left(C_{ACO_2}^* + C_{ACO_2} \right)$ is the rate of CO_2 removal from the lungs through ventilation and $b\dot{Q}C_{ACO_2}$ is the rate of transfer of CO_2 from the lungs into extrapulmonary store.

For small variation of $\overline{V}_A$ and C_{ACO_2}, the term $\overline{V}_A \cdot C_{ACO_2}$ is negligible and Eq. 4.51 becomes

$$v_L \frac{dC_{ACO_2}}{dt} + C_{ACO_2} \left(\dot{V}_A^* + b\dot{Q} \right) + \overline{V}_A C_{ACO_2}^* = 0 \qquad (4.52)$$

After a small sinusoidal disturbance, the system can come back to steady state or continue to oscillate. Francis represented this disturbance r with complex numbers. If r is a complex number, it has a real part (g) and an imaginary part (ω), that is, r=g+jω. The exponential e^{rt} can be converted in

$$e^{rt} = e^{(g+j\omega)t} = e^{gt+j\omega t} = e^{gt} e^{j\omega t} = e^{gt} \left(\cos \omega t + j \sin \omega t \right) \qquad (4.53)$$

where *egt* represents the amplitude of the oscillation and $\left(\cos \omega t + j \sin \omega t \right)$ is the oscillation with period of 2π/ω. If g>0 the amplitude of the oscillation will increase, and instability occurs, while, if g<0, the amplitude will decrease, that is, the respiration returns to a stable condition, after a transient period. Combining all terms, a final equation was obtained as

$$v_L r + \left(\dot{V}_A^* + b\dot{Q} \right) + SC_{ACO_2}^* e^{-r\tau} = 0 \qquad (4.54)$$

where S is the chemoreflex sensitivity and τ chemoreflex delay.

The only unknown variable is r. The solution of Eq. 4.54, introducing a Lambert's function (W) [45], was

$$r = \frac{1}{\tau} \left[W \left(-\frac{C_{ACO_2}^* St}{v_L} e^{\left[\left(\dot{V}_A^* + b\dot{Q} \right)t/v_L \right]} \right) - \frac{\dot{V}_A^* + \dot{Q}b}{v_L} t \right] \qquad (4.55)$$

The equation is constructed from two main components $\dfrac{C_{ACO_2}^* S\tau}{v_L}$ and $\dfrac{\dot{V}_A^* + \dot{Q}b}{v_L} t$.

Using the six physiological variables, namely, chemoreflex gain, chemoreflex delay, cardiac output, ventilation and lung volume, and composing the equation, it was possible to predict the effect of any disturbance in respiration on ventilatory stability.

The rate of growth or decay e^g and the period of oscillation $2\pi/\omega$ oscillation are shown in Fig. 4.7a, b.

These results are completely general; in fact the figures plotted have dimensionless axes and are not dependent on physical constants. Considering clinical data acquired from three different populations (ten patients with chronic heart failure without periodic breathing, ten patients with chronic heart failure and daytime periodic breathing and ten controls, all age matched), this model can correctly predict breathing stability/instability in 93.3 % of cases. In this population, the key physiological factors that mainly influence the occurrence of PB/CSR were found to be the increased chemoreflex slope and the long time delay to chemoreflex response. The observed PB/CSR cycle time in the ten patients with PB averaged 1.2 ± 0.2 min, very close to the model prediction of 1.2 ± 0.1 min (against the Mackey and Glass prediction of 2.1 ± 0.3 min).

Using the model it was possible to build a chart easily applicable to the clinical setting to predict the occurrence/disappearance of PB/CSR (Fig. 4.8a). Considering the direction of the arrows, we may immediately feel the reason why changing the chemoreflex slope is possible to easily shift from stability to instability and vice versa, whereas only changing cardiac output, or lung volume, it is more difficult to shift from one state to the other. Likewise, it is possible to predict the effect of different treatment strategies on ventilatory stability (Fig. 4.8b), since oxygen reduces the chemoreflex gain, continuous positive airway pressure increases lung volume, corrective surgery reduces circulatory delay and enhances cardiac output, and CO_2 reduces alveolar-atmospheric CO_2 difference and increases ventilation, both influencing stability.

Conclusions

Mathematical models have greatly helped in the understanding of the pathophysiology of PB/CSR. The key lesson that may be inferred from mathematical models is that PB and central apneas are produced by the interplay of multiple factors. While it is unlikely that PB in different physiological and pathophysiological scenarios has the same cause, the instability in the feedback control involved in the chemical regulation of breathing is usually caused by increased controller and plant gains and delays in information transfer. Each component of the loop gain is actually composed of several factors, and thus mathematics help to assemble complex data and allow the analysis of possible interrelationships among these multiple factors, estimating at the same time their relative impact. Apart from giving a general overview of the respiratory system, this also generates hypotheses that may be tested in experimental and clinical studies. Data arising from those studies may in turn be used to refine the model in a positive hermeneutical circle.

Another important aim of modelling is to reveal areas in which more information is required. Currently, the main limitations of most models is that they consider the controller as a black box without weighing the complexity of the neural

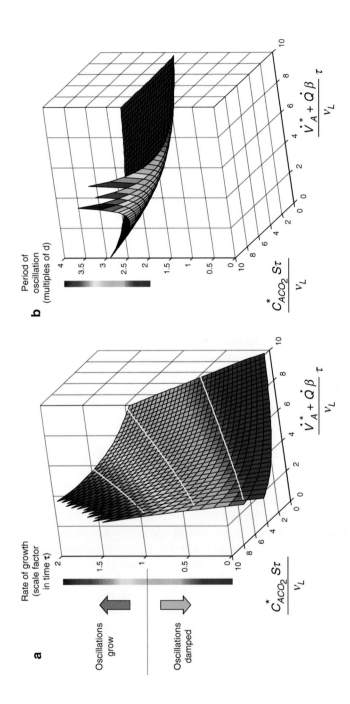

Fig. 4.7 Effect of $\dfrac{C^*_{ACO_2}\,S\tau}{v_L}$ and $\dfrac{\dot{V}^*_A + \dot{Q}\beta}{v_L}\tau$ on the growth factor (**a**) and on period of oscillation (**b**). If growth factor >1, the oscillations grows and breathing becomes periodic, while if growth factor <1, the oscillations damps and breathing returns to steady state. Gently taken and adapted with permission from Francis DP et al. Circulation. 2000 [14]

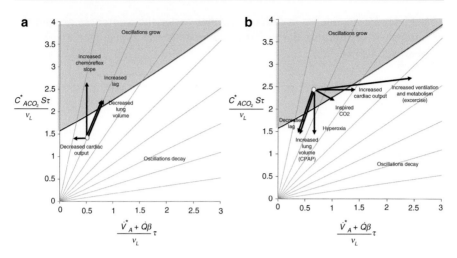

Fig. 4.8 Effects of physiological changes on stability: (**a**) shows which kind of abnormalities favours instability, while (**b**) shows which kind of treatment favours stability. Gently taken and adapted with permission from Francis DP et al. Circulation. 2000 [14]

circuits that generate the respiratory rhythm and their relationship with the chemical input mediated by peripheral and central chemoreceptors. In particular, the real mechanisms behind central chemoreception (intracellular or extracellular pH, PCO_2) are actually not known. Furthermore, among multiple central sensors, it is currently unknown which of the group/groups is/are involved in PB/CSR (see also Chap. 5), whether different groups have different CO_2/pH sensing mechanisms or apnoeic thresholds and whether different groups have different roles in different development ages or conditions (awake/asleep phases). The respiratory controller is likely not a static element, and variation in the controller gain may occur during sleep or exercise. However, in models the controller gain was usually considered as a steady component, and this belief has been translated also in an oversimplification adopted by clinical research. Another field of interest is the relationship between cardiac output and chemoreflex gain. From animal studies (see Chap. 5), we now know that decreasing cardiac output actually increases the controller gain or at least peripheral chemosensitivity, but all mathematical models have considered the two variables mainly unrelated. In addition, the potential role of other feedbacks (i.e. baroreflex and ergoreflex) has not been included in mathematical model as well as studied in the experimental setting.

While the complexity of the controller has been widely unravelled by real data (especially in animals) so to actually outdo the complexity expressed by models, there have been many schemes of the plant gain and circulatory delay proposed by different mathematical versions, but a labour shortage both in the bench and bedside is still present concerning these two topics. Therefore, we believe that future studies should focus on these neglected components in order to further foster the awareness around the control of ventilation and to better understand the appearance and disappearance of PB.

References

1. Traube L. Gesammelte Zur Theorie des Cheyne-Stokes' schen Athmungsphaenomens. Berliner Kinische Wochenschrift. 1874;11:185–209.
2. Biondi E, Cobelli C. Storia della bioingegneria. Pàtron ed.(Collana di ingegneria biomedica); 2001.
3. Cerutti S, Marchesi C, Metodi avanzati di elaborazione di segnali biomedici. Pàtron ed.(Gruppo nazionale di bioingegneria); 2004.
4. White DP. Pathogenesis of obstructive and central sleep apnea. Am J Respir Crit Care Med. 2005;172(11):1363–70.
5. Cherniack NS, Longobardo GS. Mathematical models of periodic breathing and their usefulness in understanding cardiovascular and respiratory disorders. Exp Physiol. 2006;91(2):295–305.
6. Javaheri S. A mechanism of central sleep apnea in patients with heart failure. N Engl J Med. 1999;341(13):949–54.
7. Ponikowski P, Anker SD, Chua TP, Francis D, Banasiak W, Poole-Wilson PA, et al. Oscillatory breathing patterns during wakefulness in patients with chronic heart failure: clinical implications and role of augmented peripheral chemosensitivity. Circulation. 1999;100(24):2418–24.
8. Solin P, Roebuck T, Johns DP, Walters EH, Naughton MT. Peripheral and central ventilatory responses in central sleep apnea with and without congestive heart failure. Am J Respir Crit Care Med. 2000;162(6):2194–200.
9. Hall MJ, Xie A, Rutherford R, Ando S, Floras JS, Bradley TD. Cycle length of periodic breathing in patients with and without heart failure. Am J Respir Crit Care Med. 1996;154(2 Pt 1):376–81.
10. Longobardo GS, Cherniack NS, Fishman AP. Cheyne-Stokes breathing produced by a model of the human respiratory system. J Appl Physiol. 1966;21(6):1839–46.
11. Giannoni A, Emdin M, Poletti R, Bramanti F, Prontera C, Piepoli M, et al. Clinical significance of chemosensitivity in chronic heart failure: influence on neurohormonal derangement, Cheyne-Stokes respiration and arrhythmias. Clin Sci (Lond). 2008;114(7):489–97.
12. Khoo MC, Kronauer RE, Strohl KP, Slutsky AS. Factors inducing periodic breathing in humans: a general model. J Appl Physiol. 1982;53(3):644–59.
13. Pinna GD, Maestri R, Mortara A, La Rovere MT, Fanfulla F, Sleight P. Periodic breathing in heart failure patients: testing the hypothesis of instability of the chemoreflex loop. J Appl Physiol. 2000;89(6):2147–57.
14. Francis DP, Willson K, Davies LC, Coats AJ, Piepoli M. Quantitative general theory for periodic breathing in chronic heart failure and its clinical implications. Circulation. 2000;102(18):2214–21.
15. Crowell JW, Guyton AC, Moore JW. Basic oscillating mechanism of Cheyne-Stokes breathing. Am J Physiol. 1956;187(2):395–8.
16. Szollosi I, Thompson BR, Krum H, Kaye DM, Naughton MT. Impaired pulmonary diffusing capacity and hypoxia in heart failure correlates with central sleep apnea severity. Chest. 2008;134(1):67–72.
17. Douglas CG, Haldane JS. The causes of periodic or Cheyne-Stokes breathing. J Physiol. 1909;38(5):401–19.
18. Gray JS, The Multiple Factor Theory of Respiratory Regulation. AAF School of Aviation Medicine Project Report No 386 (1 2 3);1945.
19. Grodins FS, Gray JS, Schroeder KR, Noris AL, Jones RW. Respiratory responses to CO_2 inhalation; a theoretical study of a nonlinear biological regulator. J Appl Physiol. 1954;7(3):283–308.

20. Grodins FS, Buell J, Bart AJ. Mathematical analysis and digital simulation of the respiratory control system. J Appl Physiol. 1967;22(2):260–76.
21. Horgan JD, Lange RL. Analog computer studies of periodic breathing. IRE Trans Biomed Electron. 1962;9(4):221–8.
22. Gray JS. Pulmonary ventilation and its physiological regulation. Thomas; 1949.
23. Brown HW, Plum F. The neurologic basis of Cheyne-Stokes respiration. Am J Med. 1961;30(6):849–60.
24. Lange RL, Hecht HH. The mechanism of Cheyne-Stokes respiration. J Clin Invest. 1962;41(1):42–52.
25. Cherniack NS, Longobardo GS, Levine OR, Mellins R, Fishman AP. Periodic breathing in dogs. J Appl Physiol. 1966;21(6):1847–54.
26. Farhi LE, Rahn H. Gas stores of the body and the unsteady state. J Appl Physiol. 1955;7(5):472–84.
27. Farhi LE, Rahn H. Dynamics of changes in carbon dioxide stores. Anesthesiology. 1960;21:604–14.
28. Nielsen M, Smith H. Studies on the regulation of respiration in acute hypoxia; with a appendix on respiratory control during prolonged hypoxia. Acta Physiol Scand. 1952;24(4):293–313.
29. Altman PL, Gibson JF, Wang CC. Handbook of respiration. Philadelphia: Saunders; 1958.
30. Mitchell RA, Loeschcke HH, Severinghaus JW, Richardson BW, Massion WH. Regions of respiratory chemosensitivity on the surface of medulla. Ann N Y Acad Sci. 1963;109(2): 661–81.
31. Lambertsen CJ, Factors in the stimulation of respiration by carbon dioxide. In The regulation of human respiration; D. J. C. Cunningham & B. B. Lloyd Eds.; Oxford: Blackwell Scientific Publications. Philadelphia; 1963. pp. 257–76.
32. Dejours P. Control of respiration by arterial chemoreceptors. Ann N Y Acad Sci. 1963;109(2):682–95.
33. Mackey MC, Glass L. Oscillation and chaos in physiological control systems. Science. 1977;197(4300):287–9.
34. Hill AV. The possible effects of the aggregation of the molecules of haemoglobin on its dissociation curves. J Physiol. 1910;40:iv–vii.
35. Landa P, Rosenblum M. Modified Mackey-Glass model of respiration control. Phys Rev E Stat Phys Plasmas Fluids Relat Interdiscip Topics. 1995;52(1):R36–9.
36. Phillipson EA. Control of breathing during sleep. Am Rev Respir Dis. 1978;118(5):909–39.
37. Rigatto H, Brady JP. Periodic breathing and apnea in preterm infants. II. Hypoxia as a primary event. Pediatrics. 1972;50(2):219–28.
38. Waggener TB, Brusil PJ, Kronauer RE, Gabel R. Strength and period of ventilatory oscillations in unacclimatized humans at high altitude (Abstract). Physiology 1977;20:9.
39. Lange RL, Horgan JD, Botticelli JT, Tsagaris T, Carlisle RP, Kuida H. Pulmonary to arterial circulatory transfer function: importance in respiratory control. J Appl Physiol. 1966;21(4):1284–91.
40. Faulkner E. Introduction to the theory of linear systems. London: Chapman & Hall; 1969.
41. Lugaresi E, Coccagna G, Cirignotta F, Farneti P, Gallassi R, Di Donato G, et al. Breathing during sleep in man in normal and pathological conditions. Adv Exp Med Biol. 1978;99:35–45.
42. Specht H, Fruhmann G. Incidence of periodic breathing in 2000 subjects without pulmonary or neurological disease. Bull Physiopathol Respir. (Nancy). 1972;8(5):1075–83.
43. Bulow K. Respiration and wakefulness in man. Acta Physiol Scand Suppl. 1963;209:1–110.
44. Carley DW, Shannon DC. A minimal mathematical model of human periodic breathing. J Appl Physiol. 1985;65(3):1400–9.
45. Corless RM, Gonnet GH, Hare DEG, Jeffrey DJ, Knuth DE. On the Lambert W function. Adv Comput Math. 1996;5(1):329–59.

The Importance of Visceral Feedbacks: Focus on Chemoreceptors

5

Role of Peripheral and Central Sensors of Oxygen, Carbon Dioxide, and pH

Alberto Giannoni, Alberto Aimo, Francesca Bramanti, and Massimo F. Piepoli

Abbreviations

Ang II	Angiotensin II
AT1R	AG-II receptors type 1
BBB	Blood–brain barrier
CB	Carotid body
CHF	Chronic heart failure
CNS	Central nervous system
CRG	Central respiratory generator
CSR	Cheyne–Stokes respiration
HCVR	Hypercapnic ventilatory response
HRV	Heart rate variability
HVR	Hypoxic ventilatory response
KLF2	Kruppel-like factor 2
LVEF	Left ventricular ejection fraction
NO	Nitric oxide
nNOS	Neuronal nitric oxide synthase
NREM	Non-rapid eye movement

A. Giannoni (✉) • F. Bramanti
Division of Cardiology and Cardiovascular Medicine,
Fondazione Toscana Gabriele Monasterio, Pisa, Italy
e-mail: alberto.giannoni@gmail.com; alberto.giannoni@ftgm.it

A. Aimo
Institute of Life Sciences, Scuola Superiore Sant'Anna, Pisa, Italy
e-mail: a.aimo@sssup.it

M.F. Piepoli
Heart Failure Unit, Cardiac Department, Guglielmo da Saliceto Polichirurgico Hospital,
AUSL, Piacenza, Italy
e-mail: m.piepoli@alice.it

© Springer International Publishing Switzerland 2017
M. Emdin et al. (eds.), *The Breathless Heart*,
DOI 10.1007/978-3-319-26354-0_5

125

NST	Nucleus of the solitary tract
NYHA	New York Heart Association
O_2^-	Oxygen superoxide
$PaCO_2$	Arterial partial pressure of carbon dioxide
PB	Periodic breathing
VE/VCO$_2$ slope	Ventilation/carbon dioxide output slope

5.1   Introduction

In the neurohormonal hypothesis of chronic heart failure (CHF), a crucial determinant of disease progression is represented by the general resetting of visceral feedback systems. An increased sensitivity of chemoreceptors and ergoreceptors and a reduced sensitivity of baroreceptors develop since the early stages of CHF [1, 2].

Enhanced chemosensitivity plays a key role in the genesis of periodic breathing/ Cheyne–Stokes respiration (PB/CSR) [3]. As discussed in other chapters of the book, PB/CSR can occur during both sleep and awake hours, both at rest and during exercise, and it is associated with higher perception of dyspnea, sleep disruption, ventilatory inefficiency during effort, and thus with a worse quality of life [3, 4]. Moreover, PB/ CSR is a negative prognostic factor in CHF patients, probably owing to its association with adrenergic activation and vagal withdrawal [5]. Autonomic dysfunction associated with PB/CSR is primarily the consequence of enhanced chemoreflex sensitivity; however, a potential contributor of autonomic imbalance may be also a depressed baroreflex sensitivity, which is indeed a primary aftermath of CHF, and possibly also a consequence of chemoreflex overactivity. In addition, increased ergoreflex sensitivity may contribute to ventilatory instability and autonomic dysfunction during exercise.

In this chapter, we will discuss the role of chemoreflex and the other two visceral feedback systems in the determinism of PB/CSR and the associated autonomic imbalance.

5.2   Chemoreflex Overactivity, Ventilatory Instability, and Sympatho-vagal Imbalance

5.2.1   Clinical Correlates of Enhanced Chemosensitivity in CHF

As already explained in Chap. 2, there are two types of chemoreceptors. Peripheral chemoreceptors are located in the carotid and aortic bodies; the relative functional role of carotid *versus* aortic chemoreceptor bodies is not completely known, but the carotid bodies (CBs) have been shown to play a predominant role in the chemoreception in most mammalian species [6]. The CB is organized in clusters of chemoreceptor cells (type I), in charge of sensing bloodstream stimuli, surrounded by sustentacular glial cells (type II). Peripheral chemoreceptors determine around the 20 % of the hypercapnic ventilatory response (HCVR) in conditions of normoxia; moreover, they are the sole determinants of the hypoxic ventilatory response (HVR) [7]. With respect to central chemoreceptors, they are located in several areas of the brain stem and in other scattered subcortical centers; they are not sensitive to hypoxia but accounts for about 80 % of the response to hypercapnia in condition of normoxia [7].

In animal models of CHF, an enhancement of peripheral chemosensitivity has been extensively demonstrated (as recently reviewed) [6]; by contrast, central chemoreceptors have been only characterized in healthy animals, but a thorough assessment of central chemoreceptor increase in CHF models has not been described yet.

In the first phases of CHF, enhanced chemosensitivity can be regarded as a compensatory mechanism, primarily increasing ventilation to prevent hypoxia and hypercapnia (therefore also pH changes) and secondarily augmenting sympathetic outflow to sustain hemodynamics, besides baroreflex deactivation [8]. However, on the long term, chronic chemoreflex overactivity leads to ventilatory instability and dysautonomia, resulting in more severe symptoms and worse prognosis [9].

CHF patients can display a normal chemosensitivity, an isolated increase to either hypoxia or hypercapnia, or even a combined enhancement of both chemosensitivities [9]. In different laboratories, either chemosensitivity to hypoxia or hypercapnia has been studied and correlated with several CHF-related clinical indexes. First of all, the group of Dr. Coats in London has studied the clinical characteristics of CHF patients with increased peripheral chemosensitivity to hypoxia, assessed using transient inhalation of pure nitrogen. Using two standard deviations over the mean of a control group as a cutoff for defining increased chemosensitivity to hypoxia, they found that around 40 % of CHF patients presented with increased peripheral chemosensitivity. In different studies, the same group showed also that increased chemosensitivity to hypoxia was associated with worse symptoms (higher New York Heart Association – NYHA – class), increased ventilatory inefficiency during exercise (higher ventilation/carbon dioxide output – VE/VCO$_2$ – slope) and worse exercise performance (reduced peak oxygen consumption – VO$_2$/kg) [10, 11], depressed baroreflex and impaired autonomic control (as testified by heart rate variability indexes) [12], as well as with increased non-sustained ventricular tachycardias [10]. Increased chemosensitivity to hypoxia was also associated with both PB and CSR during wakefulness by the same group [5], with modulation of the chemoreflex by either hyperoxia or dihydrocodeine able to reduce or abolish the abnormal respiratory pattern. On the other hand, in a seminal paper published in the *New England Journal of Medicine* by Javaheri in 1998, increased central chemosensitivity to hypercapnia, assessed using Read's rebreathing technique [13] (hyperoxic hypercapnic ventilatory response), was associated with nocturnal PB/CSR (central sleep apnea), even after adjustment for possible confounders as body-surface area, forced vital capacity, maximal voluntary ventilation, oxygen consumption, and carbon dioxide production [14]. A strong direct correlation between the ventilatory response to hypercapnia and the apnea–hypopnea index was also found ($R=0.6$, $p=0.01$). In the paper by Javaheri, some overlap in the ventilatory response to carbon dioxide between patients with and those without central sleep apnea was found, a finding that emphasizes the importance of other mechanisms in the development of central sleep apnea, as already discussed in Chap. 4. If we just focus on the chemoreflex gain, the missing information about the chemosensitivity to either hypoxia (for Javaheri's work) or to hypercapnia (for Coats' group) may partially account for the variability observed in autonomic and ventilatory findings. In fact, in a paper by our group, in which both chemosensitivity to hypoxia and hypercapnia were studied, we found that three possible conditions may occur: a condition of isolated increased chemosensitivity to hypoxia, a condition of isolated increased chemosensitivity to hypercapnia, and a condition of combined increased chemosensitivity to both hypoxia and hypercapnia [9]. When an isolated increase in chemosensitivity was found, there were only minor differences in clinical variables as compared to patients with normal chemosensitivity. On the contrary, when a combined increase was present, the worse clinical scenario was found, with higher NYHA class, greater ventilatory inefficiency (higher VE/VCO_2 slope) during exercise, higher incidence of both diurnal and nocturnal PB/CSR, and more severe dysautonomia with adrenergic overactivity and more frequent atrial/ventricular arrhythmias (Table 5.1), despite no differences in left ventricular volumes or ejection fraction [9]. Moreover, in a larger population from the same cohort, increased chemosensitivity to both hypoxia and hypercapnia was also shown to be an independent predictor of cardiac death and ventricular arrhythmia successfully treated by implantable cardioverter defibrillator (Fig. 5.1) [15]. At multivariate analysis, combined elevation in chemosensitivity emerged as the strongest independent prognostic marker, even when adjusted for univariate predictors (VE/VCO_2 slope, CSR, left ventricular ejection fraction, and plasma brain natriuretic peptide) [12]. This was in line with a previous report on 80 consecutive CHF patients from Coats laboratory, in which only the chemosensitivity to hypoxia was assessed, with no information collected about the chemosensitivity to hypercapnia (potentially being present in at least a subset of patients). In this study, increased chemosensitivity to hypoxia was associated with depressed baroreflex activity. Although both reflexes were indicated as univariate predictors of death, only chemoreflex finally emerged as independent predictor of survival at multivariate analysis [16].

5.2.2 Mechanisms of Increased Chemoreflex Sensitivity in CHF

In CHF, the discharge rate of fibers convoying peripheral chemosensitivity is markedly elevated under normoxic conditions, to levels that normally point to significant hypoxemia. As remarked by Schultz et al., "Because these changes in CB afferent function have been shown in at least three different models of cardiac failure (cardiac pacing, coronary ligation, genetic cardiomyopathy) in several different species, the factors responsible for enhanced CB function do not appear to be related specifically to the etiologies of cardiomyopathy, but rather, to the homeostatic imbalance of the body created by the reduced pumping ability of the heart." Three main mechanisms have been proposed. Chronic CB hypoperfusion could reduce oxygen delivery and/or alter the signaling pathways within the CBs. Increased sympathetic outflow could exacerbate CB hypoperfusion and affect CB excitability. Finally, the intermittent bouts of hypoxia during PB/CSR could enhance CB overactivity with a feed-forward mechanism [6].

Table 5.1 NYHA class, functional capacity and ventilatory efficiency, diurnal and nocturnal CSR, neurohormonal profile, and arrhythmias according to chemosensitivity

	Normal HVR and HCVR	Isolated increase in HVR	Isolated increase in HCVR	Combined increase in HVR and HCVR
Number (%)	24 (40)	8 (13)	12 (20)	16 (27)
LVEF (%)	31.4±1.4	28.3±2.9	29.8±2.3	31.4±2.0
NYHA class III (%)	16	50*	50*	56*
Peak VO2/kg (ml/min/kg)	13.4±1.1	12.0±1.5	12.6±2.3	10.5±0.6
VEVCO2 slope	35.0±1.3	42.8±2.1	38.8±2.8	46.3±2.6*
Workload (W)	97.1±9.0	82.5±8.4	89.4±21.1	69.3±5.4*
Diurnal CSR (%)	0	24	33	68*
Nocturnal AHI (events/h)	6.1±2.3	13.7±3.2	15.4±3.1	20.1±5.3*
Noradrenaline (ng/L)	427.1±69.9	619±84.5	621.7±97.9	689.0±72.3*
BNP (ng/L)	102.4±20.6	270.6±77.6	314.2±75.1*	413.2±92.7*
NT-proBNP (ng/L)	832.7±195.5	1620.7±381.9	2945.5±713.6*	3035.0±783.7*
SDANN (ms)	74.5±4.3	87.7±20.6	82.1±8.1	33.5±11.7*#§
Atrial fibrillation (%)	8	14	16	62*#§
NSVT (%)	20	38	58*	63*#

Gently taken and adapted from Giannoni et al. [9]. http://www.clinsci.org/content/114/7/489.long

AHI apnea–hypopnea index, *BNP* brain natriuretic peptide, *CSR* Cheyne–Stokes respiration, *HVR* hypoxic ventilatory response (chemosensitivity to hypoxia), *HCVR* hypercapnic ventilatory response (chemosensitivity to hypercapnia), *NYHA* New York Heart Association, *NSVT* non-sustained ventricular tachycardia, *NT-proBNP* N-terminal of the prohormone brain natriuretic peptide, *SDANN* standard deviation of sequential 5 min R-R interval means (computed only in patients in sinus rhythm, $n=34$), *VEVCO2* minute ventilation carbon dioxide production relationship, *VO2* peak oxygen consumption

$*p<0.05$ versus normal HVR and HCVR; $\#p<0.05$ versus isolated increase in HVR and HCVR; $\S p<0.05$ versus isolated increase in HVR

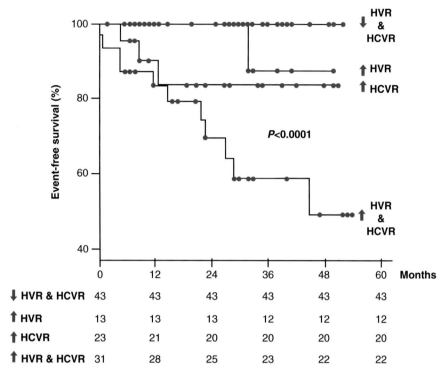

Fig. 5.1 Chemoreflex sensitivity and prognosis in chronic heart failure
Kaplan-Meier survival plot in chronic heart failure patients with normal chemosensitivity (norm HVR and HCVR) compared with patients with augmented chemosensitivity to hypoxia alone (↑ HVR), hypercapnia alone (↑ HCVR), and hypoxia and hypercapnia combined (↑ HVR and HCVR) *HCVR* hypercapnic ventilatory response, *HVR* hypoxic ventilatory response
(From Giannoni et al. [15]. Copyright agreement form attached)

The molecular mechanisms of CB overactivity have been partially disclosed through the characterization of animal models of CHF. Herein, we will provide an overview of these mechanisms, which have been recently reviewed in detail [6].

Local production of oxygen superoxide (O_2^-) is increased in CHF, inhibiting oxygen-sensitive potassium channels in CB cells, and probably also other potassium channels responsible for maintenance of the resting membrane potential [17]. O_2^- might even increase the sensitivity or expression of voltage-gated calcium channels, thus promoting the release of excitatory neurotransmitters from CB cells [6]. The main cause of increased O_2^- production seems to be angiotensin II (Ang II), either circulating or produced within the CBs, through its binding to AT1 receptors [18]. Ang II activates NADPH oxidase (NOX) to enhance O_2^- production, which in turn enhances the excitability of the CB glomus cells and central autonomic neurons via the AT1 receptor. Indeed, it has been shown that AT1R blockers effectively reduced CB afferent activity in rabbits with pacing-induced CHF [19]. Nevertheless, an effect of other prooxidant circulating mediators cannot be excluded [6]. Indeed, hydrogen sulfide (H2S) has been identified as another contributor to CB stimulation in CHF. H2S derives from cystathionine γ-lyase (CSE), whose levels are maintained in the CBs during CHF. CSE inhibition was shown to reduce CBs activity, suggesting a role for H2S levels in the sustaining of CB overactivity during CHF [6].

Local oxidative stress is exacerbated by the reduced expression of both copper/zinc O_2^- dismutase and manganese O_2^- dismutase, which are intracellular scavengers of O_2^- [20]. Other prooxidant mechanisms are represented by the downregulation of the angiotensin 1–7 nitric oxide (NO) pathway and by the reduced production of carbon monoxide, regulated by heme oxygenase-2 (HO-2) that similarly to NO reduces the CB activity [6]. The downregulation of Kruppel-like factor 2 (KLF2) seems to play a significant role in the development of these abnormalities [6]. Indeed, KLF2 downregulation results in increased expression of angiotensin-converting enzyme and reduced production of Ang 1–7 and NO within the CBs [21]. Interestingly, the expression of KLF2 is promoted by shear stress; therefore it is reduced by CB hypoperfusion [6, 17]. By contrast, it is increased by exercise (probably through increased CB perfusion) [22] and by simvastatin [23] (Fig. 5.2).

In CHF, a marked reduction in cardiac output is a common finding. Although acute changes in systemic hemodynamics have little effect on chemoreceptor activity, a sustained reduction over 3 weeks obtained with adjustable cuff occluders on the carotid arteries was actually able to increase AT1R expression and decrease nNOS expression in the CBs in rabbits, inducing an increase in CB afferent activity, similar to that observed in CHF rabbits [24].

In addition to Ang II, the expression of endothelin 1 (ET-1), another potent vasoactive peptide, together with its type A (ET-AR) and B (ET-BR) receptor, has been shown within the CBs. The enhancement in CB afferent activity following intermittent hypoxia has been partly explained by ET-1 signaling mediated by the linkage with the ET-AR [25]. Finally, a paracrine secretion of the putative neurotransmitter ATP by CB type II cells has been advocated, with a potential modulating effect on glomus cells [26].

The molecular mechanisms of increased central chemosensitivity have been less extensively explored. First, a tonic sustain of central chemoreceptors by peripheral chemoreceptors has been hypothesized. In healthy rats, "an uninterrupted chain of sensors and neurons involved in the integration of peripheral and central chemoreception" has been in fact characterized [27]. This chain includes the CBs, chemoreceptor afferents, the nucleus of the solitary tract (NST), the parafacial respiratory group, and the retrotrapezoid nucleus [28]. It is plausible that increased peripheral chemosensitivity might enhance central chemosensitivity through this pathway, as already demonstrated in some animal studies (as reviewed by Dempsey et al. [29]). In awake dogs with vascularly isolated CBs via extracorporeal perfusion, CB chemoreflex inhibition using hyperoxic, hypocapnic perfusate decreased the slope of the ventilatory response to systemic hypercapnia (acting only on central chemoreceptors) to about 20 %. On the other hand, CB chemoreflex stimulation via hypoxic, normocapnic perfusate led to more than 200 % increase in the central ventilatory response to hypercapnia (Fig. 5.3). This has relevant repercussions in the genesis of PB/CSR, as explained in detail in Sect. 5.2.3.

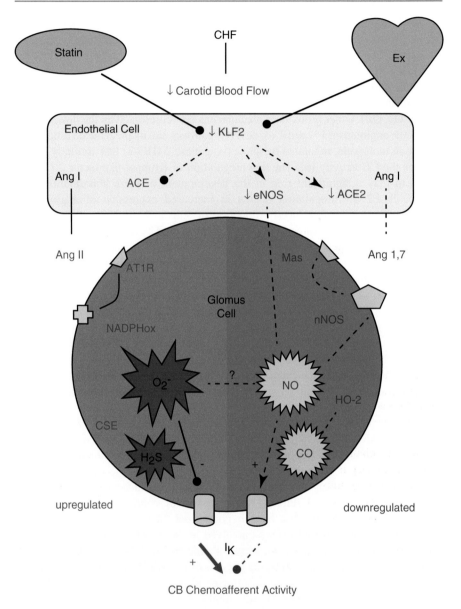

Fig. 5.2 Molecular mechanisms of carotid body sensitization in chronic heart failure
Oxygen superoxide (O_2^-), a reactive oxygen species, is upregulated by angiotensin (Ang) II; it inhibits hyperpolarizing potassium channel currents (I_K), thus increasing the excitability of glomus cells. The opposing inhibitory influence of nitric oxide (NO) and carbon monoxide (CO) on excitability is instead depressed. These changes are ascribed to carotid body hypoperfusion, reducing the expression of transcription factor Kruppel-like factor 2 (KLF2), resulting in the upregulation of angiotensin-converting enzyme (ACE) and the suppression of endothelial (e) and neural (n) nitric oxide synthase (NOS). Statins (simvastatin) and exercise (Ex) may relieve KLF2 suppression (Figure already published in the Springer book "Arterial Chemoreception: from Molecules to Systems" by Colin A. Nurse, Constancio Gonzales, Chris Peers, and Naduri R. Prabhakar. Chapter 52, Figure 52.3)

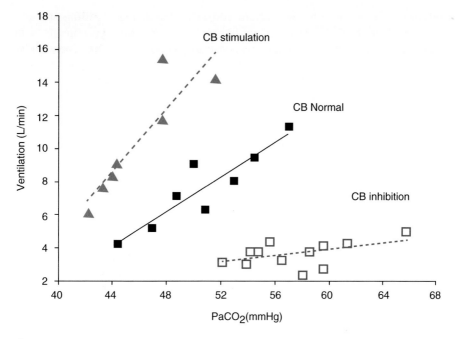

Fig. 5.3 Carotid body function and the ventilatory response to hypercapnia
CO2 carbon dioxide, *FICO2* fraction of carbon dioxide in the inspired air, *PcbCO2* partial pressure of carbon dioxide in the carotid body, *PcbO2* partial pressure of oxygen in the carotid body (From Blain et al. [40]. Figure already published in the Springer book "Arterial Chemoreception: From Molecules to Systems" by Colin A. Nurse, Constancio Gonzales, Chris Peers, and Naduri R. Prabhakar. Chapter 42, Figure 46.3)

Central chemosensitivity can be enhanced even when peripheral chemosensitivity is normal; therefore, other mechanisms of increased central chemosensitivity must be postulated, other than peripheral stimulation of central receptors. Since the α2-adrenoreceptor agonist guanfacine lowers central chemosensitivity in CHF patients, it has been proposed that chronic adrenergic stimulation contributes to central chemoreceptor overactivity [30]. AT1 receptors have been found in the rostral ventrolateral medulla, which is a chemosensitive area [20], and the local administration of Ang II causes vasomotor responses in rabbits [31]; however, the role of Ang II in the modulation of central chemosensitivity has not been explored so far. Another potential cause of central chemoreceptor sensitization, i.e., cerebral hypoperfusion leading to local CO_2 accumulation, is quite implausible. Indeed, hypercapnia results in cerebral vasodilation and thus in increased perfusion [32]; through this mechanism, cerebral perfusion is preserved even when cardiac output is severely reduced, as recently reviewed [33]. Although the reduction in cardiac output seems more important in determining peripheral, rather than central activation of chemoreceptors, another hemodynamic consequence of CHF may play a role in the sensitization of both reflexes. Indeed, in chronically instrumented, unanesthetized dog model during non-rapid eye movement (NREM) sleep, the inflation of balloon in the left atrium, mirroring the increased filling pressure associated with CHF, resulted in hyperventilation and hypocapnia, with increased gain of the ventilatory response to CO_2 below eupnea (potentially leading to ventilatory instability) [34]. It is still unclear whether the effect of increased pulmonary venous pressure would act only on either peripheral or central chemosensitivity to CO_2.

Of note, central chemoreceptors, first localized in areas on the ventral surface of the medulla, now are thought to be located in many areas within the brain stem, cerebellum, hypothalamus, and midbrain. Nowadays, we know that central chemoreception involves several neuronal groups such as the retrotrapezoid nucleus, the rostral medullary raphe (*raphe magnus*), the caudal medullary raphe (*raphe obscurus*), the region just dorsal to the caudal ventral medullary surface, the nucleus of the solitary tract (NTS), the hypothalamic orexin neurons, the *locus coeruleus*, the fastigial nucleus of the cerebellum, and the pre-Bötzinger complex [35]. Further, glial cells around chemosensitive areas may also contribute to chemoreception. The reason why there are so many putative central chemoreceptor sites and what their individual contributions might be is at present uncertain. It is currently unknown whether a diffuse overactivity of all these chemoreceptor groups occurs, or several centers are more dysregulated than others in CHF [14]. A reliable animal model enabling to assess central chemosensitivity in CHF would be crucial in order to fill this gap of knowledge, allowing to clarify the pathophysiology of the overactivity of specific group of chemoreceptors, as already done in the case of peripheral chemoreceptors.

5.2.3   From Enhanced Chemosensitivity to PB/CSR

The complex interaction between altered chemosensitivity and other mechanisms involved in the pathogenesis of PB/CSR, such as hemodynamics, pulmonary J receptors, and lung properties, is discussed in detail in Chap. 4. In this paragraph we will briefly review the relative contribution of chemoreflex overactivity to the origin of ventilatory instability in CHF.

Fluctuations in arterial partial pressure of CO_2 ($PaCO_2$) levels seem to be the main drive to the ventilatory oscillations observed in PB/CSR [5, 14]. Usually, following an increase in $PaCO_2$, a disproportionate increase in ventilation driven by the chemoreflex takes place, with a ventilatory overshoot driving down the $PaCO_2$ to the apneic threshold [26]. When this threshold is reached, the average apnea duration is around 30 s [36]. Peripheral chemoreceptors are considered to be faster than central chemoreceptors in sensing and responding to $PaCO_2$ variations. Indeed, in classic physiology, peripheral chemoreceptors, being located outside the blood–brain barrier (BBB), were believed to respond to changes in $PaCO_2$ within 30 s, with central chemoreceptors being involved after a long delay ranging from 2 to 5 min due to their location inside the BBB [7]. In the latter case, CO_2 was supposed to first diffuse inside the liquor, subsequently leading to a progressive change in liquor pH and eventually altering the firing of central chemoreceptors [28]. Therefore, peripheral chemoreceptors were considered as the primary drivers of ventilatory instability, leading to CO_2 oscillation around an average CO_2 value established by central chemoreceptors [27, 28].

In fact, it is very difficult to experimentally determine which group of chemoreceptors – either peripheral or central – is primarily responsible for PB/CSR genesis and maintenance [28]. Recent studies on both animals and healthy humans suggest that the response of central chemoreceptors is much faster than previously hypothesized, with an average delay of just 11 s of central chemoreceptors from the response to peripheral chemoreceptor stimulation [28]. Furthermore, a clear separation of early- and late-phase responses to CO_2 is not always measurable, with a plausible temporal overlap between the responses of peripheral and central chemoreceptors [37, 38]. Finally, and possibly more importantly, variations in sensory inputs from peripheral chemoreceptors could be transmitted rapidly to central chemoreceptors through the above mentioned pathway, producing the so-called chemoreceptor interdependence [27].

At present, there is a general consensus that the occurrence of PB/CSR is related to the combined response to $PaCO_2$ changes by both groups of chemoreceptors. First, in several species including dogs, goats, ponies, and humans, bilateral CB denervation results in significant hypoventilation and CO_2 retention, together with blunted responses to systemic hypercapnia under both normoxic and hyperoxic conditions [39]. Second, in awake dogs with extracorporeal perfusion of the vascularly isolated CBs, a hyperadditive response was found when increasing $PaCO_2$ and exposing peripheral chemoreceptors to hypercapnia, as already described in Sect. 5.2.2 (Fig. 5.3) [40, 41]. The functional interdependence between peripheral and central chemoreceptors has been found to exert an influence on the genesis of PB/CSR. In a study by the group of Dempsey and performed in the sleeping dog, systemic hypocapnia induced by transient hyperventilation resulted in ventilatory oscillations and apneas with an apneic threshold approximately 5 mmHg below eupneic $PaCO_2$ [42]. However, hypocapnia applied only to the isolated CBs, even at as much as 10–15 mmHg below eupnea, did not elicit apneas [34]. Even systemic hypocapnia (achieved through mechanical ventilation) when the CBs were maintained at constant normocapnia via extracorporeal perfusion did not elicit apneas [43].

Another confirmation of the interdependence of peripheral and central chemoreceptors and their role in the genesis of PB/CSR in the animal setting was found in the pacing rabbit. In this model, peripheral and central chemosensitivity were both augmented during pacing, but peripheral chemoresponse augmented earlier. However, only once central chemosensitivity was also increased, central apneas occurred [44].

In the clinical setting, several evidences suggest that enhanced central and/or peripheral chemoreflex sensitivity [9, 10, 14, 15] contributes to the pathogenesis of CSR by causing instability of the respiratory control system, confirming the prediction from mathematical modeling (please refer to Chap. 4) and animal data. Different groups of researchers have usually assessed either peripheral or central chemosensitivity in patients with CHF, invariably finding an association of increased chemosensitivity with PB/CSR [10–16]. As already evidenced in Sect. 5.2, in two reports from our group, the highest incidence of PB/CSR was found in CHF patients with a combined increased in the chemosensitivity to both hypoxia and hypercapnia

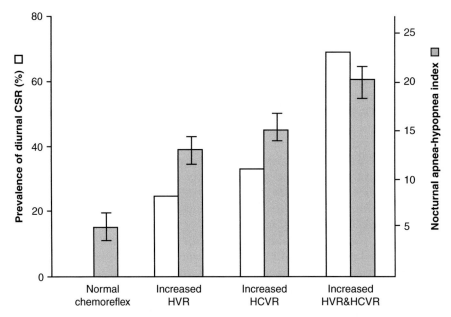

Fig. 5.4 Prevalence of diurnal CSR (%) and severity of nocturnal CSR (expressed as AHI) among patients with normal chemosensitivity, isolated increased in chemosensitivity to hypoxia (HVR), isolated increase in chemosensitivity to hypercapnia (HCVR), and combined increased in chemosensitivity to both hypoxia and hypercapnia (HVR + HCVR). * $p < 0.001$ † $p < 0.001$ versus patients with normal chemosensitivity [9]. http://www.clinsci.org/content/114/7/489.long

Authors do not usually need to contact Portland Press to request permission to reuse their own material, as long as the original work is properly credited. It is usual to provide the citation of (and where relevant a hyperlink to the original publication

(Fig. 5.4) by rebreathing technique (hypoxic normocapnic test and hypercapnic normoxic test, respectively), supporting the idea of the need of a general increase in chemosensitivity to develop breathing instability [9–15]. In another study by Solin and colleagues, the peripheral chemosensitivity to CO_2, evaluated by single breath technique, and the central chemosensitivity to CO_2 evaluated by the rebreathing technique (hyperoxic hypercapnic test), were both found increased in CHF patients with PB/CSR [45].

In summary, the two groups of chemoreceptors seem to be functionally interrelated; following a ventilatory overshoot, the hypocapnia sensed by peripheral chemoreceptors probably triggers the apneic phase, but additional inputs from central chemoreceptors could be required to produce central apneas (Fig. 5.5).

5.2.4   Chemoreflex Overactivity and Autonomic Deregulation

Peripheral and central chemoreceptors, beyond controlling ventilation, also regulate blood flow, so that arterial pressure is maintained despite the direct vasodilatory

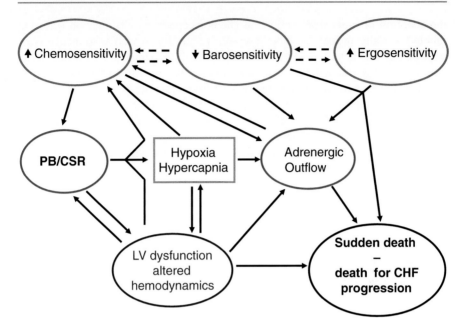

Fig. 5.5 Deregulation of feedbacks systems in CHF and their role in PB/CSR genesis, autonomic dysfunction, and disease progression. *CHF* chronic heart failure, *CSR* Cheyne–Stokes respiration, *LV* left ventricular, *PB* periodic breathing
(Taken and adapted from Giannoni et al. [73])

effects of hypoxemia and/or hypercapnia. To do this, chemoreflex activation also results in increased sympathetic outflow to the heart and the vascular bed. However, the chemoreflex can become maladaptive in disease states, such as CHF where the overactivity of sympathetic outflow is known to negatively impact on disease progression.

Under physiological conditions, selective activation of peripheral chemoreceptors, achieved, for example, through close injections of CO_2-saturated saline [46] or intermittent hypoxia [47], increases sympathetic outflow and blood pressure in animals [6]. While in the past it was generally believed that chemoreflex normally is not activated in rest conditions as normoxia/isocapnia, we now know that hyperoxic inhibition of peripheral chemoreceptors reduces the baseline sympathetic activity, underscoring a tonic effect of the chemoreflex on the sympathetic system [17].

An enhanced discharge of peripheral chemoreceptors has been demonstrated in various animal model of CHF, such as pacing-induced CHF in rabbits, myocardial infarction-induced CHF in rats, and genetic cardiomyopathy in mice [48]. In CHF animals, CB discharge at rest is elevated at rest (normoxia) to levels similar to the ones obtained after significant hypoxemia in normal animals. In animal models of CHF (rats and rabbits), heart rate variability indices were reduced at baseline (sympatho-vagal imbalance) but normalized after CB ablation. In other models of CHF, the abolition of input from peripheral chemoreceptors by CB ablation (rats and rabbits) was able to increase blood pressure variability, as well as to reduce sympathetic nervous activity and the discharge rate of presympathetic neurons in the rostral ventrolateral medulla (as reviewed in [6, 17, 49]). Even the inhibition of CBs through hyperoxia was able to improve autonomic function, as demonstrated by reduced sympathetic nerve activity in CHF sheep [49]. These findings have provided a conceptual framework for CB demolition or inhibition as potential therapeutic approaches for CHF [50].

The activation of central chemoreceptors increases sympathetic nerve activity and blood pressure, as demonstrated in animals exposed to increases in $PaCO_2$ after CB ablation [51]. A modest rise in CO_2 levels in the central nervous system (CNS) increases sympathetic vasomotor tone in bursts that are synchronous with the respiratory cycle. Activation of the central respiratory generator (CRG) probably modulates sympathetic nerve activity at several brain stem or spinal locations, but the most important site of interaction seems to be the caudal ventrolateral medulla, where CRG components periodically gate the response to baroreflex stimulation. The proposed mechanisms are periodical changes in the activity of pulmonary stretch receptors and baroreceptors and an influence of the respiratory network on the caudal ventrolateral medulla or the NST [52]. It has been observed that CNS exposure to CO_2 levels even slightly above 40 mmHg results also in a sympatho-excitatory effect that is not dependent on the respiratory network. Among the centers possibly involved, there are the retrotrapezoid nucleus, the NST, and some raphe nuclei (short loop reflexes) [52]. Other nuclei within the CNS seem to be activated only at high CO_2 levels; they would elicit aversive sensations in the waking state and arousals from sleep. The *locus coeruleus*, the raphe nuclei, and the orexinergic neurons could mediate such responses (long loop reflexes). The studies on these topic have been reviewed by Guyenet et al. [52].

With respect to humans, the selective stimulation of both peripheral and central chemoreceptors (achieved by modulating the arterial partial pressures of O_2 and CO_2) increases sympathetic outflow in healthy subjects [53, 54]. The overactivity of peripheral chemoreceptors in CHF could contribute to both baroreflex impairment and sympatho-vagal imbalance with adrenergic activation and vagal withdrawal, which is a hallmark of CHF, and it is reflected by the reduction of several indices of heart rate variability (HRV) [12]. In a small population of CHF patients, unselected for baseline chemosensitivity levels, Narkiewicz showed an increase in muscle sympathetic nerve activity (MSNA) larger than controls only after exposing patients to hypercapnia (7 % CO_2/93 % O_2), but not after hypoxia (10 % O_2 in N_2 with CO_2 titrated to maintain isocapnia). The increase in MSNA after hypercapnia in CHF patients occurs in spite of a higher increase also in ventilation, which should blunt the sympathetic response. Furthermore, in a cohort from our group, in which the chemoreflex sensitivity was instead evaluated, enhanced chemosensitivity to both hypoxia and hypercapnia was associated with a 60 % increase in mean plasma levels of norepinephrine compared with patients with normal chemosensitivity; the combined increase in chemosensitivity was associated also with a general neurohormonal impairment and some negative effect of increased sympathetic outflow on the heart, such as higher incidence of atrial and ventricular arrhythmias (Table 5.1) [9].

5.3 Altered Baroreceptor and Ergoreceptor Sensitivities: Contributors to Autonomic Dysfunction and Ventilatory Instability?

5.3.1 Baroreflex Depression, Sympatho-Vagal Imbalance, and PB/CSR

The baroreflex is a negative feedback system regulating sympathetic outflow in order to stabilize blood pressure. Its sensitivity can be assessed by increasing arterial pressure (usually via the administration of the α1-agonist phenylephrine) or performing a mechanical stimulation of the carotid sinus (via a suction or a compression on the neck) and measuring the heart rate response to these maneuvers. Its physiological function is to sustain blood pressure avoiding hypotension (especially postural hypotension) and subsequent tissue hypoperfusion [55]. In CHF, arterial baroreflex-mediated HR responses to blood pressure (BP) changes are clearly diminished, with a recognized negative impact on survival [56]. Some recent evidences have pointed out that while stimulating baroreceptor, afferent input elicits a significant fall in norepinephrine levels (paced canine model), sinoaortic denervation has no effect on the time course change in hemodynamics, and norepinephrine concentration as CHF develops, suggesting a central gating of the baroreflex, rather than a depressed baroreflex stimulation or receptor resetting [57]. Since the integrative centers and the efferent arms of the baroreflex and the chemoreflex are common [52], it is reasonable to postulate an interaction between the chemo- and the baroreflex.

In rats, bilateral denervation of carotid bodies (peripheral chemoreceptors) did not affect the baroreflex control of HR, suggesting that peripheral chemoreceptors do not exert a tonic inhibition of baroreceptor responses under basal conditions [58]. Again in rats, the contextual electric stimulation of the carotid sinus (to stimulate the baroreceptors) and the CB efferent nerve (to induce peripheral chemoreceptor activation) attenuated the reflex hypotension resulting from baroreflex stimulation alone, outlining that once stimulated the chemoreflex may blunt the baroreflex response [59]. By contrast, the stimulation of central chemoreceptors through hypercapnia did not alter baroreflex sensitivity [60]. To our knowledge, the influence of baroreflex stimulation on either peripheral and/or central chemosensitivities has not been explored so far in animal studies.

With respect to human studies, in 11 healthy humans the exposure to hypoxia had no significant effect on baroreflex sensitivity or set point, while hypercapnia did not change baroreflex sensitivity but increased its set point (i.e., mean arterial pressure) [60]; similar results have been achieved through a mathematical model of cardiorespiratory regulation [61]. In another study, baroreflex stimulation, achieved by increasing the pressure in the carotid sinus, was able to reduce the response in muscle sympathetic nerve activity during hypoxia but not during hypercapnia [62]. On the whole, there are some evidences of a functional antagonism between chemoreflex and baroreflex, but the exact manifestations of this antagonism are yet to be completely characterized.

In a study on 26 CHF patients, enhanced chemosensitivity to hypoxia was associated with blunted baroreflex sensitivity; in these patients, CB inhibition through transient hyperoxia resulted in an improvement in baroreflex sensitivity [12]. To our knowledge, only a demonstration of the cause-effect relationship between enhanced peripheral chemosensitivity and baroreflex depression has been attempted in the setting of CHF. In 18 patients with augmented peripheral chemosensitivity, the silencing of peripheral chemoreceptors through the administration of 100 % oxygen increased baroreflex sensitivity; however, it should be noted that the quantification of baroreflex sensitivity by the slope of the relationship between muscle sympathetic nerve activity and diastolic blood pressure has not been validated in literature [63].

In summary, CHF patients often display reduced baroreflex sensitivity, which could be promoted by increased peripheral chemosensitivity. It is reasonable to assume that baroreflex depression might enhance the chemoreflex contribution to autonomic dysregulation, thus worsening the sympatho-vagal imbalance that is associated with chemoreflex stimulation and with PB/CSR *per se*.

Finally, it is intriguing to speculate that baroreflex depression could contribute to ventilatory instability. Reduced baroreflex sensitivity implies a lower capacity of buffering spontaneous variations in arterial pressure [46, 64]; the parallel changes in cardiac output and circulatory time have probably never been explored, but it is reasonable to assume that the changes in these parameters are enhanced by baroreflex depression. As discussed in detail in another chapter, low cardiac output and prolonged circulatory time seem to contribute to the genesis of PB/CSR. The hypothesis of a contribution of baroreflex depression to PB/CSR development has probably never been assessed so far, with the partial exception of a study, dated 1975, in which cats undergoing total baroreflex deafferentation and blood loss developed oscillations of both systemic arterial pressure and ventilatory amplitude, with the same period [65]. Further studies are advisable in order to clarify the role of baroreflex depression in PB/CSR pathogenesis.

5.3.2   Ergoreflex Overactivity and PB/CSR During Exercise

During exercise, the control of ventilation and cardiovascular function relies partially upon the ergoreflex, a neural mechanism activated by muscle contraction. The ergoreflex has two components: the metaboreflex, activated by the accumulation of metabolites in the exercising muscles, and the mechanoreflex, triggered by the tension of muscle fibers [66]. Metaboreflex sensitivity can be evaluated by measuring ventilation and/or neurovascular parameters during post-exercise circulatory occlusion [67]; by contrast, eliciting a selective mechanoreflex response is more complex and can be achieved by passive limb movements or other protocols [68].

The main consequences of metaboreflex stimulation in healthy subjects are increases in ventilation and blood pressure [1]. Again in healthy subjects, mechanoreflex activation causes a rise in blood pressure, whereas its contribution to ventilatory control has never been demonstrated [1].

CHF patients often develop a skeletal myopathy because of muscle hypoperfusion, systemic inflammation, physical deconditioning, and other mechanisms [69]. There is a general consensus on the fact that ergoreflex sensitivity can be enhanced in CHF in parallel with muscle impairment and that only one component of the ergoreflex (i.e., the metabo- or the mechanoreflex) is overactivated [1]. The group of Dr. Piepoli and Coats provided an extensive body of evidence supporting enhanced metaboreflex sensitivity in CHF [57], although several studies reporting an overactive mechanoreflex and a blunted metaboreflex have been published [58]; the differences in experimental protocols possibly account for these discrepancies [58, 61].

In CHF patients undergoing cardiopulmonary exercise testing, metaboreflex sensitivity was inversely correlated with peak VO_2 (an index of exercise tolerance) and directly correlated with the VE/VCO_2 slope [70]; this last parameter quantifies ventilatory inefficiency during exercise and is increased by enhanced peripheral and/or central chemosensitivity [71]. An increase in chemoreflex sensitivity during exercise is plausible. A clinical trial searching for a chemoreflex gain during exercise in CHF patients was started in 2010 by Dr. Francis' group [72], but to our knowledge the results have not been published so far. Following the demonstration of a chemoreflex gain during exercise, it would be reasonable to verify whether ergoreflex overactivity during muscle activation can promote such gain and then the occurrence of PB during effort.

Conclusions

In the last few years, several animal and humans studies have evidenced that the deregulation of baro-, ergo-, and chemoreflexes in CHF patients leads to parasympathetic withdrawal and increased adrenergic outflow. In particular, chemoreflex activation is one of the key determinants of PB/CSR occurrence, which contributes to sympathetic overactivity and disease progression in patients with CHF. Animal studies have allowed to clarify the mechanisms leading to the increased peripheral chemosensitivity, while the enhancement of central chemosensitivity is still unexplained because of the lack of CHF animal models specifically designed to address this topic. A great advances in the physiology and pathophysiology of chemoreception have been represented by the recognition of the tight interlink between peripheral and central chemoreceptors, influencing each other and being both necessary to lead to ventilatory instability. While baroreceptors and ergoreceptors are known contributor to autonomic imbalance in CHF, their role in the genesis of PB/CSR both in rest condition and during exercise is still largely unknown. Likewise, the degree and meaning of central interaction between the three feedbacks (chemo-, baro-, and ergoreflex) in physiological conditions and in disease states (such as hypertension or CHF) are still far to be well known. Future research efforts should try to fill these gaps of knowledge in order to develop a rational modulation of the feedback systems in CHF patients, especially in those with adrenergic overactivity and ventilatory instability.

References

1. Piepoli MF, Crisafulli A. Pathophysiology of human heart failure: importance of skeletal muscle myopathy and reflexes. Exp Physiol. 2014;99:609–15.
2. Piepoli MF, Ponikowski PP, Volterrani M, Francis D, Coats AJ. Aetiology and pathophysiological implications of oscillatory ventilation at rest and during exercise in chronic heart failure. Do Cheyne and Stokes have an important message for modern-day patients with heart failure? Eur Heart J. 1999;20:946–53.
3. Mansukhani MP, Wang S, Somers VK. Chemoreflex physiology and implications for sleep apnoea: insights from studies in humans. Exp Physiol. 2015;100:130–5.
4. Passino C, Giannoni A, Milli M, Polettii R, Emdin M. Recenti conoscenze sulla sensibilità chemocettiva ad ipossia ed ipercapnia in patologia cardiovascolare. Recenti Prog Med. 2010;101:308–13.
5. Ponikowski P, Anker SD, Chua TP, Francis D, Banasiak W, Poole-Wilson PA, et al. Oscillatory breathing patterns during wakefulness in patients with chronic heart failure: clinical implications and role of augmented peripheral chemosensitivity. Circulation. 1999;100:2418–24.
6. Schultz HD, Marcus NJ, Del Rio R. Role of the carotid body chemoreflex in the pathophysiology of heart failure: a perspective from animal studies. Adv Exp Med Biol. 2015;860:167–85.
7. Ganong WF. Review of medical physiology. 21st ed. New York: Lange Medical Books/McGrow-Hill; 2003.
8. Schultz HD, Sun SY. Chemoreflex function in heart failure. Heart Fail Rev. 2000;5:45–56.
9. Giannoni A, Emdin M, Poletti R, Bramanti F, Prontera C, Piepoli M, et al. Clinical significance of chemosensitivity in chronic heart failure: influence on neurohormonal derangement, Cheyne-Stokes respiration and arrhythmias. Clin Sci (Lond). 2008;114:489–97.
10. Chua TP, Ponikowski P, Webb-Peploe K, Harrington D, Anker SD, Piepoli M, et al. Clinical characteristics of chronic heart failure patients with an augmented peripheral chemoreflex. Eur Heart J. 1997;18:480–6.
11. Ponikowski P, Francis DP, Piepoli MF, Davies LC, Chua TP, Davos CH, et al. Enhanced ventilatory response to exercise in patients with chronic heart failure and preserved exercise tolerance: marker of abnormal cardiorespiratory reflex control and predictor of poor prognosis. Circulation. 2001;103:967–72.
12. Ponikowski P, Chua TP, Piepoli M, Ondusova D, Webb-Peploe K, Harrington D, et al. Augmented peripheral chemosensitivity as a potential input to baroreflex impairment and autonomic imbalance in chronic heart failure. Circulation. 1997;96:2586–94.
13. Read DJC. A clinical method for assessing the ventilatory response to carbon dioxide. Australas Ann Med. 1967;16:20–32.
14. Javaheri S. A mechanism of central sleep apnea in patients with heart failure. N Engl J Med. 1999;341:949–54.
15. Giannoni A, Emdin M, Bramanti F, Iudice G, Francis DP, Barsotti A, et al. Combined increased chemosensitivity to hypoxia and hypercapnia as a prognosticator in heart failure. J Am Coll Cardiol. 2009;53:1975–80.
16. Ponikowski P, Chua TP, Anker SD, Francis DP, Doehner W, Banasiak W, et al. Peripheral chemoreceptor hypersensitivity: an ominous sign in patients with chronic heart failure. Circulation. 2001;104:544–9.

17. Schultz HD, Marcus NJ, Del Rio R. Role of the carotid body in the pathophysiology of heart failure. Curr Hypertens Rep. 2013;15:356–62.
18. Li YL, Gao L, Zucker IH, Schultz HD. NADPH oxidase-derived superoxide anion mediates angiotensin II-enhanced carotid body chemoreceptor sensitivity in heart failure rabbits. Cardiovasc Res. 2007;75:546–54.
19. Li YL, Xia XH, Zheng H, Gao L, Li YF, Liu D, et al. Angiotensin II enhances carotid body chemoreflex control of sympathetic outflow in chronic heart failure rabbits. Cardiovasc Res. 2006;71:129–38.
20. Ding Y, Li YL, Zimmerman MC, Schultz HD. Elevated mitochondrial superoxide contributes to enhanced chemoreflex in heart failure rabbits. Am J Physiol Regul Integr Comp Physiol. 2010;298:R303–311.
21. Dekker RJ, van Thienen JV, Rohlena J, de Jager SC, Elderkamp YW, Seppen J, et al. Endothelial KLF2 links local arterial shear stress levels to the expression of vascular tone-regulating genes. Am J Pathol. 2005;167:609–18.
22. van Thienen JV, Fledderus JO, Dekker RJ, Rohlena J, van Ijzendoorn GA, Kootstra NA, et al. Shear stress sustains atheroprotective endothelial KLF2 expression more potently than statins through mRNA stabilization. Cardiovasc Res. 2006;72:231–40.
23. Haack KK, Marcus NJ, Del Rio R, Zucker IH, Schultz HD. Simvastatin treatment attenuates increased respiratory variability and apnea/hypopnea index in rats with chronic heart failure. Hypertension. 2014;63:1041–9.
24. Ding Y, Li YL, Schultz HD. Role of blood flow in carotid body chemoreflex function in heart failure. J Physiol. 2011;589:245–58.
25. Del Rio R, Moya EA, Iturriaga R. Differential expression of pro-inflammatory cytokines, endothelin-1 and nitric oxide synthases in the rat carotid body exposed to intermittent hypoxia. Brain Res. 2011;1395:74–85.
26. Zhang M, Piskuric NA, Vollmer C, Nurse CA. P2Y2 receptor activation opens pannexin-1 channels in rat carotid body type II cells: potential role in amplifying the neurotransmitter ATP. J Physiol. 2012;590:4335–50.
27. Stornetta RL, Moreira TS, Takakura AC, Kang BJ, Chang DA, West GH, et al. Expression of Phox2b by neurons involved in chemosensory integration in the adult rat. J Neurosci. 2006;26:10305–14.
28. Takakura AC, Moreira TS, Colombari E, West GH, Stornetta RL, Guyenet PG. Peripheral chemoreceptor inputs to retrotrapezoid nucleus (RTN) CO2-sensitive neurons in rats. J Physiol. 2006;572:503–23.
29. Dempsey JA, Smith CA, Blain GM, Xie A, Gong Y, Teodorescu M. Role of central/peripheral chemoreceptors and their interdependence in the pathophysiology of sleep apnea. Adv Exp Med Biol. 2012;758:343–9.
30. Yamada K, Asanoi H, Ueno H, Joho S, Takagawa J, Kameyama T, et al. Role of central sympathoexcitation in enhanced hypercapnic chemosensitivity in patients with heart failure. Am Heart J. 2004;148:964–70.
31. Head GA. Role of AT1 receptors in the central control of sympathetic vasomotor function. Clin Exp Pharmacol Physiol Suppl. 1996;3:S93–98.
32. Willie CK, Macleod DB, Shaw AD, Mith KJ, Tzeng YC, Eves ND, et al. Regional brain blood flow in man during acute changes in arterial blood gases. J Physiol. 2012;590:3261–75.
33. Meng L, Hou W, Chui J, Han R, Gelb AW. Cardiac output and cerebral blood flow: the integrated regulation of brain perfusion in adult humans. Anesthesiology. 2015;123:1198–208.
34. Chenuel BJ, Smith CA, Skatrud JB, Henderson KS, Dempsey JA. Increased propensity for apnea in response to acute elevations in left atrial pressure during sleep in the dog. J Appl Physiol. 2006;101:76–83.
35. Nattie E, Li A. Central chemoreceptors: locations and functions. Compr Physiol. 2012;2:221–54.
36. Smith CA, Rodman JR, Chenuel BJ, Henderson KS, Dempsey JA. Response time and sensitivity of the ventilatory response to CO2 in unanesthetized intact dogs: central vs. peripheral chemoreceptors. J Appl Physiol. 2006;100:13–9.

37. Pedersen MEF, Fatemian M, Robbins PA. Identification of fast and slow ventilatory responses to carbon dioxide under hypoxic and hyperoxic conditions in humans. J Physiol. 1999;521:273–87.
38. Dahan A, Nieuwenhuijs D, Teppema L. Plasticity of central chemoreceptors: effect of bilateral carotid body resection on central CO2 sensitivity. PLoS Med. 2007;4:e239.
39. Smith CA, Forster HV, Blain GM, Dempsey JA. An interdependent model of central/peripheral chemoreception: evidence and implications for ventilatory control. Respir Physiol Neurobiol. 2010;173:288–97.
40. Blain GM, Smith CA, Henderson KS, Dempsey JA. Peripheral chemoreceptors determine the respiratory sensitivity of central chemoreceptors to CO(2). J Physiol. 2010;588: 2455–71.
41. Smith CA, Blain GM, Henderson KS, et al. Peripheral chemoreceptors determine the respiratory sensitivity of central chemoreceptors to CO2: role of carotid body CO2. J Physiol. 2015;593:4225–43.
42. Smith CA, Saupe KW, Henderson KS, Dempsey JA. Ventilatory effects of specific carotid body hypocapnia in dogs during wakefulness and sleep. J Appl Physiol. 1995;79:689–99.
43. Smith CA, Chenuel BJ, Henderson KS, Dempsey JA. The apneic threshold during non-REM sleep in dogs: sensitivity of carotid body vs. central chemoreceptors. J Appl Physiol. 2007;103:578–86.
44. Marcus NJ, Schultz HD. Role of carotid body chemoreflex function in the development of Cheyne-Stokes Respiration during progression of congestive heart failure. FASEB J. 2011;25:841–7.
45. Solin P, Roebuck T, Johns DP, Walters EH, Naughton MT. Peripheral and central ventilatory responses in central sleep apnea with and without congestive heart failure. Am J Respir Crit Care Med. 2000;162:2194–200.
46. McAllen RM. Actions of carotid chemoreceptors on subretrofacial bulbospinal neurons in the cat. J Auton Nerv Syst. 1992;40:181–8.
47. Del Rio R, Moya EA, Iturriaga R. Carotid body potentiation during chronic intermittent hypoxia: implication for hypertension. Front Physiol. 2014;5:434.
48. Schultz HD, Marcus NJ, Del Rio R. Mechanisms of carotid body chemoreflex dysfunction during heart failure. Exp Physiol. 2015;100:124–9.
49. Xing DT, May CN, Booth LC, Ramchandra R. Tonic arterial chemoreceptor activity contributes to cardiac sympathetic activation in mild ovine heart failure. Exp Physiol. 2014;99:1031–41.
50. Giannoni A, Passino C, Mirizzi G, Del Franco A, Aimo A, Emdin M. Treating chemoreflex in heart failure: modulation or demolition? J Physiol. 2014;592:1903–4.
51. Guyenet PG, Stornetta RL, Abbott SB, Depuy SD, Fortuna MG, Kanbar R. Central CO2 chemoreception and integrated neural mechanisms of cardiovascular and respiratory control. J Appl Physiol (1985). 2010;108:995–1002.
52. Guyenet PG. Regulation of breathing and autonomic outflows by chemoreceptors. Compr Physiol. 2014;4:1511–62.
53. Somers VK, Mark AL, Zavala DC, Abboud FM. Contrasting effects of hypoxia and hypercapnia on ventilation and sympathetic activity in humans. J Appl Physiol (1985). 1989;67:2101–6.
54. Pitsikoulis C, Bartels MN, Gates G, Rebmann RA, Layton AM, De Meersman RE. Sympathetic drive is modulated by central chemoreceptor activation. Respir Physiol Neurobiol. 2008;164:373–9.
55. Benarroch EE. The arterial baroreflex: functional organization and involvement in neurologic disease. Neurology. 2008;71:1733–8.
56. La Rovere MT, Pinna GD, Maestri R, Robbi E, Caporotondi A, Guazzotti G, et al. Prognostic implications of baroreflex sensitivity in heart failure patients in the beta-blocking era. J Am Coll Cardiol. 2009;53:193–9.
57. Floras JS. Sympathetic nervous system activation in human heart failure: clinical implications of an updated model. J Am Coll Cardiol. 2009;54:375–85.

58. Oikawa S, Hirakawa H, Kusakabe T, Nakashima Y, Hayashida Y. Autonomic cardiovascular responses to hypercapnia in conscious rats: the roles of the chemo- and baroreceptors. Auton Neurosci. 2005;117:105–14.
59. Katayama PL, Castania JA, Dias DP, Patel KP, Fazan Jr R, Salgado HC. Role of chemoreceptor activation in hemodynamic responses to electrical stimulation of the carotid sinus in conscious rats. Hypertension. 2015;66:598–603.
60. Cooper VL, Pearson SB, Bowker CM, Elliott MW, Hainsworth R. Interaction of chemoreceptor and baroreceptor reflexes by hypoxia and hypercapnia – A mechanism for promoting hypertension in obstructive sleep apnoea. J Physiol. 2005;568:677–87.
61. Lin J, Ngwompo RF, Tilley DG. Development of a cardiopulmonary mathematical model incorporating a baro-chemoreceptor reflex control system. Proc Inst Mech Eng H. 2012;226:787–803.
62. Somers VK, Mark AL, Abboud FM. Interaction of baroreceptor and chemoreceptor reflex control of sympathetic nerve activity in normal humans. J Clin Invest. 1991;87:1953–7.
63. Despas F, Lambert E, Vaccaro A, Labrunee M, Franchitto N, Lebrin M, et al. Peripheral chemoreflex activation contributes to sympathetic baroreflex impairment in chronic heart failure. J Hypertens. 2012;30:753–60.
64. van de Vooren H, Gademan MG, Swenne CA, TenVoorde BJ, Schalij MJ, Van der Wall EE. Baroreflex sensitivity, blood pressure buffering, and resonance: what are the links? Computer simulation of healthy subjects and heart failure patients. J Appl Physiol (1985). 2007;102:1348–56.
65. Preiss G, Iscoe S, Polosa C. Analysis of a periodic breathing pattern associated with Mayer waves. Am J Physiol. 1975;228:768–74.
66. Nobrega AC, O'Leary D, Silva BM, Marongiu E, Piepoli MF, Crisafulli A. Neural regulation of cardiovascular response to exercise: role of central command and peripheral afferents. Biomed Res Int. 2014;2014:478965.
67. Piepoli MF, Coats AJ. Increased metaboreceptor stimulation explains the exaggerated exercise pressor reflex seen in heart failure. J Appl Physiol (1985). 2007;102:494–6.
68. Middlekauff HR, Sinoway LI. Increased mechanoreceptor stimulation explains the exaggerated exercise pressor reflex seen in heart failure. J Appl Physiol (1985). 2007;102:492–4.
69. Doehner W, Frenneaux M, Anker SD. Metabolic impairment in heart failure: the myocardial and systemic perspective. J Am Coll Cardiol. 2014;64:1388–400.
70. Scott AC, Davies LC, Coats AJ, Piepoli M. Relationship of skeletal muscle metaboreceptors in the upper and lower limbs with the respiratory control in patients with heart failure. Clin Sci (Lond). 2002;102:23–30.
71. Chua TP, Clark AL, Amadi AA, Coats AJ. Relation between chemosensitivity and the ventilatory response to exercise in chronic heart failure. J Am Coll Cardiol. 1996;27:650–7.
72. www.patientslikeme.com/clinical_trials/NCT01050179-chemosensitivity
73. Giannoni A, Mirizzi G, Aimo A, Emdin M, Passino C. Peripheral reflex feedbacks in chronic heart failure: is it time for a direct treatment? World J Cardiol. 2015;7:824–8.

The Apneas Before and After Heart Failure

6

Obstructive Sleep Apnea (OSA) in Stage A and B; Central Sleep Apnea vs OSA in Stage C and D

Jens Spießhöfer and Olaf Oldenburg

Abbreviations

AASM	American Academy of Sleep Medicine
ADVENT-HF	Adaptive Servo Ventilation for Therapy of Sleep Apnea in Heart Failure
AF	Atrial fibrillation
AHI	Apnea-hypopnea index
AMEND	ASV Effects on Myocardial Energetics and Sympathetic Nerve Function in Heart Failure and Sleep Apnea
APAP	Automatic positive airway pressure
ASV	Adaptive servo ventilation
BP	Blood pressure
CAD	Coronary artery disease
CANPAP	Continuous Positive Airway Pressure for Central Sleep Apnea in Heart Failure
CIH	Chronic intermittent hypoxia
CO_2	Carbon dioxide
CPAP	Continuous positive airway pressure therapy
CSA	Central sleep apnea
CSR	Cheyne–Stokes respiration
HCVR	Hypercapnic ventilatory response
HF	Heart failure
HFpEF	Heart failure with preserved ejection fraction
HFrEF	Heart failure with reduced ejection fraction

J. Spießhöfer (✉) • O. Oldenburg
Department of Cardiology, Heart and Diabetes Center North Rhine-Westphalia,
Ruhr-University Bochum, Bad Oeynhausen, Germany
e-mail: jens.spiesshoefer@googlemail.com; oldenburg@hdz-nrw.de

© Springer International Publishing Switzerland 2017
M. Emdin et al. (eds.), *The Breathless Heart*,
DOI 10.1007/978-3-319-26354-0_6

hs-CRP	C-reactive protein
IPC	Ischemic preconditioning
LVEF	Left ventricular ejection fraction
OSA	Obstructive sleep apnea
NIP	Negative intrathoracic pressure
PCWP	Pulmonary capillary wedge pressure
SERVE-HF	Treatment of Sleep-Disordered Breathing with Predominant Central Sleep Apnea by Adaptive Servo Ventilation in Patients with Heart Failure
TNF-alpha	Tumor necrosis factor-alpha
VT	Ventricular tachycardia

There are two major subtypes of sleep apnea, namely, central sleep apnea (CSA) and obstructive sleep apnea (OSA). Obstructive apneas and hypopneas result from complete or partial collapse within the upper airways and are associated with increased breathing efforts, reduced oxygen saturation, increases in arterial carbon dioxide, left ventricular afterload and wall tension and myocardial oxygen needs, alterations in autonomic nervous tone, and arousals from sleep [1].

6.1   Obstructive Sleep Apnea Before and After Heart Failure

6.1.1   Prevalence

OSA is a global health problem. It has a prevalence of about 10 % in women and 20 % in men, which increases with age [2, 3]. In men, obesity (high body mass index), and neck circumference in particular, predicts the incidence and severity of OSA [4]. Tonus of pharyngeal muscles decreases and soft tissues collapse into the upper airways, especially at night and during rapid-eye movement (REM) sleep [4]. Depending on the severity of this collapse, increased upper airway resistance occurs with a flattened airflow-curve, resulting in a hypopnea or an apnea. Although obesity represents a major risk factor for OSA, obstructive events can also occur in patients with a normal body weight in whom other factors such as craniofacial abnormalities contribute to increased pharyngeal collapsibility [4].

6.1.2   Definitions

An obstructive apnea event is defined as a reduction in nasal airflow of more than 90 % occurring over 10 s or more and is usually assessed through a nasal cannula [5]. By definition, and in accordance with the pathophysiology described above, a compensatory increase in breathing effort is required for an event to be classified as obstructive; this is usually assessed using a thoraco-abdominal effort belt [5]. Figure 6.1 (bottom panel) shows several obstructive apneas that are characterized

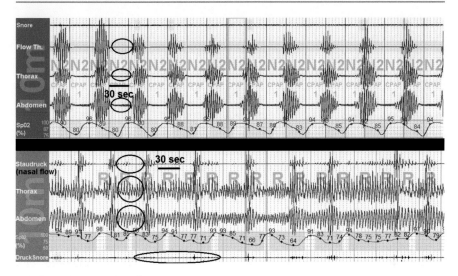

Fig. 6.1 Tracings showing the different features of obstructive sleep apnea (OSA) versus central sleep apnea-Cheyne–Stokes respiration (CSA-CSR)

by a cessation in airflow and associated breathing efforts during the apnea that eventually overcome the obstruction and may lead to snoring. Obstructive hypopneas are defined as a reduction in nasal airflow of at least 30 % occurring over at least 10 s associated with a reduction in oxygen saturation of at least 3 % [5].

6.1.3 Hemodynamics

While the exact hemodynamic changes that occur during an obstructive apnea remain a topic of debate, there is consensus that the net effect of repetitive upper airway obstruction at night is an increase in mean blood pressure (BP), heart rate, and other markers of increased sympathetic nervous activity [4]. OSA can also have detrimental effects on cardiac function. Breathing efforts during upper airways obstruction are associated with marked increases in intrathoracic pressure and an increase in right ventricular preload, while the hypoxia that follows obstructive events leads to an increase in right ventricular afterload [6]. As a consequence, there is significant hemodynamic stress on the right ventricle and the resulting increases in right ventricular pressure cause a flattening of the septum toward the left ventricle which inhibits left ventricular filling, leading to a decrease in stroke volume [4]. OSA-induced increases in cardiac stress can also contribute to the development of arrhythmias. In an animal study, Linz and colleagues showed that simulated obstructive events have a significant pro-arrhythmic potential, inducing atrial fibrillation (AF) mainly via negative tracheal and therefore high intrathoracic pressure [7]. In addition, repetitive episodes of hypoxia can induce the production of oxygen-free radicals and activate inflammatory pathways that contribute to endothelial dysfunction with significant clinical cardiovascular consequences if OSA is severe and prolonged [8]. Another consequence of repetitive upper airway obstruction is recurrent arousals during sleep, and poor sleep quality results in excessive daytime sleepiness [4]. Figure 6.2 provides an overview of the cardiovascular effects of obstructive events.

6.1.4   Severity

A variety of factors could be used to define the severity of OSA, including the number of nocturnal obstructive apneas or hypopneas, the number and extent of oxygen desaturations, [9], and time spent with suboptimal oxygen saturation (e.g., <90 %). Currently, the most commonly used marker of OSA severity is the apnea-hypopnea index (AHI), which reflects the mean number of apnea and hypopnea events per hour. Depending on the exact classification used, an AHI of >5–15/h is commonly accepted as an indicator that sleep-disordered breathing is present. However, some studies have suggested time spent with oxygen saturation <90 % is a better predictor of OSA-induced hemodynamic stress and associated cardiovascular risk than the AHI [10, 11]. This seems reasonable because long apneas with severe desaturations would paradoxically result in a low AHI (per hour), underestimating risk. Therefore, there is a high need for markers that reflect the severity of OSA in terms of predicting adverse cardiovascular events and treatment success in individual patients.

6.1.5   Metabolic and Cardiovascular Effects

The severity of untreated OSA has been shown to correlate with several inflammatory markers, such as high sensitivity C-reactive protein (hs-CRP) and tumor

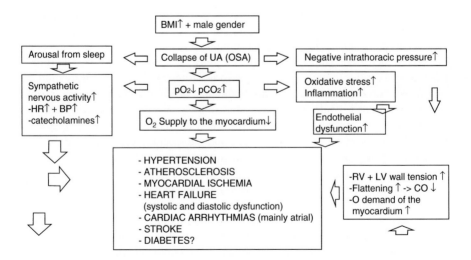

Fig. 6.2 Cardiovascular effects of obstructive sleep apnea (OSA)

necrosis factor-alpha (TNF-alpha) even after adjustment for confounding factors such as age, sex, and BMI [12, 13]. Overall, OSA appears to be an independent risk factor for metabolic disorders and various cardiovascular diseases [4]. Epidemiological data on the prevalence of OSA in patients with hypertension show significant overlap, with the prevalence of OSA in patients with hypertension ranging from 30 % to 80 % [14]. In fact, OSA is the most common cause of secondary hypertension [14]. Furthermore, OSA has been shown to contribute to the development of endothelial dysfunction, atherosclerosis, and heart failure [8, 15]. In fact, subclinical myocardial injury appears to correlate with the severity of OSA in people free of symptomatic cardiovascular diseases [16]. The results of a large prospective observational cohort study (mean follow-up ≈10 years) showed that patients with severe untreated OSA (AHI >30/h; $n = 235$) had significantly more cardiovascular events compared with healthy controls matched for age, sex, and weight [17]. Overall, available data indicate that OSA may be a modifiable determinant of the development and deterioration of various cardiovascular diseases, including heart failure (HF) [15].

6.1.6 Relationships with Heart Failure

The prevalence of OSA in HF patients with either reduced ejection fraction (HFrEF) or preserved ejection fraction (HFpEF) is 35–40 % [18, 19]. One of the issues with OSA in HF patients is the fact that this group is relatively unaffected by one of the main OSA symptoms in the general population – daytime sleepiness. This is thought to be due to increased sympathetic nervous system activation in HF patients compared with healthy subjects [20, 21] and could be an important explanation for the relative lack of recognition and detection of OSA in HF patients [22]. It also means that questionnaires determining sleepiness, such as the Epworth Sleepiness Scale (ESS), are of little value for sleep-disordered breathing (SDB) screening in HF patients [23].

It has been suggested that the relationship between the severity of HF and the severity of OSA in symptomatic HF patients is bidirectional [24]. In a cross-sectional study, Efken et al. showed a significant positive correlation between pulmonary congestion (which increases as left ventricular function worsens) and respiratory event lengths in OSA patients with heart failure [25]. An increase in circulation time, which is associated with advancing HF, was suggested as one of the main mechanisms that could have led to a prolongation of respiratory cycle lengths in HF patients [25]. Longer circulation time, as found in HF patients, could lead to delayed physiological feedback on gas tensions, thereby contributing to longer respiratory event length.

On the other hand, the recently introduced "fluid shift theory" also provides another potential mechanism that helps illustrate the more complex pathophysiological interactions that play a role in OSA patients with HF [24]. A shift of fluid from the legs to the neck when lying down was proposed to be partly responsible for the occurrence of obstructive events [24]. This is one mechanism by which HF might contribute to a worsening of OSA, especially in patients with leg edema secondary to reduced cardiac function [26]. The fact that there is little or no relationship between body mass index and the severity of OSA in HF and stroke patients supports the hypothesis that HF itself may also lead to OSA and that the pathophysiology and role of OSA in such patients is far more complex than in the general population [1, 27, 28].

There is even a plausible mechanism by which OSA could have a protective role in HF, known as ischemic preconditioning (IPC). The first study describing this phenomenon was published by Murry et al. in 1986 [29]. These authors established that intermittent periods of ischemia and reperfusion prior to an extended period of coronary artery occlusion followed by reperfusion were associated with attenuated myocardial injury. In a canine model, circumflex coronary occlusions were applied four times for 4 min each separated by 5 min of reperfusion, followed by occlusion for 40 min and then four days of reperfusion; control animals were subjected to the 40 min occlusion and prolonged reperfusion without the previous preconditioning phase. After four days, infarct size in the IPC-treated dogs was reduced to 25 % of that in controls. The authors concluded that intermittent episodes (e.g., angina, hypoxia) may have a protective effect in terms of salvaged myocardium after a subsequent significant ischemic insult (i.e., myocardial infarction). This study has been cited over 4,300 times and there are over 7,000 studies on IPC in PubMed. However, its role in patients with both OSA and HF has yet to be further investigated [30]. Nevertheless, there is a body of evidence from animal models, studies in human heart failure and epidemiological data showing that untreated OSA is a possible cause of HF, and contributes to disease progression and increased mortality [31–33].

Preclinical data show that chronic intermittent hypoxia (CIH; 8 h/day for 6 weeks) was associated with significant impairment of global left ventricular function including, but not limited to, left ventricular myocardial cellular injury, elevated mean arterial pressure and left ventricular end-diastolic pressure, and decreased cardiac output [34]. Another mechanism by which OSA could contribute to impaired cardiac function is negative intrathoracic pressure (NIP). The results of a study in 16 patients undergoing cardiac catheterization showed that NIP induced by Mueller maneuvers resulted in impaired left ventricular function [6]. Bradley et al. extended these findings, showing that Mueller maneuvers lead to an even more pronounced temporary functional impairment in the failing ventricle (patients with HF), with more time required to recover from this impairment compared to healthy subjects [35]. Longitudinal data on patients with HF and OSA support the hypothesis that OSA leads to a progression of HF and an (independent) increase in morbidity and mortality in HF patients [33, 36, 37].

6.1.7   Arrhythmia Risk

In addition to contributing to HF progression and worse outcomes, OSA has also been shown to be a risk factor for arrhythmias in HF patients. Data on the role of OSA in the development of ventricular arrhythmias are conflicting [38, 39].

A recent systematic review on the association between OSA and ventricular arrhythmias concluded that pooling studies linking OSA and ventricular arrhythmias was not possible due to heterogeneity of data [40]. However, OSA was noted to be associated with higher odds of ventricular ectopy and arrhythmias, but these findings need to be interpreted with caution based on the data limitations [40]. Therefore, although there is some indicative evidence, current data are not sufficient to prove a direct causal relationship between OSA and an increased risk of nocturnal sudden death [4].

In contrast, the body of evidence showing a correlation between atrial arrhythmias and OSA is much more substantial [41]. Mechanistically, Linz and colleagues simulated obstructive events in pigs, which were shown to result in AF [7]. A recent study (the ORBIT-AF trial) showed that 1841 of about 10,000 patients with atrial fibrillation (AF) had OSA [42]. This study also reported that, compared with AF patients without OSA, those with OSA had worse symptoms and a higher risk of hospitalization, but similar rates of mortality, major adverse cardiovascular outcomes, and AF progression [42].

6.1.8 Arteriosclerosis

OSA has also been implicated in the development of arteriosclerosis. In one study, HFpEF patients with proven coronary artery disease (CAD) proven showed a much higher prevalence of OSA and inflammation compared to those without CAD [43]. In patients with CAD, the presence of OSA has been independently associated with higher mortality, more major adverse cardiac events, and more restenosis after percutaneous coronary interventions [4, 44, 45].

6.2 Treating Obstructive Sleep Apnea Before and After Heart Failure

The most efficient therapeutic option to treat OSA is continuous positive airway pressure therapy (CPAP), which prevents the upper airways from collapsing by exerting a constant positive airway pressure. The exact pressure level during CPAP can be titrated manually and individually in a sleep laboratory environment. More recently, automatic positive airway pressure (APAP) devices have become available, which can automatically adjust the pressure level in response to obstructive events and are very useful in treating OSA.

Although there are no effective pharmacological therapies for OSA, there are a number of other treatment options apart from CPAP. These include oral appliances (OAs), electrical stimulation of the pharyngeal dilator muscles, or surgery; all tend to be less effective than CPAP [46]. According to a recent position paper by the American Academy of Sleep Medicine (AASM), OAs should be considered as a treatment option for snorers without OSA and patients with OSA who are intolerant of or unwilling to use CPAP therapy [46]. OAs are described as devices designed to protrude and stabilize the mandible to help maintain a patent airway during sleep, such as mandibular advancement devices [46]. With regard to nerve stimulation, the results of a recently published study suggest that a surgically implanted upper airway stimulation device has the potential to significantly improve the severity of OSA [47]. However, an accompanying commentary noted that the industry-sponsored study was uncontrolled, the study population was carefully selected, and residual apnea was present after treatment [48]. The study population consisted of patients who had difficulties tolerating or adhering to CPAP, did not have a significantly high BMI (≤ 32 kg/m^2) and specific locations of upper airways collapse, so that they were eligible for this type of treatment [48].

Although correlations between OSA and cardiovascular diseases (hypertension, arrhythmias, inflammation, heart failure, CAD) are quite well documented, there is much less consistent evidence for the potentially beneficial therapeutic effect of CPAP therapy in patients with OSA and cardiovascular disease, particularly for hard clinical endpoints such as mortality. This is especially the case for the treatment of OSA in HF patients [4].

6.2.1 Effects on Blood Pressure

Several randomized controlled trials (RCTs) have assessed the effects of CPAP on daytime BP; these have been reported to be very heterogeneous and any reported reductions in BP tended to be relatively small. Data from a meta-analysis suggested that the net effect of CPAP is a 2 mmHg reduction in BP [49]. A similar analysis also reported the same small but statistically significant effect of CPAP therapy in reducing blood pressure [50]. Of note, the effects of CPAP on BP were greater when the baseline AHI and arousal index were higher, and when nightly use of CPAP was higher. However, data are not consistent, and another meta-analysis failed to confirm the beneficial effects of CPAP on BP [51]. A common criticism of studies in this area is that most included normotensive patients and BP was often measured at different time points. When data from seven RCTs that enrolled patients with hypertension were combined, the reduction in BP during CPAP therapy was again about 2 mmHg, and subgroup analysis revealed that patients with high adherence to CPAP therapy, higher systolic BP at baseline, and resistant hypertension obtained the greatest benefit from CPAP therapy in terms of a decrease in 24 h in diastolic, but not systolic, BP [52].

6.2.2 Antiarrhythmic Effects

Data from the ORBIT-AF study showed that approximately one in five patients with AF also has OSA [42]. However, there were no major differences in hard clinical endpoints (i.e., hospitalization, cardiovascular outcomes) between AF patients with OSA who received CPAP treatment and those who did not. The only positive effect of OSA treatment with CPAP in AF patients was a lower rate of progression to permanent AF [42].

In a recent meta-analysis on the association between OSA and ventricular arrhythmias, only one study showed that CPAP may help reduce arrhythmogenicity [40, 53]. However, it remained unclear whether CPAP really lowered the risk of ventricular tachycardia (VT) [53].

6.2.3 Inflammation and Metabolic Effects

A recent meta-analysis on the effect of CPAP therapy on inflammation in OSA patients concluded that CPAP has some beneficial effects on inflammatory markers [13]. However, substantial differences in the effects of CPAP were observed depending on the inflammatory marker studied and the individual study design. Overall, it appeared that the beneficial effects of CPAP on inflammation were greater when usage was higher (>4 h per night) and when CPAP was used over a longer period of time (>3 months).

Although more data on the relationship between OSA, its treatment, and type 2 diabetes is required, a recent meta-analysis concluded that treating OSA with CPAP could improve control of glucose metabolism [54].

6.2.4 Use in Heart Failure

The evidence base for a beneficial effect of long-term CPAP therapy for OSA on mortality, regardless of the presence of comorbid HF, is relatively solid although it should be noted that most of the studies have a retrospective design. One of these studies looked at all-cause mortality in about 25,000 patients with a diagnosis of OSA who were partly treated with CPAP and followed for up of 10 years. In middle-aged and elderly males (but not females), CPAP therapy was associated with reduced all-cause mortality [55]. Other studies have also reported a reduction in mortality, and/or fatal and non-fatal cardiovascular events in OSA patients treated with CPAP [17, 56, 57]. However, these were all non-randomized trials and although several confounding factors were taken into account in multivariate models, there is no large-scale RCT on the effect of OSA treatment on hard clinical endpoints. One important problem is that a control group is difficult to establish given the available evidence for the benefits of CPAP treatment in OSA. In particular, the benefits of CPAP treatment in non-HF patients include decreased daytime sleepiness and improved quality of life. However, there are still issues that need to be addressed in future studies, including the effect of treating OSA with CPAP in women.

In HF patients, several randomized studies have consistently shown that CPAP treatment of OSA is associated with improvements in right and left ventricular function and a decrease in catecholamine levels, indicative of reductions in HF severity, accompanied by improvements in many cardiac function and HF symptom parameters [58–61]. Data from randomized clinical trials reporting improvements in left ventricular ejection fraction (LVEF) during CPAP treatment of OSA in HF patients are summarized in Table 6.1. What is obvious is that although several studies have

Table 6.1 Effects of CPAP treatment on left ventricular function in HFrEF patients with OSA: data from prospective RCTs. This table summarizes RCTs on the effect of OSA treatment through CPAP on LVEF in HFrEF patients. LVEF was chosen as it is a well-recognized and the most widely used marker of left ventricular function. There are more studies that are non-randomized and/or deal with other surrogate markers of HF severity and/or include different patient cohorts, e.g., patients with HFpEF. To the best of our knowledge, there is no randomized-controlled trial on the effect of OSA treatment through CPAP on mortality in patients with HFrEF

Author; year of publication	Pts completing trial, n	Treatment period	Change in LVEF during CPAP treatment
Kaneko et al. [60]	24	4 weeks	+9%
Mansfield et al. [61]	40	12 weeks	+5%
Egea et al. [58]	45	8 weeks	+3%
Hall et al. [59]	45	7 weeks	NS

CPAP continuous positive airway pressure, *HFrEF* heart failure with reduced ejection fraction, *LVEF* left ventricular ejection fraction, *NS* no significant change, *OSA* obstructive sleep apnea, *pts* patients, *RCTs* randomized controlled trials

investigated this question, most are of a relatively short duration and one in four actually failed to show an improvement in cardiac function as a result of OSA treatment [59]. Furthermore, the evidence for a reduction in mortality during CPAP treatment in OSA patients with HF is far from definitive. To date, and to the best of our knowledge, there are no large-scale randomized clinical trials showing that CPAP treatment of OSA reduces mortality in HF patients. In fact, it is important to note that any positive airway pressure (PAP) therapy may also have adverse hemodynamic effects in the failing heart [62, 63]. Therefore, there is an urgent need for more studies addressing the potential treatment effects of CPAP in patients with OSA, which will help to answer the questions of whether this will prevent the development of HF in these patients, or improve cardiac function and outcomes in those who already have HF.

6.3   Central Sleep Apnea in Heart Failure

The pathophysiology of central respiratory events and their consequences differ markedly from those of obstructive respiratory events. An altered respiratory control system is the key factor in centrally mediated apneas and hypopneas [62]. In addition to central sleep apnea (CSA) associated with drug use (opioids, sedatives), alcohol abuse or rare diseases (congenital central hypoventilation syndrome, congenital or acquired Undine-Fluch syndrome), Cheyne–Stokes respiration (CSR) is another form of central apnea. CSR is a distinct subtype of CSA with typical waxing and waning ventilation interrupted by central apneas or hypopneas [5]. This type of sleep apnea occurs mainly in patients with underlying cardiac (HF), neurologic (stroke), or nephrologic (renal failure) disease. The AASM defines CSA as CSA-CSR when both of the following are met: (1) there are episodes of ≥3 consecutive central apneas and/or central hypopneas separated by a crescendo and decrescendo change in breathing amplitude with a cycle length of at least 40 s (typically 45–90 s); and (2) there are five or more central apneas and/or central hypopneas per hour associated with the crescendo/decrescendo breathing pattern recorded over a minimum of 2 h of monitoring [5]. Figure 6.1 (top panel) shows the key characteristics of CSA-CSR, namely, periodic breathing with a crescendo-decrescendo pattern and intermittent hypoxias without associated increases in breathing efforts.

6.3.1   Pathophysiology

The pathophysiology of CSA is complex and is explained in greater detail in Chap. 4, but a brief overview of the pathophysiology of CSR in HF is provided in Fig. 6.3. It is thought that elevated pulmonary capillary wedge pressure (PCWP) due to left ventricular dysfunction leads to an activation of pulmonary J-receptors in HF patients [62]. J-receptor activation (via stimulation of pulmonary vagal afferents) and other factors result in higher sensitivity to carbon dioxide (CO_2), which can be measured by a higher hypercapnic ventilatory response (HCVR). This increase in HCVR causes a tendency to hyperventilate, with one or two deep breaths being sufficient to cause an apnea, which in turn leads to a gradual increase in CO_2 causing the patient to take deep breaths in again as CO_2 increases [64]. As a result, there is a vicious circle that sustains the periodic breathing pattern seen in CSA-CSR. In addition, a prolonged circulatory time is though to play a role in the pathophysiology of CSA-CSR in HF [65]. This prolonged circulatory time also explains why event lengths, such as the ventilatory phase, have been shown to inversely correlate with cardiac output [66]. As cardiac output decreases it takes chemoreceptors longer to react to changes in CO_2 explaining why HF severity correlations better with CSA-CSR event lengths than with the AHI [66].

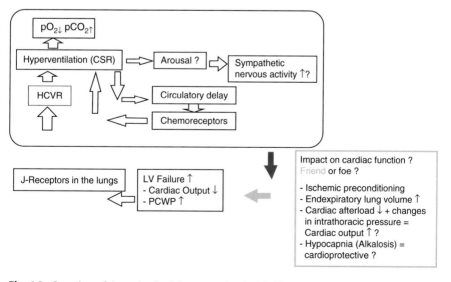

Fig. 6.3 Overview of the pathophysiology associated with CSA-CSR in HF

6.3.2   Relationships with Heart Failure

In terms of HF, and in contrast to OSA, there is currently no evidence that CSR itself can induce cardiac dysfunction or HF in particular. However, existing data do suggest that the severity of CSR mirrors the severity of cardiac dysfunction – that is, the greater the impairment of cardiac function, the greater the severity of CSR [62]. The results of two studies provide insight into this suggestion. Firstly, it has been shown that OSA can occur during the first half of the night in patients with HF, putting the heart under stress, leading to CSA being the predominant breathing pattern during the second half of the night [67]. Secondly, the fact that improvements in cardiac function are associated with improvements in CSA also supports the hypothesis that CSA is a mirror of cardiac function [66, 68]. Key risk factors for CSA include impaired cardiac function, older age, and AF [65].

The overall prevalence of CSA-CSR in patients with HFpEF or HFrEF varies between 30 % and 40 % [18, 19]. Several studies have identified CSR as an independent predictor of mortality in HFrEF patients [69–71], whereas others have suggested that CSR is a marker of HF rather than being an independent risk factor for adverse outcomes [72–74].

6.4   Treating Central Sleep Apnea in Heart Failure

A number of approaches to treating CSA-CSR in HFrEF have been investigated. Drug therapy options studied include acetazolamide and theophylline, which may have some overall effectiveness. However, the potential side effects of therapy mean that these are not appropriate in patients with heart failure [75–78]. Nocturnal oxygen is another option and has been shown to reduce the number of central respiratory events in CSA-CSR [79, 80], as can be seen with CO_2 administration or dead space breathing [78, 81–83].

6.4.1   Continuous Positive Airway Pressure

In terms of mask-based therapy, CPAP therapy was the first approach investigated for the treatment of CSA-CSR in HF patients. The Continuous Positive Airway Pressure for Central Sleep Apnea in Heart Failure (CANPAP) study, a randomized clinical trial, investigated a potential mortality benefit of CPAP therapy in HF patients with CSA-CSR [84]. This study was stopped for a variety of reasons, including unexpectedly low event rates. CPAP reduced the number of nocturnal respiratory by 50 % and improved oximetry parameters. In terms of cardiovascular function, there was a significant improvement in LVEF, but CPAP had no effect on mortality. A post-hoc analysis of the CANPAP data suggested a significant reduction in mortality in CPAP responders, defined as those in whom the AHI was reduced to <15/h during therapy [85].

6.4.2 Adaptive Servo Ventilation

Combined with the post-hoc findings of the CANPAP trial, the results of several studies showing the superiority of adaptive servo ventilation (ASV) therapy over oxygen therapy, CPAP and bilevel PAP (biPAP) for suppressing central apneas and hypopneas [86–88] provided the rationale for the first randomized clinical trial of ASV to investigate the ability of therapy to reduce morbidity and mortality in patients with HFrEF and predominant CSA [89]. The Treatment of Sleep-Disordered Breathing with Predominant Central Sleep Apnea by Adaptive Servo Ventilation in Patients with Heart Failure (SERVE-HF) trial enrolled 1325 patients who were randomly assigned to ASV added to guideline-based medical therapy compared with guideline-based medical therapy alone (control) [73]. The primary endpoint of the trial was a composite of time to first event of death from any cause, lifesaving cardiovascular intervention (transplantation, implantation of a long-term ventricular assist device, resuscitation after sudden cardiac arrest, or appropriate lifesaving shock) or unplanned hospitalization for worsening of heart failure. ASV therapy significantly reduced the number of respiratory events compared with baseline and control, but had no effect on the rate of primary endpoint events, HF symptoms, 6 min walking distance, or quality of life. Unexpectedly, rates of both all-cause and cardiovascular death were significantly increased in the ASV versus control group (by 28 % and 34 %, respectively) [73]. These results were in sharp contrast to data from previous cohort studies, small randomized trials, and meta-analyses [37, 90–94]. Data from prospective, randomized studies with hard clinical endpoints that investigated the effects of ASV on left ventricular function in HFrEF patients with proven CSR are summarized in Table 6.2.

At present, it is only possible to speculate on the mechanisms underlying the increased mortality risk observed in ASV-treated HFrEF patients with predominant

Table 6.2 Effects of ASV treatment on left ventricular function and outcomes in HFrEF patients with CSR

Author; year of publication	Pts completing trial, n	Treatment period	Treatment effect of ASV
Miyata et al. [95]	22	6 months	LVEF +6 %
Hetland et al. [96]	30	3 months	LVEF +4 %
Arzt et al. [97][a]	63	3 months	NS change in LVEF
Momomura et al. [98]	205	24 weeks	NS change in LVEF
Cowie et al. [73]	1161	31 months	NS change in LVEF Increased all-cause ($p = 0.01$) and cardiovascular ($p = 0.006$) mortality

ASV adaptive servo-ventilation, *CPAP* continuous positive airway pressure, *HFrEF* heart failure with reduced ejection fraction, *LVEF* left ventricular ejection fraction, *NS* no significant change, *OSA* obstructive sleep apnea, *pts* patients
[a]Patients could also have predominant obstructive sleep apnea (OSA)

CSA in the SERVE-HF trial. In contrast to the onset of action of efficacious and safe pharmacological therapies for HF, the treatment effects of ASV are immediate and the patient is exposed to "full-dose" positive airway pressure within hours. This could be problematic if, as has been suggested previously [74], CSA-CSR represents a compensatory mechanism in HF patients given that other HF treatments, including β-blockers, ACE inhibitors, or angiotensin receptor blockers require up-titration over several weeks. With the rapid onset of action of ASV, the potential compensatory mechanism is inactivated quickly, even if the effects of therapy may be beneficial over time. Survival curves for both all-cause and cardiovascular death in SERVE-HF did separate from the beginning of treatment, but do not appear to plateau over time. Thus, a compensatory role of CSA-CSR may not be sufficient to explain the excess mortality in ASV recipients on its own. Another contributing factor could be a rebound of CSR during the day. Cheyne–Stokes breathing and an exertional periodic breathing pattern are often seen in patients with advanced HF and are independent prognostic parameters in these patients [99]. In addition, positive airway pressure, even if not very high, might lead to a decrease in cardiac preload and, in the presence of low filling pressures, to a decrease in cardiac output [100]. This might especially be the case in HFrEF patients with impaired right ventricular function [63]. Figure 6.4 provides a simplified overview of different theories on the complex hemodynamic interplay between central apneas and ASV therapy in the failing heart.

Another possibility is that disturbance within an altered/shifted sympatho-vagal balance may cause arrhythmia and/or bradycardia. HF, and CSA-CSR in particular, are associated with increased sympathetic drive [101, 102]. On the other hand, ASV can lower sympathetic nerve activity in these patients [103, 104]. Therefore,

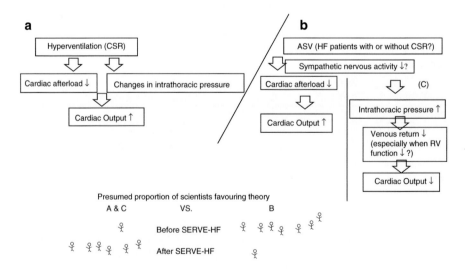

Fig. 6.4 Schematic of the complex hemodynamic interplay between central apneas and adaptive servo ventilation therapy in the failing heart

sympathetic activity might be suppressed while a patient receives ASV, but could rebound during the day. However, in HFrEF patients with CSA-CSR and implanted defibrillator (ICD) devices, appropriate ICD shocks occur randomly across throughout the 24 h day, whereas these shocks can be seen predominantly at night in HFrEF patients with OSA [105, 106]. Conversely, the number of appropriate ICD shocks was shown to be reduced by ASV in a retrospective cohort study [107] and tended to be reduced with ASV therapy even in the SERVE-HF trial. Thus, bradycardic events might be triggered. However, in the SERVE-HF trial about 55 % of patients had some kind of pacemaker implanted and should have been protected [73].

Obviously the increased mortality with ASV in the SERVE-HF trial without any clear pathophysiologic explanations creates a dilemma. Mechanistic data on the effects of ASV in HFrEF are lacking and pathophysiology needs to be investigated further. Hopefully, upcoming data from the SERVE-HF major substudy (NCT01164592) will provide some mechanistic hints. In addition, another ongoing outcome trial of ASV, the Adaptive Servo Ventilation for Therapy of Sleep Apnea in Heart Failure (ADVENT-HF) (NCT01128816) trial represents an opportunity to add new data to the SERVE-HF results but the study must be carefully monitored by their Data and Safety Monitoring Board (DSMB). An ADVENT-HF substudy will also investigate daytime left ventricular stroke work, oxidative metabolism, and sympathetic nervous system activity over 6 months (ASV Effects on Myocardial Energetics and Sympathetic Nerve Function in Heart Failure and Sleep Apnea, AMEND; NCT02116140).

6.4.3 Phrenic Nerve Stimulation

Another approach to treating CSA is unilateral phrenic nerve stimulation [108, 109] (see Chap. 13 for more detail). The results of a non-randomized pilot study showed a reduction in respiratory events of about 50 % in selected patients [110] and the findings of a first randomized clinical trial are expected in 2016. In the light of the SERVE-HF results, it is important that all of these patients are carefully followed in mandatory registries (TREAT-CSA, NCT02577445), followed by a randomized controlled outcome study.

It is important to note that the trials discussed above, including SERVE-HF, were conducted in very specific groups of patients with HFrEF. Thus, no conclusions can be drawn regarding the effects of ASV in patients with OSA, mixed or complex sleep apnea, or those with HFpEF).

References

1. Bradley TD, Floras JS. Sleep apnea and heart failure: part I: obstructive sleep apnea. Circulation. 2003;107:1671–8.
2. Peppard PE, Young T, Barnet JH, Palta M, Hagen EW, Hla KM. Increased prevalence of sleep-disordered breathing in adults. Am J Epidemiol. 2013;177:1006–14.

3. Sforza E, Chouchou F, Collet P, Pichot V, Barthelemy JC, Roche F. Sex differences in obstructive sleep apnoea in an elderly French population. Eur Respir J. 2011;37(5):1137–43.
4. Bradley TD, Floras JS. Obstructive sleep apnoea and its cardiovascular consequences. Lancet. 2009;373(9657):82–93.
5. Berry RB, Budhiraja R, Gottlieb DJ, Gozal D, Iber C, Kapur VK, Marcus CL, Mehra R, Parthasarathy S, Quan SF, Redline S, Strohl KP, Davidson Ward SL, Tangredi MM, American Academy of Sleep M. Rules for scoring respiratory events in sleep: update of the 2007 AASM Manual for the Scoring of Sleep and Associated Events. Deliberations of the Sleep Apnea Definitions Task Force of the American Academy of Sleep Medicine. J Clin Sleep Med. 2012;8:597–619.
6. Virolainen J, Ventila M, Turto H, Kupari M. Effect of negative intrathoracic pressure on left ventricular pressure dynamics and relaxation. J Appl Physiol (1985). 1995;79:455–60.
7. Linz D, Schotten U, Neuberger HR, Bohm M, Wirth K. Negative tracheal pressure during obstructive respiratory events promotes atrial fibrillation by vagal activation. Heart Rhythm. 2011;8:1436–43.
8. Ip MS, Tse HF, Lam B, Tsang KW, Lam WK. Endothelial function in obstructive sleep apnea and response to treatment. Am J Respir Crit Care Med. 2004;169:348–53.
9. Punjabi NM, Newman AB, Young TB, Resnick HE, Sanders MH. Sleep-disordered breathing and cardiovascular disease: an outcome-based definition of hypopneas. Am J Respir Crit Care Med. 2008;177:1150–5.
10. Gottlieb JD, Schwartz AR, Marshall J, Ouyang P, Kern L, Shetty V, Trois M, Punjabi NM, Brown C, Najjar SS, Gottlieb SS. Hypoxia, not the frequency of sleep apnea, induces acute hemodynamic stress in patients with chronic heart failure. J Am Coll Cardiol. 2009;54:1706–12.
11. Oldenburg O, Wellmann B, Buchholz A, Bitter T, Fox H, Thiem U, Horstkotte D, Wegscheider K. Nocturnal hypoxaemia is associated with increased mortality in stable heart failure patients. Eur Heart J. 2015;37:1695–703.
12. Lavie L. Oxidative stress in obstructive sleep apnea and intermittent hypoxia – revisited – the bad ugly and good: implications to the heart and brain. Sleep Med Rev. 2015;20:27–45.
13. Xie X, Pan L, Ren D, Du C, Guo Y. Effects of continuous positive airway pressure therapy on systemic inflammation in obstructive sleep apnea: a meta-analysis. Sleep Med. 2013;14: 1139–50.
14. Logan AG, Perlikowski SM, Mente A, Tisler A, Tkacova R, Niroumand M, Leung RS, Bradley TD. High prevalence of unrecognized sleep apnoea in drug-resistant hypertension. J Hypertens. 2001;19:2271–7.
15. Gottlieb DJ, Yenokyan G, Newman AB, O'Connor GT, Punjabi NM, Quan SF, Redline S, Resnick HE, Tong EK, Diener-West M, Shahar E. Prospective study of obstructive sleep apnea and incident coronary heart disease and heart failure: the sleep heart health study. Circulation. 2010;122:352–60.
16. Einvik G, Rosjo H, Randby A, Namtvedt SK, Hrubos-Strom H, Brynildsen J, Somers VK, Omland T. Severity of obstructive sleep apnea is associated with cardiac troponin I concentrations in a community-based sample: data from the Akershus Sleep Apnea Project. Sleep 2014;37:1111–6, 1116A–1116B.
17. Marin JM, Carrizo SJ, Vicente E, Agusti AG. Long-term cardiovascular outcomes in men with obstructive sleep apnoea-hypopnoea with or without treatment with continuous positive airway pressure: an observational study. Lancet. 2005;365:1046–53.
18. Bitter T, Faber L, Hering D, Langer C, Horstkotte D, Oldenburg O. Sleep-disordered breathing in heart failure with normal left ventricular ejection fraction. Eur J Heart Fail. 2009;11:602–8.
19. Oldenburg O, Lamp B, Faber L, Teschler H, Horstkotte D, Topfer V. Sleep-disordered breathing in patients with symptomatic heart failure: a contemporary study of prevalence in and characteristics of 700 patients. Eur J Heart Fail. 2007;9:251–7.
20. Aggarwal A, Esler MD, Lambert GW, Hastings J, Johnston L, Kaye DM. Norepinephrine turnover is increased in suprabulbar subcortical brain regions and is related to whole-body sympathetic activity in human heart failure. Circulation. 2002;105:1031–3.

21. Leimbach Jr WN, Wallin BG, Victor RG, Aylward PE, Sundlof G, Mark AL. Direct evidence from intraneural recordings for increased central sympathetic outflow in patients with heart failure. Circulation. 1986;73:913–9.
22. MacDonald M, Fang J, Pittman SD, White DP, Malhotra A. The current prevalence of sleep disordered breathing in congestive heart failure patients treated with beta-blockers. J Clin Sleep Med. 2008;4:38–42.
23. Arzt M, Young T, Finn L, Skatrud JB, Ryan CM, Newton GE, Mak S, Parker JD, Floras JS, Bradley TD. Sleepiness and sleep in patients with both systolic heart failure and obstructive sleep apnea. Arch Intern Med. 2006;166:1716–22.
24. Kasai T, Floras JS, Bradley TD. Sleep apnea and cardiovascular disease: a bidirectional relationship. Circulation. 2012;126:1495–510.
25. Efken C, Bitter T, Prib N, Horstkotte D, Oldenburg O. Obstructive sleep apnoea: longer respiratory event lengths in patients with heart failure. Eur Respir J. 2013;41:1340–6.
26. Spiesshofer J, Heinrich J, Efken C, Lehmann R, Bitter T, Horstkotte D, Oldenburg O. Changes in sleep-disordered breathing cycle lengths mirror changes in cardiac function in a patient with heart failure. Sleep Biolog Rhythms. 2014;12:145–7.
27. Kasai T, Yumino D, Redolfi S, Su MC, Ruttanaumpawan P, Mak S, Newton GE, Floras JS, Bradley TD. Overnight effects of obstructive sleep apnea and its treatment on stroke volume in patients with heart failure. Can J Cardiol. 2015;31:832–8.
28. Ryan CM, Floras JS, Logan AG, Kimoff RJ, Series F, Morrison D, Ferguson KA, Belenkie I, Pfeifer M, Fleetham J, Hanly PJ, Smilovitch M, Arzt M, Bradley TD, Investigators C. Shift in sleep apnoea type in heart failure patients in the CANPAP trial. Eur Respir J. 2010;35:592–7.
29. Murry CE, Jennings RB, Reimer KA. Preconditioning with ischemia: a delay of lethal cell injury in ischemic myocardium. Circulation. 1986;74:1124–36.
30. Lavie P, Lavie L. Unexpected survival advantage in elderly people with moderate sleep apnoea. J Sleep Res. 2009;18:397–403.
31. Khayat R, Jarjoura D, Porter K, Sow A, Wannemacher J, Dohar R, Pleister A, Abraham WT. Sleep disordered breathing and post-discharge mortality in patients with acute heart failure. Eur Heart J. 2015;36:1463–9.
32. Roca GQ, Redline S, Claggett B, Bello N, Ballantyne CM, Solomon SD, Shah AM. Sex-specific association of sleep apnea severity with subclinical myocardial injury, ventricular hypertrophy, and heart failure risk in a Community-Dwelling Cohort: the atherosclerosis risk in communities-sleep heart health study. Circulation. 2015;132:1329–37.
33. Wang H, Parker JD, Newton GE, Floras JS, Mak S, Chiu KL, Ruttanaumpawan P, Tomlinson G, Bradley TD. Influence of obstructive sleep apnea on mortality in patients with heart failure. J Am Coll Cardiol. 2007;49:1625–31.
34. Chen L, Zhang J, Gan TX, Chen-Izu Y, Hasday JD, Karmazyn M, Balke CW, Scharf SM. Left ventricular dysfunction and associated cellular injury in rats exposed to chronic intermittent hypoxia. J Appl Physiol (1985). 2008;104:218–23.
35. Bradley TD, Hall MJ, Ando S, Floras JS. Hemodynamic effects of simulated obstructive apneas in humans with and without heart failure. Chest. 2001;119:1827–35.
36. Bolona E, Hahn PY, Afessa B. Intensive care unit and hospital mortality in patients with obstructive sleep apnea. J Crit Care. 2015;30:178–80.
37. Jilek C, Krenn M, Sebah D, Obermeier R, Braune A, Kehl V, Schroll S, Montalvan S, Riegger GA, Pfeifer M, Arzt M. Prognostic impact of sleep disordered breathing and its treatment in heart failure: an observational study. Eur J Heart Fail. 2011;13:68–75.
38. Flemons WW, Remmers JE, Gillis AM. Sleep apnea and cardiac arrhythmias. Is there a relationship? Am Rev Respir Dis. 1993;148:618–21.
39. Mehra R, Benjamin EJ, Shahar E, Gottlieb DJ, Nawabit R, Kirchner HL, Sahadevan J, Redline S. Association of nocturnal arrhythmias with sleep-disordered breathing: the Sleep Heart Health Study. Am J Respir Crit Care Med. 2006;173:910–6.
40. Raghuram A, Clay R, Kumbam A, Tereshchenko LG, Khan A. A systematic review of the association between obstructive sleep apnea and ventricular arrhythmias. J Clin Sleep Med. 2014;10:1155–60.

41. Linz D, Linz B, Hohl M, Bohm M. Atrial arrhythmogenesis in obstructive sleep apnea: thera-peutic implications. Sleep Med Rev. 2015;26:87–94.
42. Holmqvist F, Guan N, Zhu Z, Kowey PR, Allen LA, Fonarow GC, Hylek EM, Mahaffey KW, Freeman JV, Chang P, Holmes DN, Peterson ED, Piccini JP, Gersh BJ, Investigators O-A. Impact of obstructive sleep apnea and continuous positive airway pressure therapy on outcomes in patients with atrial fibrillation-Results from the Outcomes Registry for Better Informed Treatment of Atrial Fibrillation (ORBIT-AF). Am Heart J. 2015;169:647–54. e2.
43. Prinz C, Bitter T, Piper C, Horstkotte D, Faber L, Oldenburg O. Sleep apnea is common in patients with coronary artery disease. Wien Med Wochenschr. 2010;160:349–55.
44. Buchner S, Satzl A, Debl K, Hetzenecker A, Luchner A, Husser O, Hamer OW, Poschenrieder F, Fellner C, Zeman F, Riegger GA, Pfeifer M, Arzt M. Impact of sleep-disordered breathing on myocardial salvage and infarct size in patients with acute myocardial infarction. Eur Heart J. 2014;35:192–9.
45. Cassar A, Morgenthaler TI, Lennon RJ, Rihal CS, Lerman A. Treatment of obstructive sleep apnea is associated with decreased cardiac death after percutaneous coronary intervention. J Am Coll Cardiol. 2007;50:1310–4.
46. Ramar K, Dort LC, Katz SG, Lettieri CJ, Harrod CG, Thomas SM, Chervin RD. Clinical practice guideline for the treatment of obstructive sleep apnea and snoring with oral appliance therapy: An update for 2015. J Clin Sleep Med. 2015;11:773–827.
47. Strollo Jr PJ, Soose RJ, Maurer JT, de Vries N, Cornelius J, Froymovich O, Hanson RD, Padhya TA, Steward DL, Gillespie MB, Woodson BT, Van de Heyning PH, Goetting MG, Vanderveken OM, Feldman N, Knaack L, Strohl KP, Group ST. Upper-airway stimulation for obstructive sleep apnea. N Engl J Med. 2014;370:139–49.
48. Malhotra A. Hypoglossal-nerve stimulation for obstructive sleep apnea. N Engl J Med. 2014;370:170–1.
49. Bazzano LA, Khan Z, Reynolds K, He J. Effect of nocturnal nasal continuous positive airway pressure on blood pressure in obstructive sleep apnea. Hypertension. 2007;50:417–23.
50. Haentjens P, Van Meerhaeghe A, Moscariello A, De Weerdt S, Poppe K, Dupont A, Velkeniers B. The impact of continuous positive airway pressure on blood pressure in patients with obstructive sleep apnea syndrome: evidence from a meta-analysis of placebo-controlled ran-domized trials. Arch Intern Med. 2007;167:757–64.
51. Alajmi M, Mulgrew AT, Fox J, Davidson W, Schulzer M, Mak E, Ryan CF, Fleetham J, Choi P, Ayas NT. Impact of continuous positive airway pressure therapy on blood pressure in patients with obstructive sleep apnea hypopnea: a meta-analysis of randomized controlled trials. Lung. 2007;185:67–72.
52. Hu X, Fan J, Chen S, Yin Y, Zrenner B. The role of continuous positive airway pressure in blood pressure control for patients with obstructive sleep apnea and hypertension: a meta-analysis of randomized controlled trials. J Clin Hypertens (Greenwich). 2015;17:215–22.
53. Ryan CM, Usui K, Floras JS, Bradley TD. Effect of continuous positive airway pressure on ventricular ectopy in heart failure patients with obstructive sleep apnoea. Thorax. 2005;60:781–5.
54. Martinez-Ceron E, Fernandez-Navarro I, Garcia-Rio F. Effects of continuous positive airway pressure treatment on glucose metabolism in patients with obstructive sleep apnea. Sleep Med Rev. 2015;25:121–30.
55. Jennum P, Tonnesen P, Ibsen R, Kjellberg J. All-cause mortality from obstructive sleep apnea in male and female patients with and without continuous positive airway pressure treatment: a registry study with 10 years of follow-up. Nat Sci Sleep. 2015;7:43–50.
56. Buchner NJ, Sanner BM, Borgel J, Rump LC. Continuous positive airway pressure treatment of mild to moderate obstructive sleep apnea reduces cardiovascular risk. Am J Respir Crit Care Med. 2007;176:1274–80.
57. Ou Q, Chen YC, Zhuo SQ, Tian XT, He CH, Lu XL, Gao XL. Continuous positive airway pressure treatment reduces mortality in elderly patients with moderate to severe obstructive severe sleep apnea: a cohort study. PLoS One. 2015;10(6):e0127775.

58. Egea CJ, Aizpuru F, Pinto JA, Ayuela JM, Ballester E, Zamarron C, Sojo A, Montserrat JM, Barbe F, Alonso-Gomez AM, Rubio R, Lobo JL, Duran-Cantolla J, Zorrilla V, Nunez R, Cortes J, Jimenez A, Cifrian J, Ortega M, Carpizo R, Sanchez A, Teran J, Iglesias L, Fernandez C, Alonso ML, Cordero J, Roig E, Perez F, Muxi A, Gude F, Amaro A, Calvo U, Masa JF, Utrabo I, Porras Y, Lanchas I, Sanchez E, Spanish Group of Sleep Breathing D. Cardiac function after CPAP therapy in patients with chronic heart failure and sleep apnea: a multicenter study. Sleep Med. 2008;9:660–6.

59. Hall AB, Ziadi MC, Leech JA, Chen SY, Burwash IG, Renaud J, deKemp RA, Haddad H, Mielniczuk LM, Yoshinaga K, Guo A, Chen L, Walter O, Garrard L, DaSilva JN, Floras JS, Beanlands RS. Effects of short-term continuous positive airway pressure on myocardial sympathetic nerve function and energetics in patients with heart failure and obstructive sleep apnea: a randomized study. Circulation. 2014;130:892–901.

60. Kaneko Y, Floras JS, Usui K, Plante J, Tkacova R, Kubo T, Ando S, Bradley TD. Cardiovascular effects of continuous positive airway pressure in patients with heart failure and obstructive sleep apnea. N Engl J Med. 2003;348:1233–41.

61. Mansfield DR, Gollogly NC, Kaye DM, Richardson M, Bergin P, Naughton MT. Controlled trial of continuous positive airway pressure in obstructive sleep apnea and heart failure. Am J Respir Crit Care Med. 2004;169:361–6.

62. Oldenburg O. Cheyne-stokes respiration in chronic heart failure. Treatment with adaptive servoventilation therapy. Circ J. 2012;76:2305–17.

63. Spiesshofer J, Fox H, Lehmann R, Efken C, Heinrich J, Bitter T, Korber B, Horstkotte D, Oldenburg O. Heterogenous haemodynamic effects of adaptive servoventilation therapy in sleeping patients with heart failure and Cheyne-Stokes respiration compared to healthy volunteers. Heart Vessels. 2015;31:1117–30.

64. Lorenzi-Filho G, Dajani HR, Leung RS, Floras JS, Bradley TD. Entrainment of blood pressure and heart rate oscillations by periodic breathing. Am J Respir Crit Care Med. 1999;159(4 Pt 1):1147–54.

65. Bradley TD, Floras JS. Sleep apnea and heart failure: part II: central sleep apnea. Circulation. 2003;107:1822–6.

66. Wedewardt J, Bitter T, Prinz C, Faber L, Horstkotte D, Oldenburg O. Cheyne-Stokes respiration in heart failure: cycle length is dependent on left ventricular ejection fraction. Sleep Med. 2010;11:137–42.

67. Tkacova R, Niroumand M, Lorenzi-Filho G, Bradley TD. Overnight shift from obstructive to central apneas in patients with heart failure: role of PCO2 and circulatory delay. Circulation. 2001;103:238–43.

68. Solin P, Bergin P, Richardson M, Kaye DM, Walters EH, Naughton MT. Influence of pulmonary capillary wedge pressure on central apnea in heart failure. Circulation. 1999;99:1574–9.

69. Bitter T, Westerheide N, Prinz C, Hossain MS, Vogt J, Langer C, Horstkotte D, Oldenburg O. Cheyne-Stokes respiration and obstructive sleep apnoea are independent risk factors for malignant ventricular arrhythmias requiring appropriate cardioverter-defibrillator therapies in patients with congestive heart failure. Eur Heart J. 2011;32:61–74.

70. Javaheri S, Shukla R, Zeigler H, Wexler L. Central sleep apnea, right ventricular dysfunction, and low diastolic blood pressure are predictors of mortality in systolic heart failure. J Am Coll Cardiol. 2007;49:2028–34.

71. Linz D, Woehrle H, Bitter T, Fox H, Cowie MR, Bohm M, Oldenburg O. The importance of sleep-disordered breathing in cardiovascular disease. Clin Res Cardiol. 2015;104:705–18.

72. Andreas S, Schulz R, Werner GS, Kreuzer H. Prevalence of obstructive sleep apnoea in patients with coronary artery disease. Coron Artery Dis. 1996;7:541–5.

73. Cowie MR, Woehrle H, Wegscheider K, Angermann C, D'Ortho MP, Erdmann E, Levy P, Simonds AK, Somers VK, Zannad F, Teschler H. Adaptive servo-ventilation for central sleep apnea in systolic heart failure. N Engl J Med. 2015;373:1095–105.

74. Naughton MT. Cheyne-Stokes respiration: friend or foe? Thorax. 2012;67:357–60.

75. Hu K, Li Q, Yang J, Hu S, Chen X. The effect of theophylline on sleep-disordered breathing in patients with stable chronic congestive heart failure. Chin Med J (Engl). 2003;116: 1711–6.

76. Javaheri S. Acetazolamide improves central sleep apnea in heart failure: a double-blind, prospective study. Am J Respir Crit Care Med. 2006;173:234–7.

77. Javaheri S, Parker TJ, Wexler L, Liming JD, Lindower P, Roselle GA. Effect of theophylline on sleep-disordered breathing in heart failure. N Engl J Med. 1996;335:562–7.

78. Andreas S, Weidel K, Hagenah G, Heindl S. Treatment of Cheyne-Stokes respiration with nasal oxygen and carbon dioxide. Eur Respir J. 1998;12:414–9.

79. Franklin KA, Eriksson P, Sahlin C, Lundgren R. Reversal of central sleep apnea with oxygen. Chest. 1997;111:163–9.

80. Sasayama S, Izumi T, Seino Y, Ueshima K, Asanoi H, Group C-HS. Effects of nocturnal oxygen therapy on outcome measures in patients with chronic heart failure and Cheyne-Stokes respiration. Circ J. 2006;70:1–7.

81. Mebrate Y, Willson K, Manisty CH, Baruah R, Mayet J, Hughes AD, Parker KH, Francis DP. Dynamic CO2 therapy in periodic breathing: a modeling study to determine optimal timing and dosage regimes. J Appl Physiol (1985). 2009;107:696–706.

82. Szollosi I, Jones M, Morrell MJ, Helfet K, Coats AJ, Simonds AK. Effect of CO2 inhalation on central sleep apnea and arousals from sleep. Respiration. 2004;71:493–8.

83. Wan ZH, Wen FJ, Hu K. Dynamic CO(2) inhalation: a novel treatment for CSR-CSA associated with CHF. Sleep Breath. 2013;17:487–93.

84. Bradley TD, Logan AG, Kimoff RJ, Series F, Morrison D, Ferguson K, Belenkie I, Pfeifer M, Fleetham J, Hanly P, Smilovitch M, Tomlinson G, Floras JS, Investigators C. Continuous positive airway pressure for central sleep apnea and heart failure. N Engl J Med. 2005;353: 2025–33.

85. Arzt M, Floras JS, Logan AG, Kimoff RJ, Series F, Morrison D, Ferguson K, Belenkie I, Pfeifer M, Fleetham J, Hanly P, Smilovitch M, Ryan C, Tomlinson G, Bradley TD. Suppression of central sleep apnea by continuous positive airway pressure and transplant-free survival in heart failure: a post hoc analysis of the Canadian Continuous Positive Airway Pressure for Patients with Central Sleep Apnea and Heart Failure Trial (CANPAP). Circulation. 2007; 115:3173–80.

86. Kasai T, Usui Y, Yoshioka T, Yanagisawa N, Takata Y, Narui K, Yamaguchi T, Yamashina A, Momomura SI, Investigators J. Effect of flow-triggered adaptive servo-ventilation compared with continuous positive airway pressure in patients with chronic heart failure with coexisting obstructive sleep apnea and Cheyne-Stokes respiration. Circ Heart Fail. 2010;3:140–8.

87. Philippe C, Stoica-Herman M, Drouot X, Raffestin B, Escourrou P, Hittinger L, Michel PL, Rouault S, D'Ortho MP. Compliance with and effectiveness of adaptive servoventilation versus continuous positive airway pressure in the treatment of Cheyne-Stokes respiration in heart failure over a six month period. Heart. 2006;92:337–42.

88. Teschler H, Dohring J, Wang YM, Berthon-Jones M. Adaptive pressure support servo-ventilation: a novel treatment for Cheyne-Stokes respiration in heart failure. Am J Respir Crit Care Med. 2001;164:614–9.

89. Cowie MR, Woehrle H, Wegscheider K, Angermann C, D'Ortho MP, Erdmann E, Levy P, Simonds A, Somers VK, Zannad F, Teschler H. Rationale and design of the SERVE-HF study: treatment of sleep-disordered breathing with predominant central sleep apnoea with adaptive servo-ventilation in patients with chronic heart failure. Eur J Heart Fail. 2013; 15:937–43.

90. Damy T, Margarit L, Noroc A, Bodez D, Guendouz S, Boyer L, Drouot X, Lamine A, Paulino A, Rappeneau S, Stoica MH, Dubois-Rande JL, Adnot S, Hittinger L, D'Ortho MP. Prognostic impact of sleep-disordered breathing and its treatment with nocturnal ventilation for chronic heart failure. Eur J Heart Fail. 2012;14:1009–19.

91. Nakamura S, Asai K, Kubota Y, Murai K, Takano H, Tsukada YT, Shimizu W. Impact of sleep-disordered breathing and efficacy of positive airway pressure on mortality in patients

with chronic heart failure and sleep-disordered breathing: a meta-analysis. Clin Res Cardiol. 2015;104(3):208–16.

92. Oldenburg O, Bitter T, Vogt J, Fischbach T, Dimitriadis Z, Bullert K, Horstkotte D. Central and obstructive sleep apnea are associated with increased mortality in patients with long-term cardiac resynchronization therapy. J Am Coll Cardiol. 2011;54(Suppl. A):E100.

93. Takama N, Kurabayashi M. Safety and efficacy of adaptive servo-ventilation in patients with severe systolic heart failure. J Cardiol. 2014;63:302–7.

94. Wu X, Fu C, Zhang S, Liu Z, Li S, Jiang L. Adaptive servoventilation improves cardiac dysfunction and prognosis in heart failure patients with sleep-disordered breathing: a meta-analysis. Clin Respir J; 2015. doi: 10.1111/crj.12390. [Epub ahead of print].

95. Miyata M, Yoshihisa A, Suzuki S, Yamada S, Kamioka M, Kamiyama Y, Yamaki T, Sugimoto K, Kunii H, Nakazato K, Suzuki H, Saitoh S, Takeishi Y. Adaptive servo ventilation improves Cheyne-Stokes respiration, cardiac function, and prognosis in chronic heart failure patients with cardiac resynchronization therapy. J Cardiol. 2012;60:222–7.

96. Hetland A, Haugaa KH, Olseng M, Gjesdal O, Ross S, Saberniak J, Jacobsen MB, Edvardsen T. Three-month treatment with adaptive servoventilation improves cardiac function and physical activity in patients with chronic heart failure and Cheyne-Stokes respiration: a prospective randomized controlled trial. Cardiology. 2013;126:81–90.

97. Arzt M, Schroll S, Series F, Lewis K, Benjamin A, Escourrou P, Luigart R, Kehl V, Pfeifer M. Auto-servoventilation in heart failure with sleep apnoea: a randomised controlled trial. Eur Respir J. 2013;42:1244–54.

98. Momomura S, Seino Y, Kihara Y, Adachi H, Yasumura Y, Yokoyama H, Wada H, Ise T, Tanaka K, investigators S-C. Adaptive servo-ventilation therapy for patients with chronic heart failure in a confirmatory, multicenter, randomized, controlled study. Circ J. 2015;79: 981–90.

99. Corra U, Pistono M, Mezzani A, Braghiroli A, Giordano A, Lanfranchi P, Bosimini E, Gnemmi M, Giannuzzi P. Sleep and exertional periodic breathing in chronic heart failure: prognostic importance and interdependence. Circulation. 2006;113:44–50.

100. Philip-Joet FF, Paganelli FF, Dutau HL, Saadjian AY. Hemodynamic effects of bilevel nasal positive airway pressure ventilation in patients with heart failure. Respiration. 1999; 66:136–43.

101. Solin P, Kaye DM, Little PJ, Bergin P, Richardson M, Naughton MT. Impact of sleep apnea on sympathetic nervous system activity in heart failure. Chest. 2003;123:1119–26.

102. van de Borne P, Oren R, Abouassaly C, Anderson E, Somers VK. Effect of Cheyne-Stokes respiration on muscle sympathetic nerve activity in severe congestive heart failure secondary to ischemic or idiopathic dilated cardiomyopathy. Am J Cardiol. 1998;81:432–6.

103. Joho S, Oda Y, Ushijima R, Hirai T, Inoue H. Effect of adaptive servoventilation on muscle sympathetic nerve activity in patients with chronic heart failure and central sleep apnea. J Card Fail. 2012;18:769–75.

104. Koyama T, Watanabe H, Tamura Y, Oguma Y, Kosaka T, Ito H. Adaptive servo-ventilation therapy improves cardiac sympathetic nerve activity in patients with heart failure. Eur J Heart Fail. 2013;15:902–9.

105. Gami AS, Howard DE, Olson EJ, Somers VK. Day-night pattern of sudden death in obstructive sleep apnea. N Engl J Med. 2005;352:1206–14.

106. Sano K, Watanabe E, Hayano J, Mieno Y, Sobue Y, Yamamoto M, Ichikawa T, Sakakibara H, Imaizumi K, Ozaki Y. Central sleep apnoea and inflammation are independently associated with arrhythmia in patients with heart failure. Eur J Heart Fail. 2013;15:1003–10.

107. Bitter T, Gutleben KJ, Nolker G, Westerheide N, Prinz C, Dimitriadis Z, Horstkotte D, Vogt J, Oldenburg O. Treatment of Cheyne-Stokes respiration reduces arrhythmic events in chronic heart failure. J Cardiovasc Electrophysiol. 2013;24:1132–40.

108. Oldenburg O, Bitter T, Fox H, Horstkotte D, Gutleben KJ. Effects of unilateral phrenic nerve stimulation on tidal volume. First case report of a patient responding to remede(R) treatment for nocturnal Cheyne-Stokes respiration. Herz. 2014;39:84–6.

109. Ponikowski P, Javaheri S, Michalkiewicz D, Bart BA, Czarnecka D, Jastrzebski M, Kusiak A, Augostini R, Jagielski D, Witkowski T, Khayat RN, Oldenburg O, Gutleben KJ, Bitter T, Karim R, Iber C, Hasan A, Hibler K, Germany R, Abraham WT. Transvenous phrenic nerve stimulation for the treatment of central sleep apnoea in heart failure. Eur Heart J. 2012;33:889–94.
110. Abraham WT, Jagielski D, Oldenburg O, Augostini R, Krueger S, Kolodziej A, Gutleben KJ, Khayat R, Merliss A, Harsch MR, Holcomb RG, Javaheri S, Ponikowski P, Remede Pilot Study I. Phrenic nerve stimulation for the treatment of central sleep apnea. JACC Heart Fail. 2015;3:360–9.

Not Only Sleep Apnea: The "Awake" Apneas of the Failing Heart

Apneas Beyond Sleep: Features and Significance

Maria Teresa La Rovere, Roberto Maestri, and Gian Domenico Pinna

Abbreviations

CSA	Central sleep apnea
CSR	Cheyne–Stokes respiration
LVEF	Left ventricular ejection fraction
PB	Periodic breathing
EEG	Electroencephalogram
EOG	Electrooculogram
NREM	Nonrapid eye movement

In its original descriptions [1], an abnormal breathing pattern characterized by episodes of hyperpnea alternating with periods of apnea and subsequently defined as Cheyne–Stokes respiration (CSR) was actually observed in the awake state, although in the preterminal condition, of patients with advanced heart failure (HF). It was more than one century later that it appeared that a periodic breathing pattern characterized by a cyclic waxing and waning of tidal volume alternating with central apneas or hypopneas can be observed during daytime in a remarkably high proportion of patients with poor left ventricular function and compensated HF. Although

M.T. La Rovere (✉)
Division of Cardiology, Fondazione "Salvatore Maugeri", IRCCS, Pavia, PV, Italy

Istituto Scientifico di Montescano, Montescano, PV, Italy
e-mail: mariateresa.larovere@fsm.it

R. Maestri • G.D. Pinna
Istituto Scientifico di Montescano, Montescano, PV, Italy

Biomedical Engineering, Fondazione "Salvatore Maugeri", IRCCS, Pavia, PV, Italy
e-mail: roberto.maestri@fsm.it; giandomenico.pinna@fsm.it

© Springer International Publishing Switzerland 2017
M. Emdin et al. (eds.), *The Breathless Heart*,
DOI 10.1007/978-3-319-26354-0_7

this abnormal pattern includes the apneic behavior of the historical description of CSR, for the sake of simplicity, in the following, we will refer to it as "apneic" or "nonapneic" periodic breathing (PB).

Whether the daytime occurrence of PB equates that these breathing abnormalities actually occur during wakefulness—as opposed to sleep—has not been definitely established.

In this chapter, we will describe the epidemiology and prognostic value of daytime PB, and we will discuss the current view on the mechanisms involved in its production.

7.1   Epidemiology and Clinical Predictors of Abnormal Breathing Patterns During Daytime in Heart Failure

Daytime PB has been observed during wakefulness in 25–66 % clinically stable HF patients [2–7]. Often, the same patient may exhibit a continuum of different patterns of breathing, ranging from normal breathing to nonapneic and apneic PB. A prolonged cycle of the breathing fluctuation—cycle lengths ranging from 35 to 100 s (0.01–0.03 Hz)—is the hallmark of the PB pattern in HF patients. This is at variance from other forms of abnormal breathing patterns of central origin such as the idiopathic form of central sleep apnea (CSA), drug-induced CSA, and the PB caused by hypoxia at high altitude. The cyclical rising and falling in ventilation characterizing PB are accompanied by phase-linked oscillations of arterial blood gases, heart rate, and blood pressure, thus producing a simultaneous involvement of the respiratory and cardiovascular systems at very low frequencies (VLF, 0.01–0.04 Hz) [8] (Fig. 7.1). The analysis of the timing relationship between respiratory and cardiovascular signals clearly indicates that the ventilatory oscillation leads the oscillation of heart rate and blood pressure and is almost opposite in phase with respect to the oscillation of oxygen saturation at carotid bodies [8]. This timing relationship suggests that central effects due to the cyclic increase in central respiratory drive and reflex effects due to mechanical stimulation of cardiopulmonary receptors are the main causes of the heart rate oscillation, while the modulation of systemic venous return brought about by the cyclic fluctuation of intrathoracic pressure is the main determinant of the blood pressure oscillation. These changes also reflect on cardiac hemodynamics [9].

Table 7.1 summarizes the epidemiological aspects of abnormal breathing patterns during daytime in HF. Although in the majority of these studies, the breathing pattern was assessed during short-term laboratory recordings in the supine position, various methodological aspects, analytical methods, and definitions may account for some of the differences.

In the study by Feld and Priest [2], including patients with mild-to-moderate congestive HF, in stable clinical conditions for at least 2 weeks before the evaluation and able to perform a cardiopulmonary exercise test, 9 out of 36 (25 %) demonstrated a cyclic breathing pattern. This study reports a lower prevalence as compared to subsequent studies likely because the respiratory pattern was studied—rather

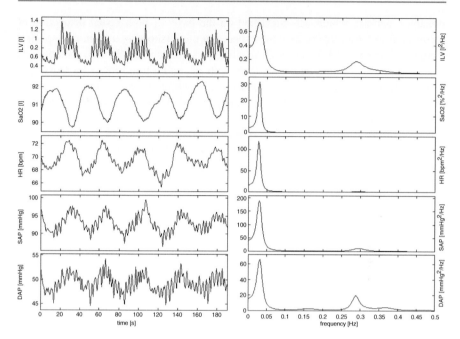

Fig. 7.1 Representative example of signals (*left*) and corresponding power spectra (*right*) from a patient with heart failure during an episode of nonapneic periodic breathing. *Top* to *bottom*: *ILV* instantaneous lung volume, *SaO₂* arterial O$_2$ saturation at the ear, *HR* heart rate, *SAP* systolic arterial pressure, *DAP* diastolic arterial pressure (Reproduced with permission from Ref. [8])

Table 7.1 Epidemiology of daytime periodic breathing

Study	No of patients	Age (years)	LVEF (%)	PB (%)
Feld and Priest [2]	36	54±14	23±9	25
Mortara et al. [3]	80	52±9	26±8	64
Ponikowski et al. [5]	74	57±10	25±10	66
La Rovere et al. [6]	380	52±9	27±8	38
Poletti et al. [7]	147	64±12	31±8	59

obtrusively—by monitoring ventilation through a mouthpiece. Variation in tidal volume ≥25 % between peak and trough values was considered to define the cyclic pattern of respiration. Cyclic respiration was confirmed on two separate occasions in each patient. Patients with a cyclic respiratory pattern had a significantly lower ejection fraction than that of patients without cyclic respiration, while no difference was present in clinical variables, exercise time, and peak exercise capacity.

With the use of a nonobtrusive monitoring of ventilation by inductance plethysmography, in the study by Mortara et al. [3], breathing disorders were observed in 51 (64 %) of 80 clinically stable patients (no changes in signs or symptoms in the 2 weeks preceding the study) undergoing a 15 min recording of ECG, beat-to-beat arterial oxygen saturation (SaO$_2$), and respiration. More specifically, the abnormal breathing pattern, which was identified on the basis of both visual inspection of recordings and the analysis of power spectrum plots (showing a dominant spectral component in the VLF band of all signals), was nonapneic PB in 30 patients and apneic PB in the remaining 21. Patients with PB had a trend toward a worse left ventricular function than patients with normal breathing. However, in a larger series of patients who underwent right heart catheterization, the same authors [4] found that a close linear relationship exists between breathing disorders and hemodynamic impairment, as assessed by cardiac output and pulmonary artery wedge pressure, particularly in those patients presenting with apneic PB, while a weaker association can be observed when only the left ventricular ejection fraction (LVEF) or maximum oxygen consumption during exercise testing is taken into account.

With a similar methodology, a high prevalence of PB during "wakefulness" (66 %) was also reported by Ponikowski et al. [5] in a series of 74 stable HF patients. In line with the previous studies, there was no difference in age, etiology, therapy, or cardiorespiratory function between patients with and without breathing disorders, apart from a more advanced NYHA functional class in patients with PB.

A lower prevalence was reported in a large series including 380 patients [6], among whom 145 (38 %) were found to have sustained PB in a 10-min recording. In this study, breathing disorders were identified as a repeated oscillation of tidal volume with a >25 % variation in peak to trough values of tidal volume and were defined as sustained if present in more than 75 % of the 10 min recording. Patients with breathing disorders (more frequently males), not only had a lower LVEF and a more advanced NYHA class, but also had a lower systolic blood pressure and worse renal function.

At variance with previous studies, Poletti et al. [7] evaluated older patients and found that age was a significant determinant of the occurrence of daytime breathing disorders that were identified in 59 % of the sample population (apneic PB in 27 %, nonapneic PB in 32 %). Again, patients with breathing disorders had a worse hemodynamic condition characterized by a more depressed LVEF, more advanced NYHA class, and increased NT-proBNP and creatinine values. In a subset of patients who also underwent, within 24 h, a nocturnal continuous polysomnographic recording, the authors [7] found that the presence of respiratory disorders during nighttime (respiratory disorder index > 20) was accurately predicted by concomitant daytime breathing abnormalities (AUC: 0.82 at receiver-operating characteristic analysis, sensitivity: 75 %, specificity: 75 %).

A more in-depth evaluation of the circadian prevalence of PB (referred to in this study as CSR) has been reported by Brack et al. [10] who recorded the breathing pattern of 60 ambulatory patients with severe stable HF continuously during 24 h, by means of a portable monitoring device incorporating a respiratory inductive plethysmograph that also allowed estimation of the apnea hypopnea index (AHI). During the day, 16 % of the patients had at least 15 periodic breathing cycles per hour while during the night, the corresponding prevalence was 62 %. PB occurred on average 10 % of daytime. Severity of daytime, but not of nighttime PB was associated with the severity of HF as assessed by the BNP value, while no significant association was found for both daytime and nighttime PB as far as age, LVEF, or NYHA class are concerned. While in previous studies patients were evaluated in the supine or in the sitting position, Brack et al. [10], by incorporating accelerometers in the monitoring device, were also able to determine that 90 % of daytime PB occurred in the upright position. The authors reasonably assumed that when the daytime PB developed in the upright position, it corresponded to the wakeful state.

In summary, these studies show that ventilatory oscillations are a common finding in patients with moderate-to-severe HF, and their occurrence is mainly related to a more severe clinical and hemodynamic impairment. These studies, however, do not establish whether daytime PB behaves as a continuum with nighttime breathing disorders or whether it is a somewhat different entity. While the study by Poletti et al. [7] showed a good predictive ability, no quantitative assessment of daytime breathing disorders was allowed by the short-term laboratory polygraphy in the study by Brack et al. [10]; by accurately computing the AHI through the entire 24 h period, the severity of nocturnal PB correlated loosely with daytime PB.

7.2   Prognostic Value of Abnormal Breathing Patterns During Daytime in Heart Failure

Although nighttime breathing disorders of central origin are generally regarded as having detrimental effects on cardiac function [11], it is still debated whether they simply reflect the HF severity or whether they are independent risk factors for increased mortality [12]. In line with the concept that PB is simply a signal that the HF is increasing in severity, some authors [13] have speculated that the occurrence of PB in patients with HF might play some compensatory role. This hypothesis has been based on the consideration that the hyperventilation phase, by increasing lung volume, may lead to an increase in oxygen stores and cardiac output while the apnea phase may represent a recovery period for the respiratory muscles. With regard to prognosis, although the majority of the studies have shown that nocturnal PB can confer, independent of other risk factors, a twofold to threefold increased risk of mortality in patients with stable severe HF [14–18], some controversial data do exist [19, 20]. In a recent study, including 267 patients (mean age 60 ± 14 years, NYHA class III 48 %, beta-blockers treatment 79 %) who were submitted to unattended overnight cardiorespiratory polysomnography, multivariate Cox analysis identified age, male sex, chronic kidney disease, and left ventricular function, but not moderate or severe PB as predictors of heart transplant-free survival [21].

Similar to nighttime PB, several studies have shown a significant association between PB occurring during the daytime and increased mortality [5–7, 10, 19]. In the study by Ponikowski et al. [5], the 2-year survival was 67 % in the presence of an oscillatory respiratory pattern versus 96 % for patients who had a normal breathing pattern ($p=0.008$); cyclical breathing predicted poor survival, independent of peak oxygen consumption. In an extended follow-up of 4 years, La Rovere et al. [6] found a cardiac mortality rate of 41 % in patients with breathing disorders and of 26 % in normal breathing patients ($p=0.002$, Fig. 7.2). Although the presence of

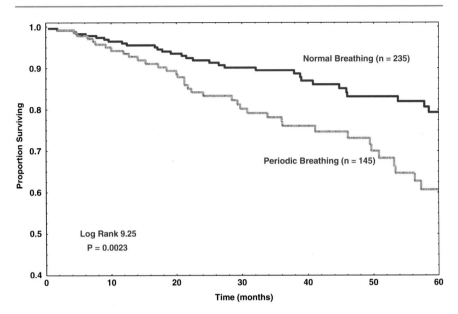

Fig. 7.2 Kaplan–Meier survival curves for the end point of total cardiac mortality. Patients with periodic breathing during a short-term daytime laboratory recording had a significant worse prognosis than patients with a normal breathing pattern (Reproduced with permission from Ref. [6])

daytime breathing abnormalities has been found to double the risk of cardiac death, independently of clinical and functional parameters, a causal role in the progression of the disease has not been definitely proven. Interestingly, in two studies that analyzed the predictive value of concomitant daytime and nighttime PB, it was only daytime but not nocturnal PB that was associated with mortality or transplantation [10, 19] after adjusting for BNP, age, and NYHA class. Brack et al. [10], who quantified the whole burden of daytime breathing abnormalities, found that mortality was higher in those patients who spent ≥10 % of their daytime with PB. Likely, as almost all of daytime PB occurred in the upright position, the prognostic importance of daytime breathing disorders in the study by Brack et al. [10] overlap with that of oscillatory ventilation during exercise (see Chap. 8). Within this context, Corrà et al. [22] suggested that exertional oscillatory ventilation is significantly associated ($p<0.01$) with sleep-disordered breathing (AHI index > 30) and that their combination represents a crucial prognostic burden in patients with HF.

In summary, on the basis of the data available in literature, the occurrence of PB during daytime significantly relates to a worse prognosis. The data suggest that this association is even stronger than that for nocturnal breathing disorders. However, the studies are few, often limited in size, and they cannot provide direct evidence that the daytime breathing abnormalities "per se" play a causal role in further worsening the progression of the disease. It has also to be underscored that the patients evaluated in these studies were enrolled more than 10 years ago; therefore, it cannot be excluded that a wider use of beta-blockers and cardiac resynchronization therapies [23] may have modified the scenario.

7.3 Pathophysiological Mechanisms of Periodic Breathing During Wakefulness

It is largely accepted that during stable wakefulness, PB may result from instability in the closed-loop, negative-feedback chemical control of ventilation [24]. In this system, peripheral and central chemoreceptors sense the changes occurring in PaO_2 and $PaCO_2/[H+]$, and project their sensory information to the medullary respiratory centers, thus leading to a change in ventilation aimed at buffering the initial disturbance. A major contribution to the understanding of the causes of respiratory instability has been provided by the application of control theory and computer modelling to the analysis of the ventilatory control system [25–27]. Three main factors determine the stability of this system [25, 27]: controller gain (i.e., the ventilatory response to changes in arterial blood gas tensions), plant gain (i.e., the responsiveness of changes in arterial blood gases to changes in ventilation), and system delays (i.e., the combined effect of circulation time from the lungs to chemoreceptors and of mixing and diffusion processes in the lungs, heart, vasculature, and brain tissues). Loop gain is the product of controller gain and plant gain, and its magnitude can be expressed as the ratio of the corrective change in ventilation to the initiating ventilatory disturbance. According to control theory, in the presence of different combinations of long circulatory delay and increased loop gain—two conditions that are common in HF patients due to impaired hemodynamics, enlarged cardiac size and enhanced chemosensitivity [24, 28–30]—any transient perturbation occurring in the respiratory control loop may trigger a self-sustaining ventilatory oscillation with the typical waxing and waning pattern of breath amplitude of classical CSR [25, 27]. Hence, it is not surprising that PB may develop during wakefulness, as previously reported in patients in the upright position during daytime activities [10] or while exercising [22].

The plausibility of the instability hypothesis during daytime nonapneic PB has been tested by Pinna et al. [31] in 37 HF patients during a short-term laboratory recording (8 min). Both time- and frequency-domain signal processing techniques were used to analyze respiratory and arterial O_2 saturation oscillations (pulse oximeter). It was found that both the estimated phase shift of the oscillation travelling around the peripheral chemoreflex loop and the response to O_2 administration showed a remarkable consistency with predictions derived from the instability hypothesis, (Fig. 7.3).

During wakefulness, a tonic, nonchemical excitation of respiratory centers commonly referred to as "wakefulness stimulus" or "wakefulness drive" [32, 33] prevents ventilation from ceasing even when there is a loss of chemical drive (e.g., during passive hyperventilation) [34]. Accordingly, apneas would not occur during waking PB. Yet, both nonapneic and apneic PB have been observed during daytime (morning hours) laboratory recordings in HF patients [3, 5, 35], despite patients were asked not to fall asleep and/or to keep their eyes open [5, 6]. Thus, these observations challenge the common belief that patients are actually awake in this experimental setting. To address this issue, it is first necessary to briefly recall current knowledge on the effects of sleep on ventilatory control in normal subjects and then extend these concepts to the patients with HF.

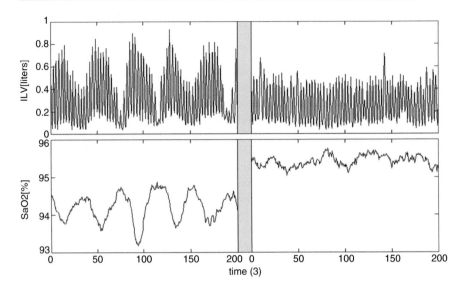

Fig. 7.3 Representative tracing of instantaneous lung volume (ILV) and arterial O_2 saturation (SaO_2) from one heart failure patient before (basal condition) and during O_2 administration. Notice the complete abolition of periodic breathing and the marked increase of SaO_2 after the therapeutic intervention (Reproduced with permission from Ref. [31])

7.4   Effects of Sleep on Ventilatory Control and Stability

During sleep, controller gain decreases [36], while plant gain increases as a result of increased $PaCO_2$, decreased metabolic rate, and increased functional residual capacity in the supine position [25, 37]. In the light stages of sleep, the reduction in controller gain is small, the increase in plant gain predominates, and overall loop gain increases, thereby increasing the propensity for ventilatory instability and periodic breathing. On the contrary, in the deeper stages of sleep, the reduction in controller gain is larger [36] and becomes the dominant factor, thus leading to a decreased loop gain and hence greater ventilatory stability [37].

A major event occurring during non-rapid eye movement (NREM) sleep is the withdrawal of the "wakefulness stimulus" and the consequent reduction in ventilation and increase in eupneic $PaCO_2$ as compared to wakefulness [33]. This is accompanied by the "unmasking" of the apneic threshold, namely the appearance of a $PaCO_2$ level below which ventilation ceases [33]. In normal subjects, the increase in $PaCO_2$ at the transition from wakefulness to NREM sleep is 2–8 mmHg, and the apneic threshold is typically 2–5 mmHg below sleeping eupneic $PaCO_2$ and close to waking eupneic level [33]. In patients with HF, on the contrary, there is little or no significant increase in $PaCO_2$, and the apnea threshold is very close to the sleeping eupneic level [38]; therefore, small increases in ventilation are likely to lower $PaCO_2$ below the threshold and induce apnea. Because of the cessation of ventilation during apneas, $PaCO_2$ steadily increases and, as soon as the apnea termination threshold is reached, the apnea is terminated and breathing resumes [33]. However, the increase in chemical drive continues well above the eupneic level due to the delays between lungs and chemoreceptors. As a result of the accumulation of a large amount of chemical stimuli, arousal often occurs, thereby restoring the awake ventilatory response in a condition of arterial hypercapnia. The occurrence of this supplemental drive to breathe contributes to further increase the ongoing, chemically driven hyperpnea, leading to a transient ventilatory overshoot and a more potent level of hypocapnia. As sleep resumes, this potentiation effect sets the stage for a new and possibly more severe apnoeic event, predisposing for a new cycle of hyperpnea and apnea.

Hence, in patients with HF, a ventilatory control system already prone to instability during wakefulness is subject, during the light stages of sleep, to a further increase in loop gain, to the destabilizing effect of a reduced difference between eupneic $PaCO_2$ and the apnea threshold, and to the exacerbating effect of sleep–wake fluctuations. These considerations therefore suggest that during light sleep, chemoreflex-mediated instability dynamically interacts with arousal-driven instability, and the two mechanisms tend to mutually reinforce one another.

7.5   Sleep or Awake Apneas?

Previous observational studies reporting the occurrence of "awake" periodic breathing in HF patients during daytime laboratory recordings have found that a remarkable proportion of respiratory events was apneic [3, 5, 8, 35]. Objective assessment of patients' vigilance level through monitoring of the electroencephalogram (EEG) and electrooculogram (EOG), however, was not performed. Since the development of apneas requires the "unmasking" of the apnoeic threshold and this, in turn, would occur during NREM sleep, the notion of "awake" apneas would be questionable. Indeed, it has long been known that episodes of apneic PB may occur during drowsiness in healthy individuals and that the ventilatory oscillation is closely linked with a fluctuation in the level of wakefulness [32, 36].

In a study involving 17 HF patients who had a daytime EEG recording during apneic and nonapneic PB in the supine resting condition, Maestri et al. [39] found that in ≈60 % of them the ventilatory oscillation was closely linked (coherence >0.70) to an oscillation in EEG activity at the same frequency. Moreover, hyperpneic and apneic phases were associated with frequency components typical of wakefulness and light sleep, respectively.

A more in-depth study on the relationship between vigilance state and apneic events was carried out by Pinna et al. [40] using a novel methodology that integrates visual scoring and automatic computer procedures in the analysis of EEG recordings, thus exploiting the strengths of each [41]. This approach allows to detect sleep–wake transitions with a high time resolution (0.25 s) and reliability, thus overcoming some limitations of traditional scoring of polysomnographic recordings. In this study, 16 HF patients underwent a polysomnographic daytime laboratory recording (25 min) in the supine resting condition during apneic PB. Ninety-two percent of the 272 central apneas observed across patients were associated with a concurrent transition from wakefulness to EEG activity typical of NREM sleep stages 1–2 (light sleep). This transition was followed by an opposite transition to wakefulness that was typically synchronous with the termination of apneas (Fig. 7.4). Hence, in the vast majority of ventilatory oscillations, wakefulness and light sleep represented the hallmark of cyclic hyperpneas and apneas, respectively. The percentages of time spent in the wakefulness, NREM 1, and NREM 2 states were (median (lower, upper quartile)) 64 [50, 80]%, 25 [20, 38]%, and 3 [0, 13]%, respectively. One possible explanation for the occasional occurrence of apneas during wakefulness in some of the patients might be that in these instances the

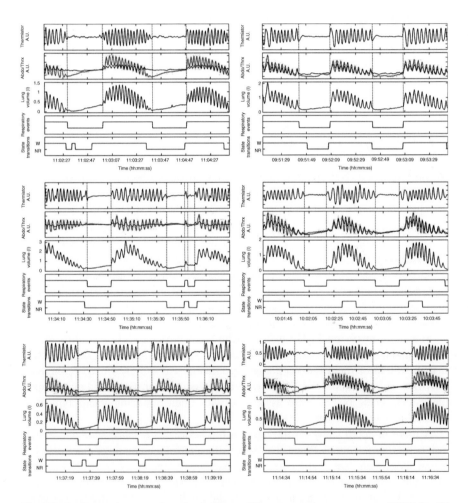

Fig. 7.4 Representative examples of wakefulness (W) → nonrapid eye movement (NREM) → W transitions concurrent with apneic events. From *top* to *bottom* in each panel: oronasal airflow by thermistor; thoraco-abdominal movements; lung volume; respiratory event diagram; and simplified state-transition diagram (NR = NREM). (Reproduced with permission from Ref. [40])

appearance of light drowsiness was enough to unmask the apneic threshold, without requiring that theta–delta dominance replaced alpha dominance. Indeed, careful analysis of EEG and EOG recordings during missing state transitions revealed that in all but one patient, there were one or more of the following signs of drowsiness: disappearance or marked attenuation of awake eye movements, appearance of slow eye movements (SEM), reduction in alpha amplitude, and mixed alpha and theta–delta activity.

These findings led the Authors to the conclusion that apneas occurring during daytime recordings in the supine resting condition are almost invariably associated with a concurrent transition to light NREM sleep, although the majority of PB occurs while the patient is in the wakefulness state. It seems therefore reasonable to refer to this phenomenon as "awake periodic breathing," while the term "awake apneas" does not faithfully reflect experimental observations.

7.6   Periodic Breathing and Body Position

As shown above, the majority of studies reporting the occurrence of PB during daytime have been performed in the supine position. The supine position, by itself, may promote ventilator instability as indicated by the beneficial effects of the lateral sleeping position on the severity of sleep apnea in HF patients with central sleep apnea [42]. Thus, it should be stressed that the prevalence of "awake" periodic breathing reported by these studies might have been biased by this experimental condition.

Conclusions

Abnormal breathing patterns are frequently observed during daytime in patients with HF and are associated with a worse prognosis. However, their appearance is related also to a worse hemodynamic condition, and their definite contribution to prognosis should be reassessed in light of the modern-treated HF population. When recordings are carried out in the supine resting condition, apneic events are almost invariably associated with a temporary transition to light sleep, although for the majority of time, periodic breathing occurs during wakefulness, thus making it reasonable to refer to the overall phenomenon as "awake PB."

References

1. Ward M. Periodic respiration. A short historical note. Ann R Coll Surg Engl. 1973;52:330–4.
2. Feld H, Priest S. A cyclic breathing pattern in patients with poor left ventricular function and compensated heart failure: a mild form of Cheyne-Stokes respiration? J Am Coll Cardiol. 1993;21:971–4.
3. Mortara A, Sleight P, Pinna GD, Maestri R, Prpa A, La Rovere MT, Cobelli F, Tavazzi L. Abnormal awake respiratory patterns are common in chronic heart failure and may prevent

evaluation of autonomic tone by measures of heart rate variability. Circulation 1997;96:246–52. Erratum in: Circulation 1997;96:4118.

4. Mortara A, Sleight P, Pinna GD, Maestri R, Capomolla S, Febo O, La Rovere MT, Cobelli F. Association between hemodynamic impairment and Cheyne-Stokes respiration and periodic breathing in chronic stable congestive heart failure secondary to ischemic or idiopathic dilated cardiomyopathy. Am J Cardiol. 1999;84:900–4.

5. Ponikowski P, Anker SD, Chua TP, Francis D, Banasiak W, Poole-Wilson PA, Coats AJ, Piepoli M. Oscillatory breathing patterns during wakefulness in patients with chronic heart failure: clinical implications and role of augmented peripheral chemosensitivity. Circulation. 1999;100:2418–24.

6. La Rovere MT, Pinna GD, Maestri R, Robbi E, Mortara A, Fanfulla F, Febo O, Sleight P. Clinical relevance of short-term day-time breathing disorders in chronic heart failure patients. Eur J Heart Fail. 2007;9:949–54.

7. Poletti R, Passino C, Giannoni A, Zyw L, Prontera C, Bramanti F, Clerico A, Piepoli M, Emdin M. Risk factors and prognostic value of daytime Cheyne-Stokes respiration in chronic heart failure patients. Int J Cardiol. 2009;137:47–53.

8. Pinna GD, Maestri R, Mortara A, La Rovere MT. Cardiorespiratory interactions during periodic breathing in awake chronic heart failure patients. Am J Physiol Heart Circ Physiol. 2000;278:H932–41.

9. Puri P, Mehra A, Elkayam U. Cheyne-Stokes respiration and cardiac hemodynamics in heart failure. Catheter Cardiovasc Interv. 2008;72:581–5.

10. Brack T, Thüer I, Clarenbach CF, Senn O, Noll G, Russi EW, Bloch KE. Daytime Cheyne-Stokes respiration in ambulatory patients with severe congestive heart failure is associated with increased mortality. Chest. 2007;132:1463–71.

11. Costanzo MR, Khayat R, Ponikowski P, Augostini R, Stellbrink C, Mianulli M, Abraham WT. Mechanisms and clinical consequences of untreated central sleep apnea in heart failure. J Am Coll Cardiol. 2015;65:72–84.

12. Sin DD, Man GC. Cheyne-Stokes respiration: a consequence of a broken heart? Chest. 2003;124:1627–8.

13. Naughton MT. Cheyne-Stokes respiration: friend or foe? Thorax. 2012;67:357–60.

14. Hanly PJ, Zuberi-Khokhar NS. Increased mortality associated with Cheyne-Stokes respiration in patients with congestive heart failure. Am J Respir Crit Care Med. 1996;153:272–6.

15. Lanfranchi PA, Braghiroli A, Bosimini E, Mazzuero G, Colombo R, Donner CF, Giannuzzi P. Prognostic value of nocturnal Cheyne-Stokes respiration in chronic heart failure. Circulation. 1999;99:1435–40.

16. Javaheri S, Shukla R, Zeigler H, Wexler L. Central sleep apnea, right ventricular dysfunction, and low diastolic blood pressure are predictors of mortality in systolic heart failure. J Am Coll Cardiol. 2007;49:2028–34.

17. Pinna GD, Maestri R, Mortara A, Johnson P, Andrews D, Ponikowski P, Witkowski T, Robbi E, La Rovere MT, Sleight P. Pathophysiological and clinical relevance of simplified monitoring of nocturnal breathing disorders in heart failure patients. Eur J Heart Fail. 2009;11:264–72.

18. Jilek C, Krenn M, Sebah D, Obermeier R, Braune A, Kehl V, Schroll S, Montalvan S, Riegger GA, Pfeifer M, Arzt M. Prognostic impact of sleep disordered breathing and its treatment in heart failure: an observational study. Eur J Heart Fail. 2011;13:68–75.

19. Andreas S, Hagenah G, Moller C, Werner GS, Kreuzer H. Cheyne-Stokes respiration and prognosis in congestive heart failure. Am J Cardiol. 1996;78:1260–4.

20. Roebuck T, Solin P, Kaye DM, Bergin P, Bailey M, Naughton MT. Increased long-term mortality in heart failure due to sleep apnoea is not yet proven. Eur Respir J. 2004;23:735–40.

21. Grimm W, Sosnovskaya A, Timmesfeld N, Hildebrandt O, Koehler U. Prognostic impact of central sleep apnea in patients with heart failure. J Card Fail. 2015;21:126–33.

22. Corrà U, Pistono M, Mezzani A, Braghiroli A, Giordano A, Lanfranchi P, Bosimini E, Gnemmi M, Giannuzzi P. Sleep and exertional periodic breathing in chronic heart failure: prognostic importance, and interdependence. Circulation. 2006;113:44–50.

23. Lamba J, Simpson CS, Redfearn DP, Michael KA, Fitzpatrick M, Baranchuk A. Cardiac resynchronization therapy for the treatment of sleep apnoea: a meta-analysis. Europace. 2011;13:1174–9.
24. Javaheri S, Dempsey JA. Mechanisms of sleep apnea and periodic breathing in systolic heart failure. Sleep Med Clin. 2007;2:623–30.
25. Khoo MC, Kronauer RE, Strohl KP, Slutsky AS. Factors inducing periodic breathing in humans: a general model. J Appl Physiol Respir Environ Exerc Physiol. 1982;53:644–59.
26. Longobardo GS, Cherniack NS, Gothe B. Factors affecting respiratory system stability. Ann Biomed Eng. 1989;17:377–96.
27. Cherniack NS, Longobardo GS. Mathematical models of periodic breathing and their usefulness in understanding cardiovascular and respiratory disorders. Exp Physiol. 2006;91:295–305.
28. Hall MJ, Xie A, Rutherford R, Ando S, Floras JS, Bradley TD. Cycle length of periodic breathing in patients with and without heart failure. Am J Respir Crit Care Med. 1996;154(2 Pt 1):376–81.
29. Solin P, Roebuck T, Johns DP, Walters EH, Naughton MT. Peripheral and central ventilatory responses in central sleep apnea with and without congestive heart failure. Am J Respir Crit Care Med. 2000;162:2194–200.
30. Giannoni A, Baruah R, Willson K, Mebrate Y, Mayet J, Emdin M, Hughes AD, Manisty CH, Francis DP. Real-time dynamic carbon dioxide administration: a novel treatment strategy for stabilization of periodic breathing with potential application to central sleep apnea. J Am Coll Cardiol. 2010;56:1832–7.
31. Pinna GD, Maestri R, Mortara A, La Rovere MT, Fanfulla F, Sleight P. Periodic breathing in heart failure patients: testing the hypothesis of instability of the chemoreflex loop. J Appl Physiol. (1985) 2000;89:2147–57.
32. Phillipson EA, Bowes G. Control of breathing during sleep. In: Cherniak NS, Widdicombe JG, editors. Handbook of physiology. The respiratory system. Control of breathing. Bethesda: American Physiological Society; 1986. p. 640–90.
33. Dempsey JA, Smith CA, Przybylowski T, Chenuel B, Xie A, Nakayama H, Skatrud JB. The ventilatory responsiveness to CO_2 below eupnoea as a determinant of ventilatory stability in sleep. J Physiol. 2004;560(Pt 1):1–11.
34. Skatrud JB, Dempsey JA. Interaction of sleep state and chemical stimuli in sustaining rhythmic ventilation. J Appl Physiol Respir Environ Exerc Physiol. 1983;55:813–22.
35. Fanfulla F, Mortara A, Maestri R, Pinna GD, Bruschi C, Cobelli F, Rampulla C. The development of hyperventilation in patients with chronic heart failure and Cheyne-Strokes respiration: a possible role of chronic hypoxia. Chest. 1998;114:1083–90.
36. Bulow K. Respiration and wakefulness in man. Acta Physiol Scand. 1963;59:1–110.
37. Khoo MC, Gottschalk A, Pack AI. Sleep-induced periodic breathing and apnea: a theoretical study. J Appl Physiol. 1991/1985;70:2014–24.
38. Xie A, Skatrud JB, Puleo DS, Rahko PS, Dempsey JA. Apnea-hypopnea threshold for CO2 in patients with congestive heart failure. Am J Respir Crit Care Med. 2002;165:1245–50.
39. Maestri R, La Rovere MT, Robbi E, Pinna GD. Fluctuations of the fractal dimension of the electroencephalogram during periodic breathing in heart failure patients. J Comput Neurosci. 2010;28:557–65.
40. Pinna GD, Robbi E, Pizza F, Caporotondi A, La Rovere MT, Maestri R. Sleep-wake fluctuations and respiratory events during Cheyne-Stokes respiration in patients with heart failure. J Sleep Res. 2014;23:347–57.
41. Pinna GD, Robbi E, La Rovere MT, Maestri R. A hybrid approach for continuous detection of sleep-wakefulness fluctuations: validation in patients with Cheyne-Stokes respiration. J Sleep Res. 2012;21:342–51.
42. Pinna GD, Robbi E, La Rovere MT, Taurino AE, Bruschi C, Guazzotti G, Maestri R. Differential impact of body position on the severity of disordered breathing in heart failure patients with obstructive vs. central sleep apnoea. Eur J Heart Fail. 2015;17:1302–9.

Exertional Oscillatory Ventilation and Central Sleep Apnea in Heart Failure: Siblings, Cousins, or What Else?

8

Piergiuseppe Agostoni, Anna Apostolo, and Ugo Corrà

Abbreviations

AHI	Apnea/hypopnea index
ASV	Adaptive servoventilation
BNP	Brain natriuretic peptide
CPET	Cardiopulmonary exercise test
CSA	Central sleep apneas
EDV/ESV	End-diastolic/systolic volume
EOV	Exertional oscillatory ventilation
EOPB	Exercise-induced periodic breathing
HF	Heart failure
LVAD	Left ventricular assist device
LVEF	Left ventricular ejection fraction
MECKI	Metabolic Exercise, Cardiac, Kidney Index
NYHA	New York Heart Association

P. Agostoni (✉)
Department of Clinical Sciences and Community Health, Cardiovascular Section, University of Milan, Milan, Italy

Heart Failure, Clinical Cardiology and Rehabilitation Unit, Centro Cardiologico Monzino IRCCS, Milan, Italy
e-mail: Piergiuseppe.Agostoni@ccfm.it

A. Apostolo
Heart Failure, Clinical Cardiology and Rehabilitation Unit, Centro Cardiologico Monzino IRCCS, Milan, Italy
e-mail: anna.apostolo@ccfm.it

U. Corrà
Divisione di Cardiologia Riabilitativa, Fondazione Salvatore Maugeri, IRCCS, Istituto Scientifico di Veruno, Veruno, Italy
e-mail: ugo.corra@fsm.it

© Springer International Publishing Switzerland 2017
M. Emdin et al. (eds.), *The Breathless Heart*,
DOI 10.1007/978-3-319-26354-0_8

PAPs	Systolic pulmonary artery pressure
pO_2/pCO_2	Partial pressure of oxygen/carbon dioxide
VCO_2	Carbon dioxide output
VE	Minute ventilation

8.1   Definition of Exertional Oscillatory Ventilation

Over the last few years, ventilation inefficiency has become an established matter of interest in heart failure (HF) patients performing a cardiopulmonary exercise test (CPET), its most remarkable aspect being exertional oscillatory ventilation (EOV), also called exercise-induced periodic breathing. EOV is a phenomenon originally described as anecdotal [1–3], and now considered as a marker of disease severity and of worse prognosis [4, 5]. EOV is a cyclic fluctuation of minute ventilation (VE) and expired gas kinetics occurring during exercise: it is a slow, prominent, consistent rather than random, fluctuation in VE that may be evanescent or transient and can follow several distinct patterns. The reported incidence of EOV ranges from 7 % to 51 % [6–14]; such a broad interval is due to the lack of universal criteria to define EOV.

Three are the main attributes for defining EOV: amplitude and interval (length) of the single VE oscillation, and duration of the abnormal VE phenomenon during exercise. The wide variability of EOV patterns is mystified by assessment methods, which include manual scoring and/or visual interpretation. A recent systemic review screened 75 studies, accounting for 17,440 patients, 4638 (26.6 %) of which presented EOV [15]; seven of these studies incorporated other populations than HF, for example, cardiac dysfunction, idiopathic dilated cardiomyopathy, total cavopulmonary connection after Fontan procedure, liver transplantation, and congenital cardiac disorder. The

Table 8.1 Definition of exertional oscillatory ventilation in heart failure

Original definition by Kremser et al. [1]: Ventilatory oscillations lasting ≥66 % of the exercise protocol, with an amplitude of each VE oscillation ≥15 % of the average value at rest
Original definition by Leite et al. [7]: ≥3 regular VE oscillations (i.e., clearly discernible from inherent data noise). Regularity was defined if the SD of three consecutive VE cycle lengths (time between two consecutive nadirs) was within 20 % of the average; minimal average amplitude of VE oscillation ≥5l (peak value minus the average of two in-between consecutive nadirs)
Original definition by Ben-Dov et al. [3]: Marked VE oscillations of 30–60 s duration. Magnitude (Δ) VE (Δ = (peak nadir)/mean over the time period of the oscillation) ≥25 % in ≥2 consecutive cycles (nadir to nadir) during exercise
Original definition by Sun et al. [16]: ≥3 consecutive cyclic fluctuations of VE: amplitude of oscillatory VE ≥30 % of concurrent mean VE with a complete oscillatory cycle within 40–140 s. VE oscillations of similar frequency must also be visible in ≥3 or more of the following variables: oxygen pulse, VO_2, VCO_2, VE/VCO_2, RER, $PetO_2$, or $PetCO_2$

VE ventilation, *VO2* oxygen consumption, *VCO2* carbon dioxide production, *VE/VCO2* relationship between VE and VCO_2, *RER* respiratory gas exchange ratio (i.e., VCO_2/VO_2), *PetO2* oxygen end-tidal pressure, *PetCO2* carbon dioxide end-tidal pressure

EOV definitions were categorized in nine subdivisions, four of which referred to an original definition as suggested by Kremser et al. [1] (n=23), Leite et al. [7] (n=13), Ben-Dov et al. [3] (n=6), and Sun et al. [16] (n=2): the original EOV definitions are summarized in Table 8.1. Other EOV definitions were combinations, relying on different oscillation quantifications, with different computational analyses [15].

8.2   Prevalence of Exercise-Induced EOV

Very few data are available as regards the prevalence of exercise-induced EOV in patients with heart failure [8, 9, 16, 17]. In ~6000 patients with systolic heart failure who underwent a maximal cardiopulmonary exercise test followed by the Metabolic Exercise, Cardiac, Kidney Index (MECKI) score research group [18–20], EOV was present in 17.5 % of cases, and mainly in those with the most impaired exercise capacity. Table 8.2 shows the incidence of exercise-induced EOV according to the severity of exercise limitation. It is of note that the number of female patients with exercise-induced EOV is particularly low, since, in the MECKI score HF population, exercise-induced EOV is present in 13.5 % of females and 18.4 % of males. This behavior is present in all the severity groups analyzed. The physiological reasons behind this finding are still unclear. However, the same observation was made with regard to EOV in HF patients during sleep and at high altitude [9, 21, 22]. In a recent report by Lombardi et al., the occurrence of EOV during sleep at high altitude has been evaluated at different altitudes and up to 5400 m (Mount Everest South Base Camp) [21]. Female gender was associated to a lower presence of EOV during sleep, regardless of the altitude and acclimatization time. Lombardi et al. proposed that differences in peripheral muscle CO_2 production, apneic CO_2 threshold, or in the chemoreflex response to pO_2 and pCO_2 (related to the effect of sex hormones) are likely responsible for the observed gender differences in high-altitude EOV.

8.3   Physiology of Exercise-Induced Periodic Breathing in Heart Failure

The physiology of exercise-induced EOV is still poorly understood. The main concepts have been derived from central sleep apneas (CSA) in HF, but there is no definite proof that these concepts apply also to exercise-induced EOV. Indeed, just as in

Table 8.2 Heart failure population grouped by VO_2 class

	$VO_2 < 50$ $n = 2199$ $m = 1955\,f = 244$	VO_2 50–80 % $n = 2926$ $m = 2314\,f = 612$	$VO_2 > 80$ $n = 541$ $m = 362\,f = 179$
All	528 (24 %)	419 (14.3 %)	45 (8.3 %)
Males	488 (25 %)	336 (14.5 %)	28 (7.7 %)
Females	40 (16.4 %)	83 (13.6 %)	17 (9.5 %)

VO2 oxygen consumption expressed by percentage of predicted value, *m* males, *f* females

Table 8.3 Mechanisms underlying CSA in heart failure

Chronic hyperventilation
1. Pulmonary interstitial congestion due to rostral fluid displacement
2. Exaggerated peripheral chemoreceptor activity
3. Upper airway resistance
Circulatory delay (it delays detection of changes in blood gases between the peripheral and the central chemoreceptors)
1. Low cardiac output
Cerebrovascular reactivity
1. Respiratory-induced changes in the $PaCO_2$ do alter the regulatory circulation of the cerebral district
2. The normal buffering action to changes in central hydrogen ion concentration is impaired (as a consequence)
3. Depressed ability of the central respiratory control center to dampen ventilatory undershoots or overshoots, such as those seen during apnea or at apnea termination

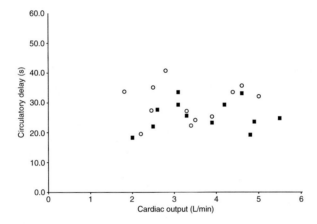

Fig. 8.1 Circulatory delay and cardiac output at Jarvik 2000 pump speed 2 (*white circles*) and at speed 4 (*black squares*). R^2 of the correlation = 0.001

CSA, it is believed that at least three factors have a pivotal role in exercise-induced EOV in HF, specifically hyperventilation, low cardiac output leading to increased circulatory delay, and cerebrovascular reactivity to CO_2 [23] (Table 8.3). Hyperventilation is part of the increased sympathetic activity frequently observed in HF, and it is mainly the consequence of an enhanced stimulation of intrapulmonary receptors, including the so-called J-receptors, and of chemoreceptors and metaboreceptors [24]. As a result of hyperventilation, $PaCO_2$ falls below the threshold level needed to stimulate breathing, so that the central drive to respiratory muscles ceases, and breathing ceases until an increase of $PaCO_2$ promotes a further period of hyperventilation. Moreover, HF patients have a reduced cerebrovascular reactivity to CO_2, further increasing breathing instability [23]. The increased circulatory delay, which is a direct consequence of reduced cardiac output, is considered as another

Table 8.4 Exercise parameters and periodic breathing in a heart failure population bearing a left ventricular assist device (Jarvik 2000) at speed 2 and 4

	All	Without PB	With PB
2 VO_2 peak	782±174	779±158	783±188
4 VO_2 peak	844±157	845±113	844±178
Delta VO_2 peak 2–4	62.6±68.3	66±103.8	61.3±56.1
% of change	9±11	10±17	9±9
2 VO_2/kg peak	10.00±1.69	10.0±2.03	10.01±1.66
4 VO_2/kg peak	10.93±2.11	11.09±2.91	10.87±1.90
Delta VO_2/kg peak	0.93±1.03	1.10±1.60	0.86±0.81
% of change	9.3±11.0	10.6±16.8	8.8±9.0
2 CO rest	3.40±0.97	3.87±0.75	3.24±1.02
4 CO rest	3.70±1.05	4.17±1.02	3.54±1.07
Delta CO rest	0.30±0.58	0.30±0.61	0.30±0.61
% of change	10.7±19.1	7.5±15.8	11.8±20.8
2 CO peak	5.23±1.38	5.53±0.93	5.11±1.55
4 CO peak	5.74±1.32	5.98±0.93	5.65±1.48
Delta CO peak	0.51±0.63	0.45±0.30	0.54±0.74
% of change	11.6±14.9	8.4±5.8	12.9±17.5

VO_2 oxygen consumption, *CO* carbon monoxide

key factor in the occurrence of exercise-induced EOV, since it leads to a temporary misalignment of the chemical signals (low or high $PaCO_2$) to the respiratory response (increased or reduced ventilation) [23, 25]. Albeit frequently suggested, the role of low cardiac output in the pathogenesis of exercise-induced EOV, as well as in that of CSA, presently has little scientific evidence. As a matter of fact, no significant differences in cardiac output or in the circulatory delay from lungs to peripheral receptors have been found between HF patients with and without exercise-induced EOV [26, 27]. Similarly, no correlation exists between cardiac output and circulatory delay at rest in patients with severe HF. In a recent series of HF patients who successfully underwent implantation of a left ventricular assist device (LVAD) (Jarvik 2000), resting cardiac output and circulatory delay resulted unrelated with each other, both at low LVAD pump speed and at high pump speed (Fig. 8.1). Moreover, in the same series of HF patients with LVAD, exercise-induced EOV occurred in 9 out of 15 patients with LVAD at pump speed = 2, and in 5 patients at pump speed = 4. It is of note that exercise evaluations were done only few hours after pump speed changes and that pump speed changes are associated to cardiac output changes both at rest and during effort. Indeed, peak VO_2 and peak cardiac output increased in the total population, in patients without exercise-induced EOV, in patients in whom EOV disappeared with higher LVAD pump speed, and in those in whom exercise-induced EOV remained with both LVAD pump speeds (Table 8.4); the presence of exercise-induced EOV in this series of patients was associated to a lower cardiac output at rest. It is of note that a reduction of exercise-induced EOV due to HF improvement has been reported, starting with the pioneering work of Ribeiro et al., who showed that exercise-induced EOV disappeared after HF improvement in a series of five patients [2]. Many different interpretations are mentioned, regarding cycle length, amplitude of single VE oscillation, and duration of oscillatory phenomenon during exercise. Concerning cycle length, many descriptions are given, such as the distance between two nadirs, the period of observed oscillation divided by the number of oscillations, and the interval from peak to peak for each cycle at rest expressed as mean value [15]. As regards the duration of the VE cycle, definitions vary significantly: approximately 60 s, 40–140 s, 30–60 s, or it is calculated as a percentage of the average [15]. Furthermore, the amplitude of the VE oscillations is described as the difference between the peak VE of the oscillation and the average of the VE of the two surrounding nadirs, by calculating the variation coefficient of VE by assessing the correlation coefficient of VE, or it is expressed as a percentage of the mean of the rest VE [15]. Finally, the total duration of the EOV also varies. For the definition of EOV presence, a duration of at least >66 % of the exercise protocol, >60 % or $\geq$60 %, or $\geq$50 % has been proposed [15]. Therefore, no gold standard has been proposed so far [28]. In addition, cardiac output increase during exercise has been suggested as the cause of the disappearance of exercise-induced EOV frequently observed in a progressive effort. Indeed, approximately in 60 % of cases, exercise-induced EOV ceases during a progressive effort before exhaustion. In Fig. 8.2, the examples of a patient with exercise-induced EOV persisting throughout the exercise and of a patient in whom EOV ceased with a greater effort are reported. In this regard, Schmid et al. showed that, in 52 % of patients in whom exercise-induced EOV ceased, the VO_2 versus work relationship increased after EOV cessation; it was still in 24 % of cases; and it decreased in 24 % of cases (Figs. 8.3 and 8.4) [29]. Notably, the evaluation of the VO_2 versus work relationship allows to understand the amount of O_2 delivery to the working muscle, since a reduction of this relationship during exercise is suggestive of a reduction of cardiac output, either due to exercise-induced cardiac ischemia or to mitral insufficiency [30, 31]. An increase of the VO_2 versus work relationship during exercise was reported only in patients in whom EOV ceased during exercise, and specifically in ~50 % of cases. This implies a higher O_2 delivery to the working muscles, and it suggests a negative effect of exercise-induced EOV on exercise performance, likely due to an increased work of breathing. However, it is still unclear why exercise-induced EOV persists throughout a progressive exercise session in some and not in other patients. Actually, the main unsolved question is what oscillates first; in other words, whether it is ventilation or circulation that leads oscillation. A few pieces of evidence suggest that oscillation in blood flow is the first initiating mechanism. Pioneering studies by Ben Dov [3] demonstrated that, when aligning VO_2, VCO_2, and VE, VO_2 oscillation anticipates VCO_2 and VE oscillations (Fig. 8.5). However, we reevaluated this finding in our population of HF patients and found that this specific behavior was present in some, but not in all of the studied patients. Moreover, Francis [32] showed that exercise-induced EOV can be voluntarily induced by acting on ventilation (Fig. 8.6).

We have got further relevant, albeit spotty, information about the physiology of exercise-induced EOV, but the complete physiological image of this mosaic is still not appreciable. As reported above, we do know that exercise-induced EOV is

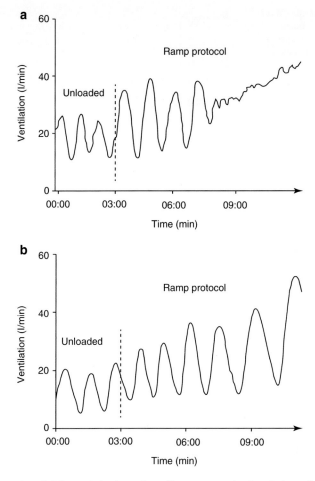

Fig. 8.2 Examples of different behaviors of ventilatory pattern in chronic heart failure patients during exercise: (**a**) disappearance of oscillatory ventilation; (**b**) persistence of oscillatory ventilation (From Ref. [29])

mainly associated with severe HF, and that it disappears if severe HF is successfully treated. This seems to link the disappearance of exercise-induced EOV to an improvement in lung mechanics and also to an increased cardiac output. However, the temporal relationship between the disappearance of EOV and the improvement of HF is not defined, so that the disappearance of exercise-induced EOV may possibly occur later than the hemodynamic improvement. The following case suggests this.

Male patient, 74 years old, referred to our center in April 2008 with a long-term clinical history of severe HF due to dilated cardiomyopathy and low left ventricular ejection fraction. The patient had few emergency hospitalizations in the previous years due to acute decompensated heart failure.

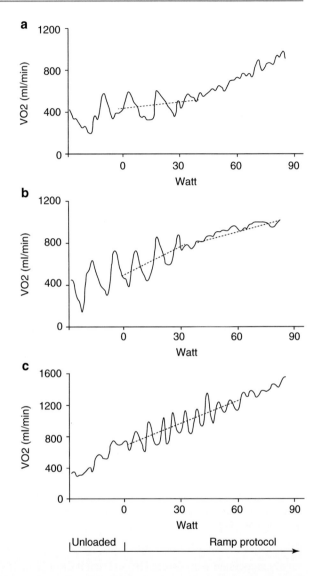

Fig. 8.3 Examples of an increase (**a**), a decrease (**b**), and a lack of change (**c**) of the VO_2/workload slope in patients with EOV disappearing during the exercise test. *Dashed lines* indicate the change of VO_2/workload slope from the EOV phase to the phase after EOV disappearance (From Ref. [29])

In April 2008, the patient was in New York Heart Association (NYHA) class III with no clinical signs of fluid retention and high brain natriuretic peptide (BNP) levels (2500 pg/ml). Electrocardiogram showed sinus rhythm and left branch bundle block, and chest x-rays showed a marked cardiac enlargement and pulmonary congestion. Echocardiography confirmed severe left ventricular dilation (end-diastolic/systolic volumes—EDV/ESV—278/232 ml) with reduced ejection fraction (LVEF 16.5 %) and severe mitral valve regurgitation with increased pulmonary pressure (PAPs, 52 mmHg). A coronary angiography confirmed the absence of atherosclerotic coronary lesions.

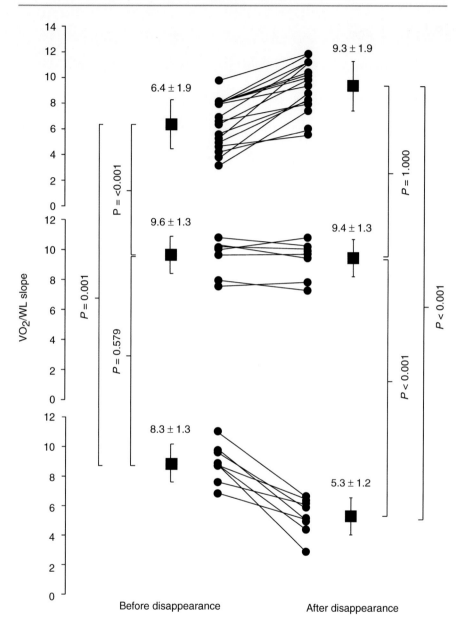

Fig. 8.4 Individual behavior of VO_2/workload slope in 33 patients in which EOV disappeared. During exercise, the disappearance of EOV was accompanied by an increase of VO_2/workload slope in 17 patients, a decrease in 8 patients, and no change in 8 patients (From Ref. [29])

Ramp protocol cardiopulmonary exercise test showed low exercise tolerance (peak VO_2 9.3 ml/kg/min, 40 % of the predicted value) with low VO_2 work slope and

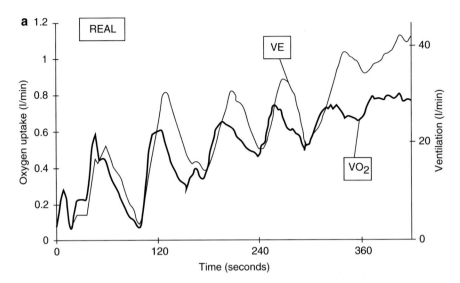

Fig. 8.5 When aligning VO₂, VCO₂, and VE, VO₂ oscillation anticipates VCO₂ and VE oscillations (From Ref. [3])

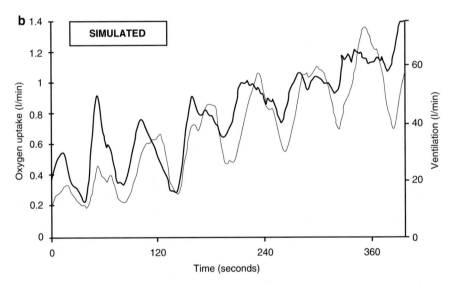

Fig. 8.6 Exertional oscillatory ventilation voluntarily obtained by acting on ventilation (From Ref. [32])

O₂ pulse and an elevated value of VE/VCO₂ slope (=47). Moreover, the cardiopulmonary exercise test showed EOV throughout the test (Fig. 8.7).

At polysomnography, the patient had a high rate of events with an apnea/hypopnea index (AHI) of 50.7/h.

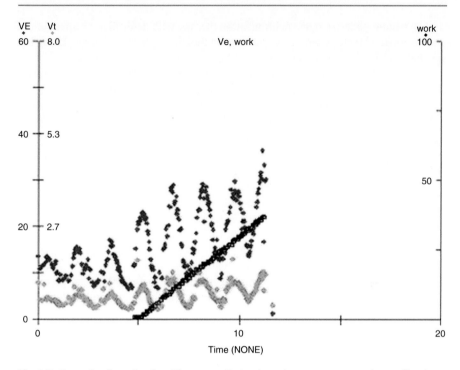

Fig. 8.7 Example of exertional oscillatory ventilation throughout a ramp protocol at cardiopulmonary exercise test

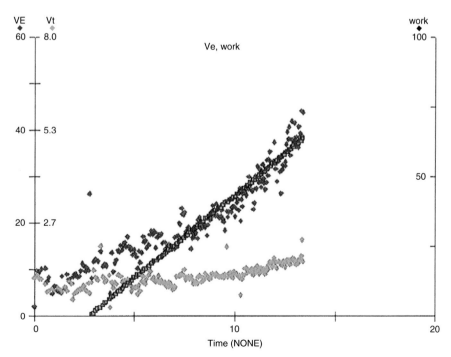

Fig. 8.8 Example of exertional oscillatory ventilation ceasing during a ramp protocol at cardiopulmonary exercise test

The patient underwent resynchronization therapy with defibrillator implantation, and his medical therapy was optimized (carvedilol 25 mg bd, furosemide 25 mg bd, spironolactone 25 mg od, amiodarone 200 mg od, perindopril 2.5 mg bd).

In May 2008, the patient showed a relevant clinical improvement (NYHA class II), and he underwent a cardiopulmonary exercise test in which EOV ceased earlier than in the previous one (Fig. 8.8) (peak VO_2 13 ml/min/kg, BNP 572 pg/ml). Echocardiography showed EDV/ESV 275/220 ml, LVEF 20 %, moderate–severe mitral valve regurgitation, PAPS 31 mmHg.

In November 2008, the patient underwent a further clinical evaluation. He was still in NYHA class II with no signs of pulmonary or peripheral congestion. BNP was 242 pg/ml, and reduction of left ventricular volumes (EDV/ESV 238/155 ml), LVEF 35 %, moderate mitral valve regurgitation, PAPS 29 mmHg were observed at echocardiography. At cardiopulmonary test, exercise tolerance was similar to that observed few months earlier (peak VO_2 14.2 ml/kg/min, 54 % of the predicted value), with a normal VE/VCO_2 slope [29], but EOV was no more detectable (Fig. 8.9). At polysomnography, AHI decreased to 43.1/h.

Besides the reduction of EOV through treatment, there are several pieces of evidence that exercise-induced EOV can be eliminated by adding a further

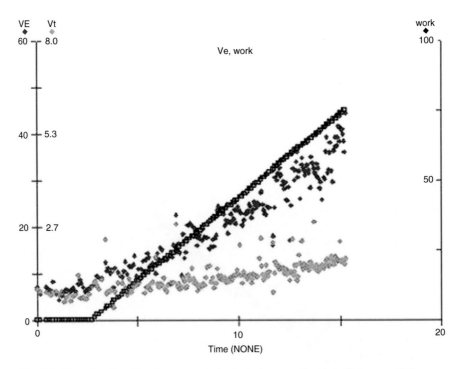

Fig. 8.9 Example of cardiopulmonary exercise test where exertional oscillatory ventilation was no more detectable after optimization of treatment and therapy of the patient

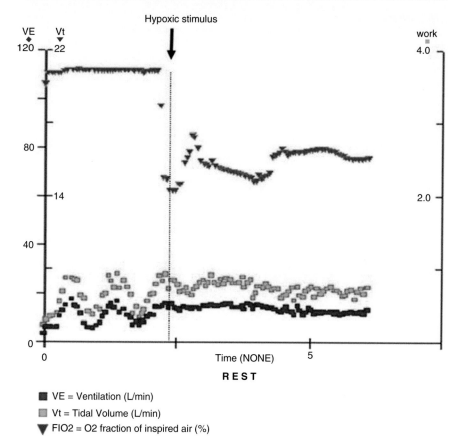

Fig. 8.10 Exertional oscillatory ventilation disappears during a constant low workload exercise if a hypoxic stimulus is suddenly added

ventilation stimulus. For example, if a hypoxic stimulus is suddenly added during constant low workload exercise (Fig. 8.10), EOV disappears. Similarly, Apostolo et al. [33] showed that when 2 % CO_2 is added into the breathing air during constant workload exercise in a subject with exercise-induced EOV, EOV ceases. An example is shown in Fig. 8.11. However, if the added respiratory stimulus is lower, like with 1 % CO_2 instead of 2 % CO_2, periodic breathing persists. A rather complicated interplay between O_2- and CO_2-dependent chemoreceptors is likely the basis of this finding. Indeed, the tendency to periodic breathing may arise from an augmentation in the summed chemoreceptor inputs to respiratory drive, which are O_2- (peripheral) and CO_2-dependent (peripheral and central). While the slight rise in PCO_2 stimulates the ventilatory drive, the concurrent rise in PO_2 (higher with 2 % CO_2 and lower with 1 % CO_2) may exert a counter-inhibitory effect via withdrawal of peripheral chemoreceptor afferent signaling. Although O_2-sensitive

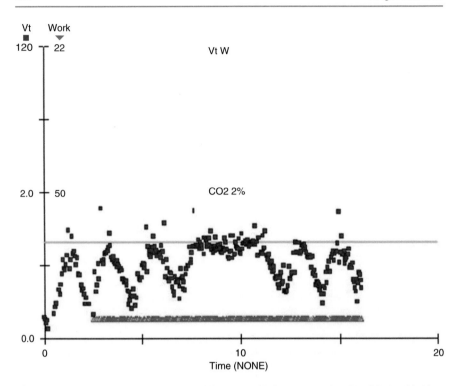

Fig. 8.11 Exercise-induced exertional oscillatory ventilation ceases when 2% CO_2 is added into the breathing air during a constant workload exercise

carotid body output is not generally thought to be important when PaO_2 is greater than 70 mmHg due to the very hyperbolic nature of the hypoxic ventilatory response, some peripheral chemoreceptor activity is still present at normal physiological PaO_2 (and more so in HF patients), and it can be suppressed with further elevation of PaO_2 beyond 100 mmHg [34].

Finally, when an external dead space is added, EOV disappears early during exercise, or it does not appear at all, according to the amount of added dead space, 250 ml and 500 ml, respectively (Fig. 8.12). Interestingly, these experiments supported the concept of the presence of the "thoracic cage" in patients with HF and exercise-induced EOV. Indeed, when adding a further ventilatory stimulus in patients with EOV, the increase in ventilation is due to a respiratory rate increase, and mostly to an increase of the tidal volume of the breaths with a low volume.

8.4   Sleep Disorders in HF Patients with EOV

Since the underlying mechanisms of CSA with Cheyne–Stokes respiration (CSR) resemble (partially) those of EOV, it was assumed that both respiratory disorders may cohabit in HF patients. Nonetheless, the relationship between EOV and CSA

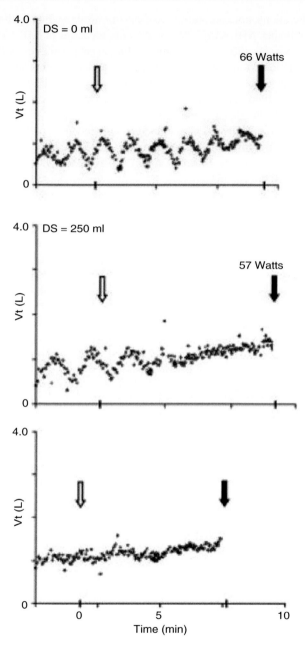

Fig. 8.12 Exertional oscillatory ventilation disappearance after addition of an external dead space (DS) of 0 ml, 250 ml, and 500 ml, respectively. *Vt* tidal volume

with CSR in HF has been scantily studied. In 2006, 133 HF patients were studied during the night and during a symptom-limited CPET [9], and one-third showed respiratory alterations, both during exercise and during sleep. EOV patients showed a significantly higher AHI, and EOV was the only predictor of AHI >30/h. During follow-up, 31 patients (23 %) had major cardiac events (cardiac death or urgent heart transplantation): total mortality was 9 % in patients without EOV and AHI ≤30/h, 17 % in those with EOV alone, 31 % in those with AHI >30/h alone, and 54 % in those with combined EOV and AHI >30/h. Thus, the combination of EOV and significant CSA heralds a worse prognosis [9].

The management of EOV and CSA should be individualized and specialized. The presentation of these atypical breathing patterns is an indication for a more aggressive therapy: servoventilation [35], sildenafil intake [36], inhalation of acetazolamide and carbon dioxide [33], milrinone application, and heart transplantation [2] proved to be effective in blunting EOV and CSA. Supporting the idea of deconditioning, physical activity in the form of aerobic exercise leads to a remarkable 71.2 % disappearance of EOV [37], and supervised home care rehabilitation, adjustments in daily living and coaching could be useful adjuvant therapies in this deconditioned population. Nocturnal continuous positive airway pressure alleviates CSA and improves ventilatory efficiency [38]. Adaptive servoventilation (ASV), which can almost eliminate CSA and normalize breathing, has become applicable in HF [39]: ASV can improve cardiac function, ventilatory inefficiency, and hypercapnic chemosensitivity in HF patients with CSA [40, 41]. Of note, EOV patients show higher norepinephrine levels and burst rate than those without EOV [35]. Changes of VE/VCO$_2$ slope and amplitude of EOV are correlated with muscle sympathetic nerve activity modifications and norepinephrine levels, but not with changes in LVEF. Modifications of VE/VCO$_2$ slope and amplitude of EOV are correlated with changes of AHI [35]. Thus, ASV improves exercise tolerance and ventilatory efficiency in HF patients with CSA.

Overall, the evidence raises several provocative questions about further steps. For example, how long will benefits persist after training cessation or nocturnal ventilation therapy? Is a high-intensity aerobic training program the add-on approach for nonresponder subjects? Is the reversal of EOV and CSA an on/off phenomenon or a progressive dose–response process? Most importantly, how might reverse changes in EOV and CSA really bear prognostic implications reflecting a true improvement in the natural history of the disease?

8.5 Prognostic Role of Exercise-Induced Periodic Breathing

EOV is a robust CPET risk index in distinct HF cohorts [7–14, 16], including heart transplantation candidates, and in patients chronically treated with beta-blockers. EOV and numerous CPET-derived parameters have proven to be predictive in HF [42], but most have been studied in a binary analysis, considering risk indexes in isolation, disregarding the potential value of combining variables. In addition, few observations have been validated yet. So far, only peak VO$_2$, VE/VCO$_2$ slope, and EOV (representing the so-called 2008 European Society of Cardiology—ESC— model) have been validated [43]: the 2008 ESC multiparametric model was superior to other predictive prototypes, created by adding, in isolation, predicted peak VO$_2$, peak oxygen pulse, peak respiratory exchange ratio, peak circulatory power, peak VE/VCO_2, VE/VCO_2 slope normalized by peak VO_2, VO_2 efficiency slope, ventilatory anaerobic threshold detection, peak end-tidal CO_2 partial pressure, peak heart rate, and peak systolic arterial blood pressure. Hence, although difficult to properly compute, EOV should always be taken into account during CPET, if macroscopically evident at visual or analytical inspection.

Conclusions

Exercise-induced EOV is a relatively frequent observation in males, but not in females, with chronic HF. It is associated with a negative prognosis, particularly if concomitant with EOV during sleep. The physiology behind it is complex and still not clearly defined. However, hyperventilation due to an increased sympathetic activity and associated to an enhanced stimulation of intrapulmonary chemoreceptors and metaboreceptors, low cardiac output leading to increased circulatory delay, and cerebrovascular reactivity to CO_2 all have a definite role.

References

1. Kremser CB, O'Toole MF, Leff AR. Oscillatory hyperventilation in severe congestive heart failure secondary to idiopathic dilated cardiomyopathy or to ischemic cardiomyopathy. Am J Cardiol. 1987;59:900–5.
2. Ribeiro JP, Knutzen A, Rocco MB, Hartley LH, Colucci WS. Periodic breathing during exercise in severe heart failure. Reversal with milrinone or cardiac transplantation. Chest. 1987;92:555–6.
3. Ben-Dov I, Sietsema KE, Casaburi R, Wasserman K. Evidence that circulatory oscillations accompany ventilatory oscillations during exercise in patients with heart failure. Am Rev Respir Dis. 1992;145:776–81.
4. Dickstein K, Cohen-Solal A, Filippatos G, McMurray JJ, Ponikowski P, Poole-Wilson PA, Stromberg A, van Veldhuisen DJ, Atar D, Hoes AW, Keren A, Mebazaa A, Nieminen M, Priori SG, Swedberg K. ESC Guidelines for the diagnosis and treatment of acute and chronic heart failure 2008: the Task Force for the diagnosis and treatment of acute and chronic heart failure 2008 of the European Society of Cardiology. Developed in collaboration with the Heart Failure Association of the ESC (HFA) and endorsed by the European Society of Intensive Care Medicine (ESICM). Eur Heart J. 2008;29:2388–442.
5. Cornelis J, Taeymans J, Hens W, Beckers P, Vrints C, Vissers D. Prognostic respiratory parameters in heart failure patients with and without exercise oscillatory ventilation – a systematic review and descriptive meta-analysis. Int J Cardiol. 2015;182:476–86.
6. Feld H, Priest S. A cyclic breathing pattern in patients with poor left ventricular function and compensated heart failure: a mild form of Cheyne-Stokes respiration? J Am Coll Cardiol. 1993;21:971–4.
7. Leite JJ, Mansur AJ, de Freitas HF, Chizola PR, Bocchi EA, Terra-Filho M, Neder JA, Lorenzi-Filho G. Periodic breathing during incremental exercise predicts mortality in patients with chronic heart failure evaluated for cardiac transplantation. J Am Coll Cardiol. 2003;41:2175–81.
8. Corra U, Giordano A, Bosimini E, Mezzani A, Piepoli M, Coats AJ, Giannuzzi P. Oscillatory ventilation during exercise in patients with chronic heart failure: clinical correlates and prognostic implications. Chest. 2002;121:1572–80.

9. Corra U, Pistono M, Mezzani A, Braghiroli A, Giordano A, Lanfranchi P, Bosimini E, Gnemmi M, Giannuzzi P. Sleep and exertional periodic breathing in chronic heart failure: prognostic importance and interdependence. Circulation. 2006;113:44–50.

10. Guazzi M, Arena R, Ascione A, Piepoli M, Guazzi MD. Exercise oscillatory breathing and increased ventilation to carbon dioxide production slope in heart failure: an unfavorable combination with high prognostic value. Am Heart J. 2007;153:859–67.

11. Guazzi M, Raimondo R, Vicenzi M, Arena R, Proserpio C, Sarzi Braga S, Pedretti R. Exercise oscillatory ventilation may predict sudden cardiac death in heart failure patients. J Am Coll Cardiol. 2007;50:299–308.

12. Guazzi M, Boracchi P, Arena R, Myers J, Vicenzi M, Peberdy MA, Bensimhon D, Chase P, Reina G. Development of a cardiopulmonary exercise prognostic score for optimizing risk stratification in heart failure: the (P)e(R)i(O)dic (B)reathing during (E)xercise (PROBE) study. J Card Fail. 2010;16:799–805.

13. Arena R, Myers J, Abella J, Peberdy MA, Pinkstaff S, Bensimhon D, Chase P, Guazzi M. Prognostic value of timing and duration characteristics of exercise oscillatory ventilation in patients with heart failure. J Heart Lung Transplant. 2008;27:341–7.

14. Corra U, Mezzani A, Giordano A, Bosimini E, Giannuzzi P. Exercise haemodynamic variables rather than ventilatory efficiency indexes contribute to risk assessment in chronic heart failure patients treated with carvedilol. Eur Heart J. 2009;30:3000–6.

15. Cornelis J, Beckers P, Vanroy C, Volckaerts T, Vrints C, Vissers D. An overview of the applied definitions and diagnostic methods to assess exercise oscillatory ventilation – a systematic review. Int J Cardiol. 2015;190:161–9.

16. Sun XG, Hansen JE, Beshai JF, Wasserman K. Oscillatory breathing and exercise gas exchange abnormalities prognosticate early mortality and morbidity in heart failure. J Am Coll Cardiol. 2010;55:1814–23.

17. Francis DP, Davies LC, Piepoli M, Rauchhaus M, Ponikowski P, Coats AJ. Origin of oscillatory kinetics of respiratory gas exchange in chronic heart failure. Circulation. 1999;100:1065–70.

18. Agostoni P, Corra U, Cattadori G, Veglia F, La Gioia R, Scardovi AB, Emdin M, Metra M, Sinagra G, Limongelli G, Raimondo R, Re F, Guazzi M, Belardinelli R, Parati G, Magri D, Fiorentini C, Mezzani A, Salvioni E, Scrutinio D, Ricci R, Bettari L, Di Lenarda A, Pastormerlo LE, Pacileo G, Vaninetti R, Apostolo A, Iorio A, Paolillo S, Palermo P, Contini M, Confalonieri M, Giannuzzi P, Passantino A, Cas LD, Piepoli MF, Passino C. Metabolic exercise test data combined with cardiac and kidney indexes, the MECKI score: a multiparametric approach to heart failure prognosis. Int J Cardiol. 2013;167:2710–8.

19. Carubelli V, Metra M, Corra U, Magri D, Passino C, Lombardi C, Scrutinio D, Correale M, Cattadori G, Piepoli MF, Salvioni E, Giovannardi M, Raimondo R, Cicoira M, Belardinelli R, Guazzi M, Limongelli G, Clemenza F, Parati G, Scardovi AB, Di Lenarda A, Bussotti M, La Gioia R, Agostoni P. Exercise performance is a prognostic indicator in elderly patients with chronic heart failure – application of metabolic exercise cardiac kidney indexes score. Circ J. 2015;79(12):2608–15.

20. Scrutinio D, Agostoni P, Gesualdo L, Corra U, Mezzani A, Piepoli M, Di Lenarda A, Iorio A, Passino C, Magri D, Masarone D, Battaia E, Girola D, Re F, Cattadori G, Parati G, Sinagra G, Villani GQ, Limongelli G, Pacileo G, Guazzi M, Metra M, Frigerio M, Cicoira M, Mina C, Malfatto G, Caravita S, Bussotti M, Salvioni E, Veglia F, Correale M, Scardovi AB, Emdin M, Giannuzzi P, Gargiulo P, Giovannardi M, Perrone-Filardi P, Raimondo R, Ricci R, Paolillo S, Farina S, Belardinelli R, Passantino A, La Gioia R. Renal function and peak exercise oxygen consumption in chronic heart failure with reduced left ventricular ejection fraction. Circ J. 2015;79:583–91.

21. Lombardi C, Meriggi P, Agostoni P, Faini A, Bilo G, Revera M, Caldara G, Di Rienzo M, Castiglioni P, Maurizio B, Gregorini F, Mancia G, Parati G. High-altitude hypoxia and periodic breathing during sleep: gender-related differences. J Sleep Res. 2013;22:322–30.

22. Sin DD, Fitzgerald F, Parker JD, Newton G, Floras JS, Bradley TD. Risk factors for central and obstructive sleep apnea in 450 men and women with congestive heart failure. Am J Respir Crit Care Med. 1999;160:1101–6.

23. Costanzo MR, Khayat R, Ponikowski P, Augostini R, Stellbrink C, Mianulli M, Abraham WT. Mechanisms and clinical consequences of untreated central sleep apnea in heart failure. J Am Coll Cardiol. 2015;65:72–84.
24. Yu J, Zhang JF, Fletcher EC. Stimulation of breathing by activation of pulmonary peripheral afferents in rabbits. J Appl Physiol. 1998;85:1485–92.
25. Pryor WW. Cheyne-Stokes respiration in patients with cardiac enlargement and prolonged circulation time. Circulation. 1951;4:233–8.
26. Javaheri S, Parker TJ, Liming JD, Corbett WS, Nishiyama H, Wexler L, Roselle GA. Sleep apnea in 81 ambulatory male patients with stable heart failure. Types and their prevalences, consequences, and presentations. Circulation. 1998;97:2154–9.
27. Bradley TD, Floras JS. Sleep apnea and heart failure: part II: central sleep apnea. Circulation. 2003;107:1822–6.
28. Dhakal BP, Murphy RM, Lewis GD. Exercise oscillatory ventilation in heart failure. Trends in Cardiovascular Medicine. 2012;22:185–91.
29. Schmid JP, Apostolo A, Antonioli L, Cattadori G, Zurek M, Contini M, Agostoni P. Influence of exertional oscillatory ventilation on exercise performance in heart failure. Eur J Cardiovasc Prev Rehabil. 2008;15:688–92.
30. Bussotti M, Apostolo A, Andreini D, Palermo P, Contini M, Agostoni P. Cardiopulmonary evidence of exercise-induced silent ischaemia. Eur J Cardiovasc Prev Rehabil. 2006;13:249–53.
31. Belardinelli R, Lacalaprice F, Carle F, Minnucci A, Cianci G, Perna G, D'Eusanio G. Exercise-induced myocardial ischaemia detected by cardiopulmonary exercise testing. Eur Heart J. 2003;24:1304–13.
32. Francis DP, Davies LC, Willson K, Wensel R, Ponikowski P, Coats AJ, Piepoli M. Impact of periodic breathing on measurement of oxygen uptake and respiratory exchange ratio during cardiopulmonary exercise testing. Clin Sci (Lond). 2002;103:543–52.
33. Apostolo A, Agostoni P, Contini M, Antonioli L, Swenson ER. Acetazolamide and inhaled carbon dioxide reduce periodic breathing during exercise in patients with chronic heart failure. J Card Fail. 2014;20:278–88.
34. Schultz HD, Marcus NJ. Heart failure and carotid body chemoreception. In: Nurse C, editor. Arterial chemoreception: from molecules to systems, Advances in experimental medicine and biology. New York: Springer; 2012. p. 387–95.
35. Joho S, Ushijima R, Akabane T, Oda Y, Inoue H. Adaptive servo-ventilation improves exercise oscillatory ventilation and ventilatory inefficiency in patients with heart failure and central sleep apnea. IJC Metab Endocrine. 2013;1:20–6.
36. Guazzi M, Vicenzi M, Arena R. Phosphodiesterase 5 inhibition with sildenafil reverses exercise oscillatory breathing in chronic heart failure: a long-term cardiopulmonary exercise testing placebo-controlled study. Eur J Heart Fail. 2012;14:82–90.
37. Zurek M, Corra U, Piepoli MF, Binder RK, Saner H, Schmid JP. Exercise training reverses exertional oscillatory ventilation in heart failure patients. Eur Respir J. 2012;40:1238–44.
38. Arzt M, Schulz M, Wensel R, Montalvan S, Blumberg FC, Riegger GA, Pfeifer M. Nocturnal continuous positive airway pressure improves ventilatory efficiency during exercise in patients with chronic heart failure. Chest. 2005;127:794–802.
39. Teschler H, Dohring J, Wang YM, Berthon-Jones M. Adaptive pressure support servo-ventilation: a novel treatment for Cheyne-Stokes respiration in heart failure. Am J Respir Crit Care Med. 2001;164:614–9.
40. Philippe C, Stoica-Herman M, Drouot X, Raffestin B, Escourrou P, Hittinger L, Michel PL, Rouault S, d'Ortho MP. Compliance with and effectiveness of adaptive servoventilation versus continuous positive airway pressure in the treatment of Cheyne-Stokes respiration in heart failure over a six month period. Heart. 2006;92:337–42.
41. Oldenburg O, Schmidt A, Lamp B, Bitter T, Muntean BG, Langer C, Horstkotte D. Adaptive servoventilation improves cardiac function in patients with chronic heart failure and Cheyne-Stokes respiration. Eur J Heart Fail. 2008;10:581–6.
42. Corra U, Piepoli MF, Adamopoulos S, Agostoni P, Coats AJ, Conraads V, Lambrinou E, Pieske B, Piotrowicz E, Schmid JP, Seferovic PM, Anker SD, Filippatos G, Ponikowski

PP. Cardiopulmonary exercise testing in systolic heart failure in 2014: the evolving prognostic role: a position paper from the committee on exercise physiology and training of the heart failure association of the ESC. Eur J Heart Fail. 2014;16:929–41.

43. Corra U, Giordano A, Mezzani A, Gnemmi M, Pistono M, Caruso R, Giannuzzi P. Cardiopulmonary exercise testing and prognosis in heart failure due to systolic left ventricular dysfunction: a validation study of the European Society of Cardiology Guidelines and Recommendations (2008) and further developments. Eur J Prev Cardiol. 2012;19:32–40.

To Breathe, or Not to Breathe: That Is the Question

9

Gianluca Mirizzi, Alberto Giannoni, Claudio Passino, and Michele Emdin

Abbreviations

ACE	Angiotensin converting enzyme
AHI	Apnea-hypopnea index
AT-1	Angiotensin receptor 1
CPAP	Continuous positive airway pressure
CSR	Cheyne-Stokes respiration
HF	Heart failure
LA	Left atrium
LVEF	Left ventricular ejection fraction
MRA	Mineralocorticoid receptor antagonist
MSNA	Muscle sympathetic nerve activity
NE	Norepinephrine
NT-proBNP	N-terminal fragment of pro-brain natriuretic peptide
NYHA	New York Heart Association
OSA	Obstructive sleep apnea
PSG	Polysomnography

G. Mirizzi, MD (✉) • C. Passino, MD • M. Emdin, MD, PhD
Institute of Life Sciences, Scuola Superiore Sant'Anna, Pisa, Italy

Division of Cardiology and Cardiovascular Medicine, Fondazione Toscana G. Monasterio, Pisa, Italy
e-mail: gianluca.mirizzi@ftgm.it; passino@ftgm.it; emdin@ftgm.it, m.emdin@sssup.it

A. Giannoni, MD, PhD
Division of Cardiology and Cardiovascular Medicine, Fondazione Toscana G. Monasterio, Pisa, Italy
e-mail: alberto.giannoni@ftgm.it

© Springer International Publishing Switzerland 2017
M. Emdin et al. (eds.), *The Breathless Heart*,
DOI 10.1007/978-3-319-26354-0_9

9.1   Introduction

Despite the unquestionable achievements of medical and device therapy, the substantial morbidity and mortality still associated with HF have stimulated the search for new therapeutic targets through a careful pathophysiological investigation. In this setting, one of the most promising fields is represented by the study of cardiorespiratory interaction and, in particular, the investigation of the role of altered breathing patterns in HF. Several research contributions have described a significant incidence of both obstructive and central apnea in patients with heart failure (HF), as already outlined in Chaps. 5 and 6. While obstructive sleep apneas (OSA) seems mainly a risk factor leading to the development of HF [1], central apneas or Cheyne-Stokes respiration (CSR) are thought to be a real contributor to HF progression and mortality once HF is established. While the majority of studies actually identified CSR as a prognosticator in HF [2–5], there are a few studies in which at least nocturnal CSR was not associated with mortality [6, 7]. Moreover, the only two therapeutic trials, which have challenged the impact of continuous positive airway pressure (CPAP) and assisted servo ventilation (ASV) on HF mortality, actually failed to show any benefit in treating central apneas and rather harmed some patients [8, 9]. These conflicting results have finally led to dispute the detrimental significance of CSR against a putative protective connotation of the phenomenon. Indeed, while the majority of researchers still consider CSR as a negative player in HF, the group of Naughton has raised some conceptual points in favor of a protective role of CSR in HF [10].

The aim of this chapter is thus to discuss the evidences supporting both sides of the question, elucidating the supposedly protective or detrimental effect of CSR in systolic HF.

9.2   To Take Arms Against a Sea of Troubles and by Opposing End Them. *Periodic Breathing as a Compensatory Phenomenon. The Naughton's Hypothesis* (Hyperpnea Versus Apnea; Beneficial Effects on Hemodynamics, Ventilation and Other)

9.2.1   Is Really Cheyne-Stokes Respiration Detrimental?

The original description of the waxing and waning oscillation of breathing made by John Cheyne and Willam Stokes was actually made in patients with presumably heart failure during the day (see Chap. 1); since then, the occurrence of the phenomenon was assumed to be linked to the severity of the underlying disease, thus acquiring a negative connotation still present today. As we will see, CSR in HF is actually linked to a worse clinical phenotype and increasing evidences point to the prognostic significance of its occurrence in HF patients. Given these premises, several attempts, both pharmacological and device based, have been made in order to correct this respiratory disturbance and prove the survival advantage of these interventions (see Chaps. 12 and 13). Despite the supportive pathophysiological background and encouraging results from small pivotal studies, much of the efforts have resulted in neutral outcomes and, in some occasions, they showed an actual harm of the new approaches so far. Following these delusional outcomes, alternative explanations have been proposed to resolve this paradox; one of these points to the possibility of an actual *protective* role of CSR in HF, or at least of a compensatory one. This argument has been named "Naughton's hypothesis" according to the principal researcher that proposed it. The Naughton's hypothesis is based on the evidence that the common detrimental effects usually related to central apnea are based on speculative associations and not on causative correlation.

Central apnea and CSR derive from the summation of a periodic oscillator on an already oscillatory phenomenon, that is, respiration with its alternation of inspiratory and expiratory movements mediated by a set of respiratory muscles. These are composed of inspiratory muscles (diaphragm, external intercostal muscles, sternocleidomastoids, and *anterior serratii*) and expiratory muscles (abdominal *recti*, internal intercostal muscles); during quiet respiration only the first set of muscles works, while during effort and frequent respiration also the second set intervenes, in order to support the elastic recoil that normally suffices for quiet expiration. Increased respiratory frequency leads to an increase in respiratory muscles blood oxygen consumption, with inspiratory muscles recruitment followed by expiratory muscles during hyperventilation [11]; this redistribution of blood flow in a condition of reduced cardiac output could be either insufficient to support muscles work or impair perfusion to other vital organs. Thus cyclic periods of rest could redistribute this altered supply of blood flow from essential organs to less noble ones and provide a period of rest to the respiratory muscles, which in turn could translate in a reduction of the perception of dyspnea [12] (Fig. 9.1).

CSR imposes also oscillations in intrathoracic pressures and hence in transmural left ventricular pressure; these swings are estimated to be in the range of 25 mmHg; however, comparing these to that imposed by obstructive sleep apnea events, CSR intrathoracic pressure swings are less significant both in magnitude and variability, the obstructive swings being estimated in the range of 30–120 mmHg [13].

CSR imposes also oscillations in preload and afterload. Hyperventilation seems a consequence of increased venous pressure in the pulmonary circulation with consequent stimulation of J-receptors; the resultant hypocapnia, combined with reduced cardiac output and hence increased circulatory time, drives the respiratory control under the "apneic threshold", thus destabilizing respiration and paving the way to the appearance of CSR. Hemodynamic effects of voluntary hyperventilation have been investigated by Oldenburg et al. [14] in individuals either volunteers or affected by systolic heart failure (mean left ventricular ejection fraction – LVEF – $32\pm7\%$, NYHA class 2.6 ± 0.6). Both groups (15 vs 20 individuals, respectively) underwent hemodynamic monitoring either noninvasively (volunteers' group) or by right and left cardiac catheterization (HF group). Irrespective of the group evaluated, hyperventilation induced an increase in cardiac output driven mainly by an increase in heart rate (despite beta-blockers) and a decrease in systemic vascular resistance while stroke volume was not affected. The authors

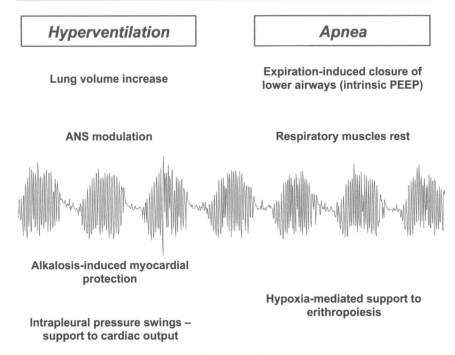

Fig. 9.1 Proposed compensatory and beneficial effects of Cheyne-Stokes respiration in heart failure. On the *left*, the consequences of hyperventilation phase, on the *right* those of the apnea. *PEEP* positive end-expiratory pressure

conclude that these effects, being part of a "quick reaction" response to reduced cardiac output, might be compensatory and "cardioprotective" in CSR but prove themselves deleterious in the long run, mainly due to the tachycardia [15–19]. Yumino et al. [20] also compared the effect of central events (apnea or hypopneas) versus obstructive events in HF patients, using a noninvasive method of stroke volume and cardiac output measure, based on digital photoplethysmographic determination and comparing the last 5 s before apnea and the last 5 s of the apneic events. They found that cardiac output and stroke volume are reduced in obstructive events (6.8 % and 5.0 % decrease, respectively) compared to central events in which the two parameters actually grew (2.6 % and 2.5 % increase, respectively); these observations were made both in patients with solely obstructive or central apnea and with a combination of the two patterns.

A known feature of central apnea is that it goes together with increased adrenergic activity. In a cohort of patients with congestive HF with and without CSR, adrenergic activation, estimated with plasma norepinephrine (NE) levels and overnight urinary NE levels, resulted significantly higher in the former group; correction of the breathing pattern during sleep with nasal continuous positive airway pressure (CPAP) resulted in a drop on urinary and plasma levels of norepinephrine [21]. However, it should be noted that this study was undertaken in a pre-beta-blockers era and that CPAP also augmented left ventricular ejection fraction, a possible contributor to the reduction of adrenergic activity in the treated group. In fact, as demonstrated by the same author in a subsequent study in HF patients without CSR, spontaneous breathing is associated with muscles sympathetic nerve activity (MSNA) but the magnitude of the effect is little [22]; moreover, as shown by Solin [23], increased sympathetic activity is an hallmark of congestive HF and is further increased by the presence of obstructive or central sleep apnea; however, when considering the predictors of sympathetic activity in HF, the degree of hemodynamic compromise is a much more potent contributor than the disordered breathing itself. This latter observation has been elegantly confirmed in a study performed on HF patients with and without CSR and obstructive sleep apnea using right heart catheterization and cardiac NE spillover; sympathetic nerve activity and cardiac NE spillover were shown to be greater in patients with CSR but only pulmonary artery pressure and pulmonary capillary wedge pressure were associated either with plasma NE and total and cardiac NE spillovers [24].

9.2.2   Is Cheyne-Stokes Respiration Compensatory?

The arguments just showed corroborate the hypothesis that CSR could prove itself less harmful than commonly thought; however, could CSR prove itself actually *protective* in the setting of HF? In a seminal contribution, Naughton enumerated a sequence of eight arguments to support this hypothesis [10]; because CSR is constituted by the alternation of two moments, hyperpnoea and apnea, the arguments are also related some to the former and others to the latter.

First, during the hyperventilatory phase, lung volume increases to the extent of 400 ml [25]; the magnitude of the increase is boosted during concomitant hypoxia, albeit at the cost of increased respiratory muscles activity. This adaptation could, on one side, augment the oxygen storage and on the other increase the end expiratory pressure thus ameliorating pulmonary gas exchange.

Second, ventilatory swings and alternations between inspiration and expiration exert a modulatory effect on cardiovascular autonomic control. Increases in lung volume and in respiratory depth reduce MSNA in normal humans [26]. In patients with HF and CSR, there is an increase in MSNA with respect to controls; however, the magnitude is modest and there is a trend toward the reduction of MSNA during the hyperpneic phases [27] and, as already shown, sympathetic activity contribution in CSR patients is related at least in part to HF hemodynamic severity [23].

Third, the metabolic consequences of hyperventilation, that is the variation of pH toward alkalosis, may positively impact on myocardial function due to the positive effects of hypocapnia and alkalosis on cardiotoxic left ventricular dysfunction [28]. Other reports support a myocardial "protective" effect of alkalosis: in an in vitro preparation of myocardial cells, exposure to hypoxia and acid pH resulted in a reduction of contractile force, while no effect on contractility was elicited by alkalosis; however, on restoration of oxygenation only acid-exposed cells regained contractility [29]. These observations reflect the effects of hypocapnia on canine model of pulmonary edema, where no effect on cardiac output was recorded in comparison with normocapnia [30].

As mentioned, hyperpnea-induced variations in intrapleural pressure during central apnea are significantly less than during obstructive events [13]; however, even these small variations could act as a supporting pump for heart with reduced cardiac output. In support to this, the variations of intrapleural pressure induced during cough have been reported to be even better in terms of produced aortic pressure variations than standard cardiac compressions [31]. Using Doppler indirect evaluation of cardiac hemodynamic changes during alternations of apnea and hyperpnea during CSR, Maze et al. [32] showed that left ventricular outflow tract velocities, approximations of stroke volume, were higher at the end of the hyperpneic phase.

Another argument in support of a compensatory role for CSR in HF comes from the observation that the apneic phase results in a prolonged expiration that leads to the closure of the lower airways, thus providing a spontaneous positive end-expiratory pressure to prevent alveolar closure and thus preserving blood-air interface. This supporting pressure, like CPAP, may be useful for the failing heart in reducing venous return to an overloaded left ventricle, improving oxygenation and thus hemodynamic profile [33, 34].

Eventually, CSR may prove protective against anemia-related consequences in HF patients [35]. This theoretical relationship is based on the observation of the disappearance of CSR during treatment with erythropoietin and iron in anemic HF patients [36]; ideally, CSR may act as compensation against HF-induced anemia stimulating, by hypoxia, bone marrow and erythropoiesis.

9.2.3 To Die, to Sleep: *Periodic Breathing Is Bad for You* (Detrimental Effects on Hemodynamics, Neurohormonal Activation, and Prognostic Value of Apneas in Heart Failure)

Against the just-mentioned evidences of potential compensatory influences of CSR in HF stands a long series of arguments that suggest otherwise.

Behind the points just evaluated stands a pitfall: each argument is associated with a particular phase of the CSR, that is, hyperpnoea or apnea, so one could argument that every positive phenomenon associated with one phase could be counteracted by the opposite phenomenon acting during the subsequent phase.

Furthermore, recurring verifications of results in pre- and post-beta-blockers era and the consistency of the data coming from series of numerous patients suggest that CSR play a negative role in HF.

The general theory behind the development of apnea of central origin is that an initial destabilization of the normally stable breathing oscillator, instead of completely deranging the breathing pattern, leads to the development of another superimposed oscillatory breathing rhythm characterized by alternating periods of apnea and hyperpnoea. The sustaining mechanism behind this phenomenon lays in the development of hypocapnia, typically the result of initial hyperventilation due to stimulation of pulmonary J receptors. The drop in CO_2 tension in the blood might then go under the so-called *apneic threshold*, thus stopping ventilation. The consequent increase in CO_2 and the increased sensitivity of central chemoreceptor in HF [37, 38] cause rebound hyperventilation and hence the loop is instituted [39] (Fig. 9.2).

The initial observations of CSR in HF pointed prevalently to the description of the clinical features of the disordered breathing pattern; Hanly et al. [40] first noted, in a small cohort of ten HF patients, that CSR, detected with polysomnography (PSG) during sleep, was associated with some features like hypoxemia and sleep arousals/disruption, and suggested a possible negative role of these findings on overall health status of these patients. This issue has been subsequently reinforced by several observations trying to explain the possible impact of CSR on prognosis in HF patients.

In a cohort of 16 patients with ischemic heart disease and HF, again Hanly [3] showed that the patients with CSR had worse prognosis on Kaplan-Meier analysis despite similar LVEF and oxygen saturation at sleep study. Andreas [41] studied 36 patients (5 women) with congestive HF (mean LVEF $20 \pm 8\,\%$) prevalently of idiopathic dilated origin with overnight PSG and showed that the single parameter that differentiated patients regarding their prognosis was left ventricular systolic function. Patients with CSR during sleep had similar prognosis in comparison of those without; however, as the authors noted, the only two patients with daytime CSR died, suggesting a prognostic impact of daytime respiratory disturbances. The number of the patients evaluated greatly limits the reliability of the results regarding prognostic significance of the parameters evaluated; however, the patients with CSR had increased left atrial diameter, reduced vital capacity, and increased transit time (estimated from the difference in time between the increase of respiration and the nadir of oxygen saturation).

A later contribution from the study of Lanfranchi, which evaluated 54 patients with systolic HF, found at multivariate analysis that night-time apnea-hypopnea

Mechanism of Periodic Breathing

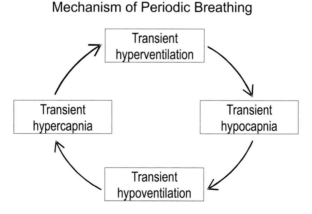

Fig. 9.2 Feedback loop at the basis of Cheyne-Stokes respiration institution. Alternation of period of reduced ventilation and consequent hypocapnia

index (AHI) was associated, together with left atrial (LA) volume, with increased risk of cardiac mortality; this translated in a worse outcome at Kaplan-Meyer analysis, especially when the two factors acted together. Despite the limited number of patients and a therapy not comparable to that of actual guideline-directed therapy (no patient was on beta-blocker or had received implantable cardioverter-defibrillator), this work for the first time documented a relationship between a measure of the incidence of the apnea phenomenon and cardiac mortality and set an arbitrary cut-point to define patients with severe forms of CSR who are at high risk of cardiac events. In this work, in fact, patients with AHI > 30 events/h had lower LVEF, worse diastolic function, reduced functional capacity during exercise and, notably, an autonomic function profile indicating adrenergic activation (lower baroreflex sensitivity, reduced heart rate variability both during 24 h and during night time) [42].

The first objection to the alleged prognostic significance of CSR in HF came from the contribution of Roebuck [7] who showed, in a population of 77 patients with HF, that the presence of sleep apnea, irrespective of its central or obstructive origin, did not actually increase the risk of death. Despite this conclusion, they showed that patients with central apnea (33 patients) had worse pulmonary capillary wedge pressure compared to obstructive sleep apnea patients and no-apnea patients (22.4±7.1 vs. 13.0±5.7 and 11.5±7.1 mmHg, respectively), albeit they had similar LVEF.

The quest for a definitive answer to the issue of the prognostic significance of CSR in HF is still ongoing; after these initial reports, in fact, a rarefaction of studies on this field was observed, probably as a consequence of the negative findings stemming from the Canadian Continuous Positive Airway Pressure (CANPAP) trial [8] that did not find an advantage of noninvasive ventilation with continuous positive pressure on survival. Since then, three subsequent studies investigated the role of nocturnal CSR in HF, and again inconclusive results came from these observations. Jilek et al. evaluated a population of 275 patients with systolic left ventricular dysfunction who underwent nocturnal PSG and were under adequate therapy regarding neurohormonal antagonism (>85 % on beta-blockers, >90 % on ACE-inhibitors/AT-1 blockers, >40 % on MRA). They found that patients with severe sleep disordered breathing, defined as AHI > 22.5 ev/h, irrespective of central or obstructive origin, had worse outcome; a subanalysis showed that patients with severe central sleep apnea had worse prognosis (38 % mortality vs. 16 % in those with mild central apnea) while no differences in mortality were observed in those with severe obstructive sleep apnea [4]. Damy et al. also evaluated a population of systolic HF patients (n=384) with nocturnal PSG and again found that those with sleep disordered breathing (AHI > 5 ev/h, irrespective of their obstructive or central origin) where associated with worse outcomes, especially those with central apneas, who experienced an outcome rate of 24 % in the first year compared to 13 % in those with OSA [2]. Recently, Grimm et al. studied a large population (n=267) of systolic HF patients who were searched for central apnea during night and found that its presence did not predict a worse outcome [6].

Apart from the association between CSR and markers of disease severity, CSR might be associated, by means of the alternations themselves of cycles of hyperpnea and apnea, to unfavorable consequences. These effects, some of which are speculative (as for the Naughton hypothesis) and need confirmation, are hence proposed as hypotheses generating and are listed below (Fig. 9.3):

1. Hyperventilation is associated with increase in dead space [43] and might induce, by the effect of the summation of subsequent very rapid shallow inspirations, an increase in functional dead space, reducing air circulation in the lungs.
2. Just as apnea might facilitate respiratory muscles rest, hyperventilation might produce excessive and futile contractions, thus augmenting the net oxygen consumption.
3. intrapleural pressure swings might result in too fast and possibly uncoordinated pre- and afterload fluctuations which might actually reduce cardiac output.
4. Period of apnea might produce an excess in adrenergic activation, especially in a context of an already heightened tone, not compensated by autonomic nervous system modulation induced by respiration; this could lead, in turn, to an excess in ventricular and supraventricular arrhythmias [37].
5. Oscillations of oxygen saturation between too low or too high values might predispose to cellular damage similar to that of reperfusion injury [44].
6. During apnea, hypoxia could also lead to transient acidosis and cellular damage [45].

Altogether, the collection of the above-mentioned evidences does not allow to clear completely the clouds that surround the impact of central apnea on the life

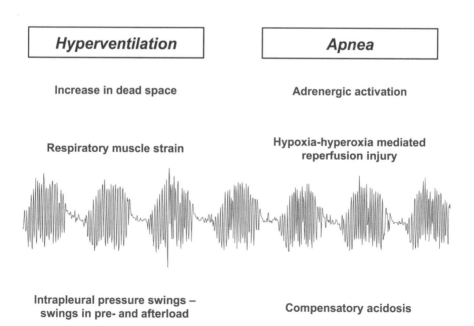

Fig. 9.3 Proposed detrimental effects of Cheyne-Stokes respiration in heart failure. On the *left*, the consequences of hyperventilation phase, on the *right* those of the apnea

span of patients with systolic HF, despite its rather strong association with markers of disease severity or progression. One reason, as Olbenburg noted [14] and as already shown in this chapter, might rely on a compensatory role of the phenomenon in the first moments of its development or alternatively in less severe and earlier forms of cardiac failure.

Another plausible reason that lacks widespread acknowledgment and adds further negative connotation to CSR is the recognition that central apnea, albeit more frequent during night due to the shift of the ventilatory control from partially voluntary efforts to metabolic influences, may not be relegated only in this period, but may also continue during daytime. To date, only three studies addressed this topic [46–48] but, significantly and despite the different methods used to evaluate daytime CSR, all showed a prognostic significance of daytime CSR in HF. One of the most significant contribution on this topic comes from Brack et al., who showed, in a population of 60 ambulatory systolic HF patients, monitored with 24-h cardiorespiratory recordings, that daytime CSR was observable in 16 % of the population (Fig. 9.4) and, in those where CSR was present in more than 10 % of the time, CSR predicted a worse prognosis. In the attempt to characterize the possible predictors of

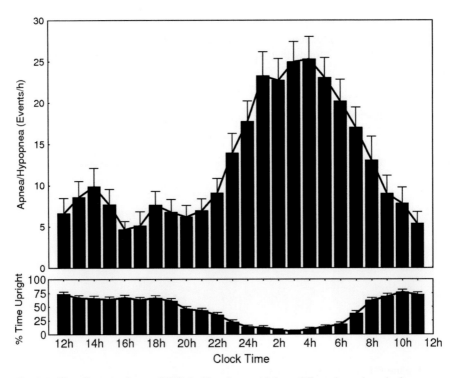

Fig. 9.4 Circadian prevalence of CSR in 60 patients with heart failure shown hour by hour over 24 h. *Upper panel*: number of events per hour (*bars*) with the respective SE (*whiskers*); *lower panel*: mean percentage of time spent upright (*bars*; SE, *whiskers*) (Reproduced with permission from Ref. [46])

daytime CSR, the authors considered several variables but the only one that correlated with daytime CSR at multivariate regression analysis was the plasma levels on brain natriuretic peptide; they also showed a similar level of LVEF. These observations were similar to those of Poletti et al., who evaluated a wider population (n = 147) finding as independent predictors of CSR only age and levels of NT-proBNP; significantly, patients underwent a complete neurohormonal characterization that showed that CSR patients had an activation of neurohormonal systems, in particular of the adrenergic and natriuretic peptides and worse indexes of left ventricular function. This latter point is further stressed by the work of La Rovere et al., who showed, in a population of systolic HF patients, that the presence of periodic breathing was associated with worse LVEF and increased left ventricular diameters, alongside with more advanced mitral regurgitation and reduced heart rate variability; it is of note that, in this study, only 26 % of patients were on beta-blocker therapy vs. 74 % of patients in the work of Poletti and 85 % of patients in the work of Brack. Following this reasoning, a possible explanation of the different results might be the protective role of neurohormonal antagonism on left ventricular function that however fails to prevent completely the development of CSR, which is only favored but not exclusively determined by left ventricular dysfunction. From this point of view, we must recall the impact of two other factors that lead to CSR development, that is, activation of chemoreflexes and pulmonary congestion.

Chemoreflex sensitivity to hypoxia or hypercapnia are two established companions in the HF cohort of altered feedback loops, alongside baroreflex sensitivity and ergoreceptor activation [38, 49–51]. CSR is one of the possible consequences of activation of chemoreceptor sensitivity to hypercapnia due to the induced shift in plasma tension of CO_2 toward lower levels, possibly under the apneic threshold [38]; however, peripheral chemosensitivity to hypoxia could participate in CSR induction, as suggested by the observation that increased hypoxic ventilatory response, a measure of hypoxic chemosensitivity, is associated with increased prevalence of daytime CSR; the respiratory disturbance is further enhanced by the combined activation of hypoxic and hypercapnic chemosensitivity [37].

Most importantly, apnea episodes are triggers of chemosensitivity: each time a drop in arterial oxygen saturation or an increase in carbon dioxide tension occurs there is a stimulation of, respectively, peripheral and central chemoreceptors. Activation of peripheral and/or central chemosensitivities are associated with markers of disease severity like arrhythmic burden, both supraventricular and ventricular, and activation of both the adrenergic and natriuretic peptides axes [37]; by means of these associations, repetitive episodes of apnea, by inducing phasic activation of the reflexes [38] may thus impact on prognosis in patients with HF.

Pulmonary congestion could promote CSR development in several ways. First, congestion could increase pulmonary J receptors and hence ventilation; one of the hypothesis behind this association is that of "rostral fluid shift", which states that during night time, the supine position favors the shift of fluid from the legs to more cranial position, inducing either mechanical restriction of upper airways and hence obstructive events or pulmonary congestion and hence hyperventilation and hypocapnia, thus favoring central apneic events [52]. Another possibility is that chemoreflex-induced cycles of hypoxia/hypercapnia, determined by cycles of apnea/hyperventilation during CSR, may lead to increased pulmonary resistance and consequent increase in pulmonary arterial pressures. Giannoni et al. demonstrated this link by observing, in HF patients with CSR, an association between the perturbed respiratory pattern and indexes of right ventricular remodeling and pulmonary pressures; determinants of increased pulmonary pressures were activation of peripheral and central chemosensitivity and activation of adrenergic system [53].

Conclusions

CSR is a chief feature of systolic HF, but whether it is detrimental for itself is still a matter of debate. Numerous contributions highlight the prognostic weight that it carries, either when developing during night or daytime, and different experiences stress the unfavorable features that go alongside this kind of periodic breathing pattern.

Apart from this point of view stands another suggestion, that CSR may be not as dangerous as commonly thought; rather, some studies underline a possible compensatory role for CSR, others even a beneficial one. The explanation of this fascinating dilemma stays, as always, in the meaningful and continuous examination of the problem from different perspectives, for example, considering the phenomenon in all of its integrity (CSR spanning throughout the 24 h and not only night-time vs. daytime) and considering always the mechanisms that may determine it (chemoreflex sensitivity).

Moreover, further task are needed to clarify the impact of CSR in different phases of disease progression, for different momentum or even different kind of it are supposable whether it occurs in patients with asymptomatic left ventricular dysfunction, clinically evident heart failure or terminal cardiac failure. In fact, while CSR might act as compensatory in the first stages of the disease, in the long run the compensations, when persistently activated, could provoke deleterious effect and produce progression of cardiac failure. These achievements might shed some light on this argument thus impacting on clinical practice and treatment modalities.

References

1. Shahar E, Whitney CW, Redline S, Lee ET, Newman AB, Nieto FJ, O'Connor GT, Boland LL, Schwartz JE, Samet JM. Sleep-disordered breathing and cardiovascular disease: cross-sectional results of the Sleep Heart Health Study. Am J Respir Crit Care Med. 2001;163:19–25.
2. Damy T, Margarit L, Noroc A, Bodez D, Guendouz S, Boyer L, Drouot X, Lamine A, Paulino A, Rappeneau S, Stoica MH, Dubois-Rande JL, Adnot S, Hittinger L, d'Ortho MP. Prognostic impact of sleep-disordered breathing and its treatment with nocturnal ventilation for chronic heart failure. Eur J Heart Fail. 2012;14:1009–19.
3. Hanly PJ, Zuberi-Khokhar NS. Increased mortality associated with Cheyne-Stokes respiration in patients with congestive heart failure. Am J Respir Crit Care Med. 1996;153:272–6.

4. Jilek C, Krenn M, Sebah D, Obermeier R, Braune A, Kehl V, Schroll S, Montalvan S, Riegger GA, Pfeifer M, Arzt M. Prognostic impact of sleep disordered breathing and its treatment in heart failure: an observational study. Eur J Heart Fail. 2011;13:68–75.
5. Sin DD, Logan AG, Fitzgerald FS, Liu PP, Bradley TD. Effects of continuous positive airway pressure on cardiovascular outcomes in heart failure patients with and without Cheyne-Stokes respiration. Circulation. 2000;102:61–6.
6. Grimm W, Sosnovskaya A, Timmesfeld N, Hildebrandt O, Koehler U. Prognostic impact of central sleep apnea in patients with heart failure. J Card Fail. 2015;21:126–33.
7. Roebuck T, Solin P, Kaye DM, Bergin P, Bailey M, Naughton MT. Increased long-term mortality in heart failure due to sleep apnoea is not yet proven. Eur Respir J. 2004;23:735–40.
8. Bradley TD, Logan AG, Kimoff RJ, Series F, Morrison D, Ferguson K, Belenkie I, Pfeifer M, Fleetham J, Hanly P, Smilovitch M, Tomlinson G, Floras JS, Investigators C. Continuous positive airway pressure for central sleep apnea and heart failure. N Engl J Med. 2005;353:2025–33.
9. Cowie MR, Woehrle H, Wegscheider K, Angermann C, d'Ortho MP, Erdmann E, Levy P, Simonds AK, Somers VK, Zannad F, Teschler H. Adaptive servo-ventilation for central sleep apnea in systolic heart failure. N Engl J Med. 2015;373:1095–105.
10. Naughton MT. Cheyne-Stokes respiration: friend or foe? Thorax. 2012;67:357–60.
11. Robertson Jr CH, Pagel MA, Johnson Jr RL. The distribution of blood flow, oxygen consumption, and work output among the respiratory muscles during unobstructed hyperventilation. J Clin Invest. 1977;59:43–50.
12. Killian KJ, Jones NL. Respiratory muscles and dyspnea. Clin Chest Med. 1988;9:237–48.
13. Tkacova R, Rankin F, Fitzgerald FS, Floras JS, Bradley TD. Effects of continuous positive airway pressure on obstructive sleep apnea and left ventricular afterload in patients with heart failure. Circulation. 1998;98:2269–75.
14. Oldenburg O, Spiesshofer J, Fox H, Bitter T, Horstkotte D. Cheyne-Stokes respiration in heart failure: friend or foe? Hemodynamic effects of hyperventilation in heart failure patients and healthy volunteers. Clin Res Cardiol. 2015;104:328–33.
15. Bohm M, Borer J, Ford I, Gonzalez-Juanatey JR, Komajda M, Lopez-Sendon J, Reil JC, Swedberg K, Tavazzi L. Heart rate at baseline influences the effect of ivabradine on cardiovascular outcomes in chronic heart failure: analysis from the SHIFT study. Clin Res Cardiol. 2013;102:11–22.
16. Bohm M, Swedberg K, Komajda M, Borer JS, Ford I, Dubost-Brama A, Lerebours G, Tavazzi L, Investigators S. Heart rate as a risk factor in chronic heart failure (SHIFT): the association between heart rate and outcomes in a randomised placebo-controlled trial. Lancet. 2010;376:886–94.
17. Castagno D, Skali H, Takeuchi M, Swedberg K, Yusuf S, Granger CB, Michelson EL, Pfeffer MA, McMurray JJ, Solomon SD, Investigators C. Association of heart rate and outcomes in a broad spectrum of patients with chronic heart failure: results from the CHARM (Candesartan in Heart Failure: Assessment of Reduction in Mortality and morbidity) program. J Am Coll Cardiol. 2012;59:1785–95.
18. Fujita B, Franz M, Goebel B, Fritzenwanger M, Figulla HR, Kuethe F, Ferrari M, Jung C. Prognostic relevance of heart rate at rest for survival and the quality of life in patients with dilated cardiomyopathy. Clin Res Cardiol. 2012;101:701–7.
19. Lonn EM, Rambihar S, Gao P, Custodis FF, Sliwa K, Teo KK, Yusuf S, Bohm M. Heart rate is associated with increased risk of major cardiovascular events, cardiovascular and all-cause death in patients with stable chronic cardiovascular disease: an analysis of ONTARGET/TRANSCEND. Clin Res Cardiol. 2014;103:149–59.
20. Yumino D, Kasai T, Kimmerly D, Amirthalingam V, Floras JS, Bradley TD. Differing effects of obstructive and central sleep apneas on stroke volume in patients with heart failure. Am J Respir Crit Care Med. 2013;187:433–8.
21. Naughton MT, Benard DC, Liu PP, Rutherford R, Rankin F, Bradley TD. Effects of nasal CPAP on sympathetic activity in patients with heart failure and central sleep apnea. Am J Respir Crit Care Med. 1995;152:473–9.

22. Naughton MT, Floras JS, Rahman MA, Jamal M, Bradley TD. Respiratory correlates of muscle sympathetic nerve activity in heart failure. Clin Sci (Lond). 1998;95:277–85.
23. Solin P, Kaye DM, Little PJ, Bergin P, Richardson M, Naughton MT. Impact of sleep apnea on sympathetic nervous system activity in heart failure. Chest. 2003;123:1119–26.
24. Mansfield D, Kaye DM, Brunner La Rocca H, Solin P, Esler MD, Naughton MT. Raised sympathetic nerve activity in heart failure and central sleep apnea is due to heart failure severity. Circulation. 2003;107:1396–400.
25. Brack T, Jubran A, Laghi F, Tobin MJ. Fluctuations in end-expiratory lung volume during Cheyne-Stokes respiration. Am J Respir Crit Care Med. 2005;171:1408–13.
26. Seals DR, Suwarno NO, Dempsey JA. Influence of lung volume on sympathetic nerve discharge in normal humans. Circ Res. 1990;67:130–41.
27. van de Borne P, Oren R, Abouassaly C, Anderson E, Somers VK. Effect of Cheyne-Stokes respiration on muscle sympathetic nerve activity in severe congestive heart failure secondary to ischemic or idiopathic dilated cardiomyopathy. Am J Cardiol. 1998;81:432–6.
28. Porter JM, Markos F, Snow HM, Shorten GD. Effects of respiratory and metabolic pH changes and hypoxia on ropivacaine-induced cardiotoxicity in dogs. Br J Anaesth. 2000;84:92–4.
29. Bing OH, Brooks WW, Messer JV. Heart muscle viability following hypoxia: protective effect of acidosis. Science. 1973;180:1297–8.
30. Domino KB, Lu Y, Eisenstein BL, Hlastala MP. Hypocapnia worsens arterial blood oxygenation and increases VA/Q heterogeneity in canine pulmonary edema. Anesthesiology. 1993;78:91–9.
31. Criley JM, Blaufuss AH, Kissel GL. Cough-induced cardiac compression. Self-administered from of cardiopulmonary resuscitation. JAMA. 1976;236:1246–50.
32. Maze SS, Kotler MN, Parry WR. Doppler evaluation of changing cardiac dynamics during Cheyne-Stokes respiration. Chest. 1989;95:525–9.
33. Peters J. Mechanical ventilation with PEEP – a unique therapy for failing hearts. Intensive Care Med. 1999;25:778–80.
34. Wiesen J, Ornstein M, Tonelli AR, Menon V, Ashton RW. State of the evidence: mechanical ventilation with PEEP in patients with cardiogenic shock. Heart. 2013;99:1812–7.
35. Groenveld HF, Januzzi JL, Damman K, van Wijngaarden J, Hillege HL, van Veldhuisen DJ, van der Meer P. Anemia and mortality in heart failure patients a systematic review and meta-analysis. J Am Coll Cardiol. 2008;52:818–27.
36. Zilberman M, Silverberg DS, Bits I, Steinbruch S, Wexler D, Sheps D, Schwartz D, Oksenberg A. Improvement of anemia with erythropoietin and intravenous iron reduces sleep-related breathing disorders and improves daytime sleepiness in anemic patients with congestive heart failure. Am Heart J. 2007;154:870–6.
37. Giannoni A, Emdin M, Poletti R, Bramanti F, Prontera C, Piepoli M, Passino C. Clinical significance of chemosensitivity in chronic heart failure: influence on neurohormonal derangement, Cheyne-Stokes respiration and arrhythmias. Clin Sci (Lond). 2008;114:489–97.
38. Javaheri S. A mechanism of central sleep apnea in patients with heart failure. N Engl J Med. 1999;341:949–54.
39. Francis DP, Willson K, Davies LC, Coats AJ, Piepoli M. Quantitative general theory for periodic breathing in chronic heart failure and its clinical implications. Circulation. 2000;102:2214–21.
40. Hanly PJ, Millar TW, Steljes DG, Baert R, Frais MA, Kryger MH. Respiration and abnormal sleep in patients with congestive heart failure. Chest. 1989;96:480–8.
41. Andreas S, Hagenah G, Moller C, Werner GS, Kreuzer H. Cheyne-Stokes respiration and prognosis in congestive heart failure. Am J Cardiol. 1996;78:1260–4.
42. Lanfranchi PA, Braghiroli A, Bosimini E, Mazzuero G, Colombo R, Donner CF, Giannuzzi P. Prognostic value of nocturnal Cheyne-Stokes respiration in chronic heart failure. Circulation. 1999;99:1435–40.
43. Metra M, Dei Cas L, Panina G, Visioli O. Exercise hyperventilation chronic congestive heart failure, and its relation to functional capacity and hemodynamics. Am J Cardiol. 1992;70:622–8.

44. Park AM, Suzuki YJ. Effects of intermittent hypoxia on oxidative stress-induced myocardial damage in mice. J Appl Physiol. 2007/1985;102: 1806–14
45. Wang T, Eskandari D, Zou D, Grote L, Hedner J. Increased carbonic anhydrase activity is associated with sleep apnea severity and related hypoxemia. Sleep. 2015;38:1067–73.
46. Brack T, Thuer I, Clarenbach CF, Senn O, Noll G, Russi EW, Bloch KE. Daytime Cheyne-Stokes respiration in ambulatory patients with severe congestive heart failure is associated with increased mortality. Chest. 2007;132:1463–71.
47. La Rovere MT, Pinna GD, Maestri R, Robbi E, Mortara A, Fanfulla F, Febo O, Sleight P. Clinical relevance of short-term day-time breathing disorders in chronic heart failure patients. Eur J Heart Fail. 2007;9:949–54.
48. Poletti R, Passino C, Giannoni A, Zyw L, Prontera C, Bramanti F, Clerico A, Piepoli M, Emdin M. Risk factors and prognostic value of daytime Cheyne-Stokes respiration in chronic heart failure patients. Int J Cardiol. 2009;137:47–53.
49. Giannoni A, Emdin M, Bramanti F, Iudice G, Francis DP, Barsotti A, Piepoli M, Passino C. Combined increased chemosensitivity to hypoxia and hypercapnia as a prognosticator in heart failure. J Am Coll Cardiol. 2009;53:1975–80.
50. Piepoli MF, Kaczmarek A, Francis DP, Davies LC, Rauchhaus M, Jankowska EA, Anker SD, Capucci A, Banasiak W, Ponikowski P. Reduced peripheral skeletal muscle mass and abnormal reflex physiology in chronic heart failure. Circulation. 2006;114:126–34.
51. Ponikowski P, Chua TP, Anker SD, Francis DP, Doehner W, Banasiak W, Poole-Wilson PA, Piepoli MF, Coats AJ. Peripheral chemoreceptor hypersensitivity: an ominous sign in patients with chronic heart failure. Circulation. 2001;104:544–9.
52. Kasai T, Motwani SS, Yumino D, Gabriel JM, Montemurro LT, Amirthalingam V, Floras JS, Bradley TD. Contrasting effects of lower body positive pressure on upper airways resistance and partial pressure of carbon dioxide in men with heart failure and obstructive or central sleep apnea. J Am Coll Cardiol. 2013;61:1157–66.
53. Giannoni A, Raglianti V, Mirizzi G, Taddei C, Del Franco A, Iudice G, Bramanti F, Aimo A, Pasanisi E, Emdin M, Passino C. Influence of central apneas and chemoreflex activation on pulmonary artery pressure in chronic heart failure. Int J Cardiol. 2016;202:200–6.

Diagnostic Tools: The Easier, the Better

10

Roberta Poletti, Alberto Aimo, Vincenzo Castiglione, Alessandro Di Gangi, Giovanni Iudice, Mauro Micalizzi, Claudio Passino, and Michele Emdin

Abbreviations

AHI	Apnea-hypopnea index
AASM	American Academy of Sleep Medicine
ASDA	American Sleep Disorders Association
BDs	Breathing disturbances
CHF	Chronic heart failure
CPAP	Continuous positive airway pressure
CR	Cardiorespiratory
CSR	Cheyne-Stokes respiration
ECG	Electrocardiogram
EMG	Electromyogram
EOG	Electrooculogram
FNE	First-night effect
in-lab	In laboratory

Polysomnography and Beyond

R. Poletti (✉) • G. Iudice
Division of Cardiology and Cardiovascular Medicine, Fondazione Toscana G. Monasterio, Pisa, Italy
e-mail: poletti@ftgm.it; iudice@ftgm.it

A. Aimo • V. Castiglione • A. Di Gangi
Institute of Life Sciences, Scuola Superiore Sant'Anna, Pisa, Italy
e-mail: a.aimo@sssup.it

M. Micalizzi
Fondazione Toscana G. Monasterio, Pisa, Italy
e-mail: micalizzi@ftgm.it

C. Passino • M. Emdin
Institute of Life Sciences, Scuola Superiore Sant'Anna, Pisa, Italy

Division of Cardiology and Cardiovascular Medicine, Fondazione Toscana G. Monasterio, Pisa, Italy
e-mail: passino@ftgm.it; c.passino@sssup.it; emdin@ftgm.it; m.emdin@sssup.it

© Springer International Publishing Switzerland 2017
M. Emdin et al. (eds.), *The Breathless Heart*,
DOI 10.1007/978-3-319-26354-0_10

MD	Medicine doctor
OSAS	Obstructive sleep apnea syndrome
PB	Periodic breathing
PSG	Polysomnography
RDI	Respiratory disturbance index
REM	Rapid eye movement
SaO_2	Arterial oxygen saturation

10.1 Introduction

Breathing disturbances (BDs) affect a large proportion of chronic heart failure (CHF) patients; they have a significant impact on patients' outcome and are currently evaluated as potential therapeutic targets [1, 2].

BDs can occur during both nocturnal and diurnal hours [3] and are represented by apneas and/or hypopneas. In adults, an apnea is scored when there is a $\geq 90\%$ reduction of airflow compared to baseline for ≥ 10 s; apneas are central in case of the simultaneous absence of nasal airflow and respiratory movements, while they are obstructive when the absence of airflow is associated to the presence of thoracic and abdominal movements; finally, mixed apneas are combinations of the previous two forms, usually beginning as central apneas and ending as obstructive ones [3]. According to the more recent definition, a hypopnea is scored when the airflow drops by $\geq 30\%$ of preevent baseline for ≥ 10 s, in association with either $\geq 3\%$ arterial oxygen desaturation or an arousal; [3] a distinction between central and obstructive hypopneas is not usually performed [3].

The severity of BDs can be quantified through the respiratory disturbance index (RDI) or the apnea-hypopnea index (AHI). The RDI expresses the average number of apneas, hypopneas, and respiratory event-related arousals per hour of sleep, whereas the AHI is calculated as the number of apneas and hypopneas per hour of estimated sleep time. AHI values are categorized as normal (0–4), mild sleep apnea (5–14), moderate sleep apnea (15–29), and severe sleep apnea (≥ 30) [4]. Significant periodic breathing (PB) is a pattern of waxing and waning of tidal volume characterized by hypopneas and an AHI ≥ 15; when central apneas are present, PB should be defined as Cheyne-Stokes respiration (CSR) [5].

The diagnostic techniques for BDs have been developed in the setting of sleep medicine [6]. The American Sleep Disorders Association (ASDA), now American Academy of Sleep Medicine (AASM), has classified sleep study systems into four categories:

- Level 1: standard (namely in-laboratory, attended) polysomnography (PSG)
- Level 2: unattended home sleep study with comprehensive portable devices incorporating the same channels as the in-laboratory standard PSG
- Level 3: unattended devices, which measure at least four cardiorespiratory (CR) parameters
- Level 4: unattended devices recording one or two parameters [6]

There appears to be a trade-off between the amount of information provided and the simplicity of the device [1]. To evaluate the relevance of such trade-off in the setting of CHF, it is worth recapitulating the advantages and drawbacks of the different diagnostic techniques. The current gold standard for the diagnosis of BDs, i.e. traditional PSG, will be analyzed in Sect. 10.2, whereas alternative diagnostic techniques will be presented in Sect. 10.3. Short-term in-lab monitoring and implanted devices do not fit completely into one of the AASM classes, but they represent promising approaches for the diagnosis of BD; they will be discussed in Sects. 10.3 and 10.4, respectively. Finally, we will try to draw some conclusions about the diagnosis of BDs in CHF patients.

10.2   Standard PSG

In-laboratory (in-lab), attended PSG is a multiparametric, nocturnal, laboratory-based sleep study that represents the gold standard for the diagnosis of several sleep-related BDs, most notably the obstructive sleep apnea syndrome (OSAS) [7].

As stated in a review on the technical aspects of PSG, this technique "has developed from our understanding of sleep and its associated physiologic processes" [7]. In 1929, Berger managed to record the human brain activity, thus performing the first electroencephalographic (EEG) recording [8]. In the following years, Kleitman identified the rapid eye movement (REM) sleep stage by simultaneous recordings of EEG and electrooculogram (EOG) [8], and in 1957, Kleitman and Dement described the entire human sleep cycle [8]. During the 60s, Gastaut et al. evaluated three patients complaining of disrupted sleep and diurnal drowsiness; by recording several signals (EEG, chest movements, airflow, and heart rate) during sleep, they were able to conclude that these patients experienced recurrent collapses of the airways, thus unraveling the pathogenesis of OSAS. Finally, in 1974, Holland coined the term "polysomnography" to describe this comprehensive sleep study [8].

Until the 90s, performing a PSG required constant calibration, large amounts of paper and ink, and a cumbersome instrumentation; moreover, the interpretation and storage of data were daunting tasks. Therefore, only short or intermittent periods of sleep were usually recorded [8]. The introduction of computer-based PSG markedly improved the cost-effectiveness of the procedure and allowed an exponential increase in the number of sleep study centers [8].

At present, the main diagnostic indications of PSG can be summarized as follows:

1. Sleep-related BDs, most notably OSAS
2. Narcolepsy
3. Several parasomnias, such as sleep behavior disorders and periodic limb movements
4. Some sleep related seizure disorders that do not respond to conventional therapies [9]

Another crucial application of PSG is the titration of continuous positive airway pressure (CPAP) in OSAS patients [9].

The minimum set of parameters monitored during PSG may vary in relation to the pathology being considered [9]. For the diagnosis of OSAS and other sleep-related BDs, EEG, EOG, and chin electromyogram (EMG) are required for the evaluation of the sleep state, whereas the recording of airflow, arterial oxygen saturation (SaO_2), thoracoabdominal movements, and the electrocardiogram (ECG) allow to characterize the cardiorespiratory function during sleep (Fig. 10.1) [9].

As discussed in other chapters, a substantial proportion of CHF patients display sleep-related BDs, which have a significant impact on morbidity and mortality. The opportunity of a sleep study in CHF patients without sleep symptoms is currently debated [10, 11]. A sleep study is recommended when these symptoms are present; however, a cardiorespiratory monitoring is more frequently performed than PSG since it has a high diagnostic value and is probably more cost-effective than PSG (see below) [10, 11].

During PSG, the controlled environment, the standardized recording techniques, and the presence of a sleep technician allow an accurate evaluation of the sleep period [12]. On the other hand, the cost of PSG in terms of human resources is high: "The workload comprises admitting the patient by the medical specialist

POLYSOMNOGRAPHY

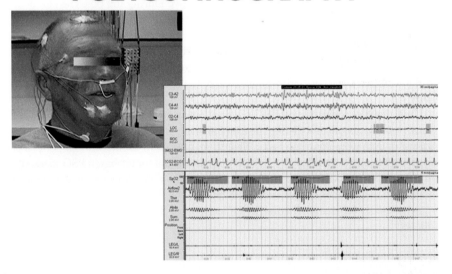

Fig. 10.1 The minimum set of parameters monitored during polysomnigraphy display of simultaneous recording of electroencefalogram (*EEG*), electrooculogram (*EOG*), electrocardiogram (*ECG*), electromyogram (*EMG*), airflow, thoracoabdominal movements, allowing the identification of central apnea

[…] (1 h). Preparation of the equipment, patient hook-up, disconnecting (1.5 h), and scoring the record (1.5 h) is performed by the technician. The medicine doctor (MD) subsequently reviews the scoring, creates the report, and gives feedback to the patient (1 h). These procedures require a total time for the licensed MD of 2 h and for the trained technician of 3.0 h. Attended PSG requires continuous monitoring by trained technical and nursing staff for the duration of recording, i.e. 8 h" [12].

Another potential problem of PSG is that the results may be biased by the unfamiliar environment. A first-night effect (FNE) in PSG is known since 1964; its main characteristics include less total sleep time and REM sleep, reduced sleep efficiency index, more intermittent wake time, and longer latency to REM sleep [13]. The FNE has been ascribed to the discomfort caused by electrodes, the limitation of movements by gauges and cables, and the sheer fact of being under scrutiny [13]. According to a study, the FNE could last up to four consecutive nights [14]; moreover, the relevance of FNE in the assessment of sleep-related BDs is uncertain [13, 14].

The limitations of in-lab PSG have prompted the search for other, possibly more cost-effective, methods for sleep assessment.

PSG for a diagnostic tool may obviously be applied to CHF patients with PB/CSR occurring during daytime; polygraphic recordings allow to demonstrate the occurrence of Cheyne-Stokes respiration during wakefulness as indicated by the electroencephalographic display (Fig. 10.2).

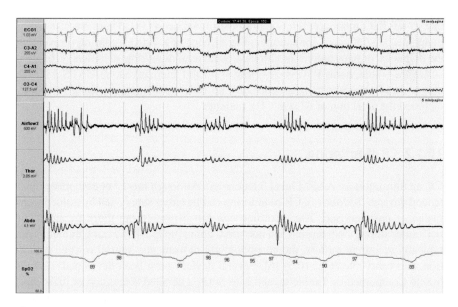

Fig. 10.2 A polygraphic recording demonstrating the occurrence of Cheyne-Stokes respiration during wakefulness as indicated by the electroencephalographic display

10.3 "Ambulatory" Sleep Recordings

10.3.1 Home Polysomnography

Home PSG is an AASM level 2 technique. The same signals registered in standard PSG are recorded at the patient's home [15]. The set-up can be performed either at home, by a sleep technician, or in a sleep laboratory; in the second case, the patient has to travel home with a fitted PSG equipment [15]. As demonstrated very recently, the two types of set-up have similar efficiency, with home set-up being more convenient for the patient but also more expensive [15].

Home PSG allows a complete assessment of sleep; therefore, it could be used for the diagnosis (as well as the grading) of various types of sleep disorders [16]. Nevertheless, the unique application of home PSG is currently the diagnosis of OSAS [16]. Even in this field, the AASM considers that there remain insufficient data to recommend routine use of home PSG, although a recent analysis of six prospective, randomized, crossover trials comparing home PSG and standard PSG conclude that the first is reliable and accurate to diagnose OSAS [16]. Home PSG seems to be more economic than in-lab PSG [16]. Furthermore, the sleep quality (as reflected by total sleep time, amount of REM sleep, and sleep fragmentation) was higher at home; it has been postulated that the first-night effect would be absent in home PSG [15], but this hypothesis has been challenged [17].

It should be remarked that in a study a majority of patients expressed a preference for in-lab PSG over home PSG, for several reasons (fewer wires, technician taking care of recording, no need to carry home the equipment) [18]. Patients thought also that in-lab PSG more accurately represented their sleep [18]. There are also other, more specialistic issues, for example, the absence of a video recording (preventing the diagnosis of parasomnias or complex behavioral night-time disorders) [16].

On the whole, home PSG is emerging as a valid alternative to in-lab PSG for the diagnosis of OSAS, but it has currently no other indications in sleep medicine, included the detection of BDs in CHF patients.

10.3.2 CR Monitoring

CR monitoring is an AASM level 3 technique. Although this level comprises unattended devices (see above), CR monitoring can be either supervised by a sleep technician or unsupervised. The recording can last overnight but more frequently is performed during both diurnal and nocturnal hours (up to 24 h). Four parameters are typically recorded: airflow, thoracoabdominal movements, arterial oxygen saturation, and heart rate (Fig. 10.3) [6]. Several devices have been developed, such as Somté Compumedics, Embletta, and Life Shirt; a detailed discussion of their characteristics goes beyond the scopes of the present section, which focuses instead on their diagnostic reliability.

CR monitoring is currently evaluated as a potential alternative to in-lab PSG for the diagnosis of OSAS [19]. Indeed, compared to in-lab PSG, CR monitoring is

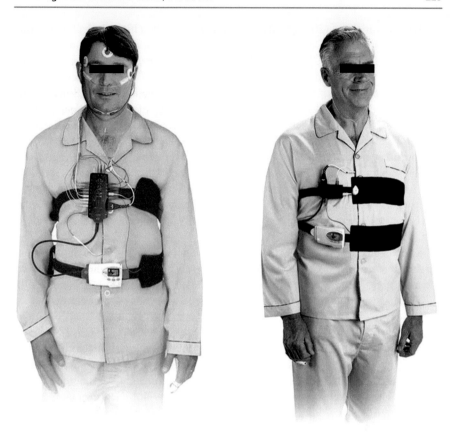

Fig. 10.3 Polysomnography and cardiorespiratory monitoring. *Left*: polysomnographic set. *Right*: devices for cardiorespiratory monitoring. In the second case, note the absence of electrocardiographic, electromyographic, and electrooculographic leads (From: www.compumedics.com.au)

cheaper and requires less time for biosensor placement and data processing [20]. The reduced number of channels and the possibility to sleep at home increase patient's comfort, possibly preventing the first-night effect, which is a concern with in-lab PSG (see above) [19, 21].

Attended CR monitoring and in-lab PSG displayed a fair agreement in the classification of OSAS patients [20]. When considering PSG as the gold standard technique, attended CR monitoring had a false negative rate of 4–8 % (as reviewed in [20]). By contrast, false negatives were up to 15 % in unattended recordings [20], at least in part because of a range of data loss estimated between 3 % and 18 % in the unsupervised setting [19].

In 1994, the ASDA recommendations stated that attended CR monitoring could be used to diagnose OSAS in two situations: (1) symptoms highly suggestive of OSAS (in order to speed up the diagnostic process and the establishment of an appropriate therapy) and (2) health problems limiting the possibility to perform an in-lab PSG (for example, immobility, or severe illnesses) [6].

AASM guidelines (2007) added that, in patients with a high clinical probability of moderate-to-severe OSAS, unattended CR monitoring could represent an alternative to in-lab PSG [19]. The AASM advised standardized procedures for sensor application, scoring and interpretation of data, as well as a comprehensive sleep evaluation under the supervision of a specialist in sleep medicine [19]. Since several studies have demonstrated that manual scoring is superior to automated scoring, the AASM suggested that devices for CR monitoring should allow the manual scoring of raw data or the editing of the automated scoring [19]. A sleep technician or an appropriately trained healthcare professional should instruct the patient on the correct biosensor application, or even directly apply them; the other potential source of data loss, namely channel displacement during sleep, cannot clearly be obviated in an unsupervised setting [19]. Finally, the AASM recommended to perform an in-lab PSG in cases where CR monitoring is technically inadequate or nondiagnostic in patients with high clinical probability [19].

AASM guidelines specifically address the adult population [19]. Their application in the female sex is perhaps questionable, since they rely on studies in which women were often largely underrepresented or were not included [20, 21]. More importantly, the AASM suggested caution when approaching patients >65 years of age, because they are more likely to suffer from sleep-related BDs other than OSAS and also from comorbidities that can influence the breathing pattern during sleep, such as CHF [19, 22].

The prevalence of BDs amongst CHF patients has been estimated to be about 40–50 % [23]; however, it could represent a large underestimation due to the limited availability of in-lab PSG and above all the lack of a screening evaluation of sleep in CHF. The cost-effectiveness of such screening has not been evaluated so far, partly because of the limited possibility to detect on a clinical basis the CHF patients more likely to present sleep-related BDs. Unattended CR monitoring could offer a cost-effective, quicker, and more accessible alternative to in-lab PSG for a sleep screening of all CHF patients, or a subgroup of them. The first step in this direction is the validation of CR monitoring against in-lab PSG.

In a study by Quintana-Gallego et al., unattended CR monitoring was successful in 68 out of 75 patients, with a sensitivity of 68.4–82.5 % and a specificity of 88.6–97.8 % (ranges related to the different AHI cut-offs considered) compared to in-lab PSG [24]. The area under the ROC curve for AHI ≥ 5, ≥ 10 and ≥ 15 was 0.896, 0.907 and 0.862, respectively [24]. Moreover, the obstructive or central nature of sleep-related BDs was correctly determined in all patients [24], as confirmed by another study [25].

A potential limitation of CR monitoring, namely the impossibility to detect the respiratory events resulting only in arousals, has been considered in the setting of OSAS [22] but never in CHF. Again in OSAS patients, it has been pointed out that the effective sleep period is not measured during the CR monitoring, because the EEG, EOG, and EMG signals are not recorded; instead, a reasonable sleep period is selected (for example, from 10 p.m. to 6 a.m.) in order to calculate the AHI, potentially resulting in the underestimation of the AHI when the effective sleep period is reduced [26]. Several solutions have been proposed, such as sleep diaries, body position detectors, and recorders of wrist movements [22, 26]. However, this problem could have relatively little relevance in CHF. In fact, Pinna et al. examined a population of 75 stable CHF patients with both in-lab PSG and overnight attended CR monitoring and demonstrated that the discordance between the two approaches regarding AHI values was not clinically relevant. The two methods concordantly classified most of the patients (87 %) in the same risk class (AHI< 5, $5 \leq$ AHI ≤ 15, $15 \leq$ AHI< 30 or AHI$\geq$30), and the disagreements always occurred in contiguous classes [25].

In contrast with Pinna et al., who evaluated only the nocturnal period [25], other authors performed daytime and night-time recordings. For example, in a cohort of 60 patients with stable CHF undergoing unattended CR monitoring, Brack et al. demonstrated that CSR occurred in 62 % of patients during night-time and 16 % during daytime [27]. Interestingly, 18 patients with CSR during >10 % of the day-time lived shorter without heart transplantation than 42 patients with <10 % of day-time CSR ($p < 0.05$) during a follow-up of 836 ± 27 days; CSR during >10 % of the daytime was also an independent predictor of mortality (hazard ratio 3.8; 95 % confidence interval, 1.1–12.7; $p < 0.05$) when controlling for age, sex, brain natriuretic peptide, left ventricular ejection fraction, and NYHA class [27]. The clinical correlates of breathing disturbances in CHF patients are discussed in detail in other chapters.

Significant night-to-night intrasubject variation in AHI values have been reported in CHF patients using unattended CR monitoring [25, 28]. However, such variability seems not to impair the possibility to categorize patients in different AHI classes with a single-night recording [28]. By contrast, poor data signals and data loss is a concern also in the setting of CHF, although its impact seems quite limited (for example, 9 % of recorded excluded in the study by Quintana-Gallego et al. [24], 8 % in the study by Pinna et al.) [25].

To conclude, in-lab PSG is currently the gold standard for confirming the presence of sleep-related BDs, both in OSAS and in CHF, but its use is limited by its high cost, limited accessibility, and excessive professional workload. CR monitoring can reduce costs and times of evaluation, is less cumbersome for the patient, and can be performed also at home. The main concerns are the impossibility to determine total sleep time, the inability to detect arousals, and the risk of data loss in case of unattended monitoring. CR monitoring should be used for OSAS diagnosis only in patients with high clinical probability of disease and in absence of potentially confounding factors. A sleep screening is currently not recommended in all patients with CHF, despite the high prevalence of BDs in this population, their probable underestimation, and their potential clinical relevance. CR monitoring is emerging as a valid alternative to in-lab PSG; moreover, it offers the unique possibility to explore the respiratory pattern even during daytime.

10.3.3 Single or Double Channel Recordings

When the clinical probability of OSAS is high, the use of devices measuring one or two channels is emerging as an acceptable alternative to standard PSG [29]. These devices can be composed by: (1) a nasal cannula, (2) an oximeter, (3) a nasal cannula plus an oximeter, or (4) an arterial tonometer. They allow to estimate the incidence of apneas and hypopneas, without distinction between central and obstructive events [29]. Their use in the diagnosis of OSAS is currently debated, and they cannot play any role in the detection of PB/CSR in CHF patients. Nevertheless, a brief description of these devices will be provided in order to illustrate the full spectrum of the diagnostic tools for BDs.

According to a very recent study, an automatic single-channel nasal pressure recorder can correctly recommend CPAP treatment in the more symptomatic patients with clinical suspicion of OSAS [30]. This device notice the occurrence of apneas and hypopneas from the reductions in nasal flow, and computes an AHI value based on valid recording time as the denominator [30]. The data were inadequate for analysis in almost 21 % of patients, and the device probably underestimate the AHI, and the error seems progressively more relevant with increasing OSAS severity [29, 30]. By contrast, oxymetry alone tends to overestimate the occurrence of BDs, and its specificity is poor [31]. When nasal flow is measured together with arterial oxygen saturation, the quantification of AHI is quite accurate, and a good agreement with standard PSG is reached [32].

Finally, the detection of apneic and hypopneic events through the associated increases in sympathetic activity has been proposed. A single device measures peripheral arterial tone, as well as heart rate, SaO_2, and body movements [33] (therefore, the inclusion of this device in the AASM level 4 is not completely accurate). The signals are integrated, and an AHI value is calculated; a strong correlation with the AHI obtained through standard PSG has been reported [33]. Peripheral vasculopathy, treatment with α-blocker medications, and severe autonomic neuropathy are the main limitations of this device [33].

10.4   Short-term In-lab Polygraphy

In addition to the previously mentioned devices, several forms of short-term in-lab polygraphy have been recently proposed; these techniques cannot be classified according to the AASM and yield particular interest in the assessment of BDs in CHF patients.

Short-term assisted recordings last up to a few hours, but less than an entire night. They can be represented by split-night PSG, PSG during daytime sleep, or assisted CR monitoring. The first two techniques have been evaluated exclusively as potential approaches for the diagnosis of OSAS, although conceptually they could be used for detecting central apneas and hypopneas as well. By contrast, short-term assisted CR monitoring has been used in several studies for the detection of central events.

In split-night PSG, the patient undergoes a routine in-laboratory polysomnography; if a diagnosis of OSAS is established, the patient is awakened, and the titration of continuous positive airway pressure (CPAP) commences during the same night [34]. This approach has appeared an attractive option since it allows a substantial reduction in waiting times, time to prescription of CPAP therapy, and resources expended [34]; for example, it has been estimated that the waiting time for CPAP therapy would be decreased by 7 months if a split-night paradigm were applied [35].

The main concern about split-night PSG is its short duration, which could prevent an accurate assessment of OSAS severity, especially for a short time spent in REM sleep, a stage associated with more depressed muscle tone in the upper airways [36]. Moreover, the potential occurrence of a first-night effect (see Sect. 10.2) is not considered in the split-night paradigm. Finally, performing CPAP titration on the same night of the diagnosis of OSAS might reduce patient acceptance and adherence to CPAP therapy (as reviewed in [34]). These issues have been addressed in several studies, which seem to demonstrate that split-night PSG represents a valid alternative to standard PSG [37]; the same position has been adopted by the AASM [9]. As stated above, split-night PSG has never been used for the detection of central events.

Another approach to the diagnosis of OSAS is PSG during daytime sleep. Limited evidences suggest the accuracy of this technique, provided that the duration of recording is sufficient and that the monitoring is not preceded by sleep deprivation [38, 39].

As discussed above, central events (apneas and/or hypopneas) can occur during both sleep and awake hours and can be detected through long-term CR monitoring. Short-term assisted CR recording has been used in CHF patients during wakefulness, to screen for central events. This approach was firstly proposed in 1997 by Mortara et al.; the authors were interested in the influence of PB/CSR on the assessment of heart rate variability, which is related to autonomic function. After 30 min of supine rest, which allowed for stabilization of the signals, recordings were performed during 15 min of spontaneous respiration and 5 min of controlled breathing at 0.25 Hz. Electrocardiogram (ECG), instantaneous lung volumes by inductance plethysmography, and beat-to-beat SaO_2 were recorded simultaneously. Baseline recordings were split in three 5-min epochs, and the results of at least two epochs were averaged; epochs with >5 % ectopic beats and artifacts were excluded. This simple method allowed the authors to demonstrate that PB/CSR is common in awake CHF patients and can interfere with the assessment of heart rate variability [40].

Two years later, a similar protocol was adopted by Ponikowski et al. to assess 74 stable CHF patients. After a 20-min supine rest, oronasal airflow, thoracoabdominal movements, SaO_2, ECG, and blood pressure were recorded continuously for 30 min; subjects breathed spontaneously and were asked to relax but not to fall asleep during the test. A significant proportion (66 %) of patients displayed PB/CSR; the oscillatory ventilation pattern was associated with autonomic dysfunction, and a worse outcome [3].

More recently, in Pisa laboratory, 147 CHF patients underwent 20-min daytime recording, using the same signals assessed by Ponikowski et al., together with carbon dioxide end-tidal pressure: Poletti et al. detected daytime CSR in 59 % of CHF patients, studied while awake and was associated with adrenergic activation, overexpression of natriuretic peptides, and cardiac mortality [41] (Fig. 10.4). Again, by

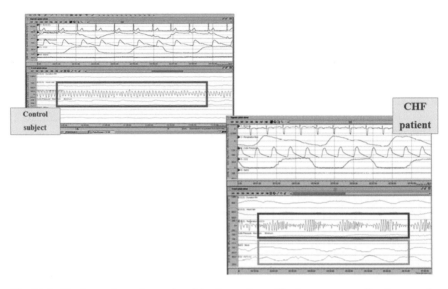

Fig. 10.4 The figure shows the results of daytime polygraphic short-term recording in an awake healthy subject (*left panel*) presenting with a normal breathing pattern, and in an awake patient with chronic heart failure (CHF) (*right panel*), with the identification of the presence of Cheyne-Stokes respiration, characterized by repetitive apnea and hyperpnea phases and related oscillation in heart rate, arterial pressure, oxygen saturation, and PETCO2

using 20-min daytime monitoring, another study demonstrated an association between the occurrence of CSR and enhanced chemosensitivity [42] in the same Pisa laboratory.

On summary, short-term assisted CR monitoring is a simple and rapid method to screen for the presence of diurnal PB/CSR in CHF patients. A potential limitation is the very limited number of studies having employed this technique and the heterogeneity of their protocols. Furthermore, this method provides a merely qualitative assessment of diurnal PB/CSR (presence or absence), and its sensitivity in the detection of diurnal PB/CSR is probably limited in less severely affected patients. A comparison between short-term in-lab CR monitoring and unassisted, long-term CR monitoring deserves some consideration.

Conclusions

An overview of diagnostic tools, signals recorded, advantages, and drawbacks is given in Table 10.1. Within certain limits, it can be said that "the easier, the better" for the diagnosis of BDs in CHF. Compared to PSG, CR monitoring limits the costs and times of evaluation, is less cumbersome for the patient, and can be performed at home; more importantly, it provides all the relevant information in the setting of CHF (namely the presence, number, and type of BDs). Contrary to PSG, CR monitoring allows to search for BDs also during the daytime. CR monitoring is thus emerging as a valid diagnostic technique. By contrast, single- or

Table 10.1 Diagnostic tools: signals recorded, advantages, and drawbacks

Recording system	AASM level	Signals recorded	Advantages	Drawbacks	Relevance in CHF
In-lab PSG	I	EEG, EOG, EMG, ECG, SaO$_2$, thoracoabdominal movements, airflow	High diagnostic accuracy, technical assistance	High professional workload, first-night effect	Possible use for diagnosis of sleep-related BDs
Home PSG	II	Same as in-lab PSG	Familiar environment More economic than in-lab PSG	Few studies, not always preferred to in-lab PSG	Possible use for diagnosis
CR monitoring	III	ECG, SaO$_2$, thoracoabdominal movements, airflow	Low costs, low professional workload, familiar environment, day and night-time monitoring	No information on sleep time and arousals, possible underestimation of AHI, data loss	Possible role for diagnosis (day and night-time BDs)
Split-night PSG	/	Same as in-lab PSG	Rapidity, low costs, low professional workload	No accurate assessment of OSAS severity, unfamiliar environment	Not useful
PSG during daytime sleep	/	Same as in-lab PSG	Rapidity	Insufficient evidence for routine clinical use	Not useful
Short-term assisted CR	/	Same as CR monitoring	Simplicity, rapidity	Qualitative assessment of diurnal PB/CSR, few studies	Possible use for diagnosis
1 or 2 channels	IV	Air flow or SaO$_2$ or arterial tonometer or Air flow + SaO$_2$	Low costs	No distinction between central and obstructive events, underestimation (airflow alone) or overestimation (SaO$_2$ alone) of AHI	Not useful

AHI apnea-hypopnea index, *BDs* breathing disturbances, *CHF* chronic heart failure, *CR* cardiorespiratory, *CSR* Cheyne-Stokes respiration, *ECG* electrocardiogram, *EOG* electrooculogram, *FNE* first-night effect, *in-lab* in laboratory, *OSAS* obstructive sleep apnea syndrome, *PB* periodic breathing, *PSG* polysomnography, *SaO2* arterial oxygen saturation double-channel recordings seem too "easy" to be useful, mostly because they do not allow to distinguish between central and obstructive apneas. Finally, short-term CR monitoring is a simple and rapid method to screen for the presence of diurnal BDs, although its sensitivity is limited because of the short recording time.

References

1. Pinna GD, La Rovere MT, Robbi E, Sioufi A, Racine-Poon A, Howald H. Assessing the severity and improving the understanding of sleep-related breathing disorders in heart failure patients. Conf Proc IEEE Eng Med Biol Soc. 2010;2010:3571–4.
2. Costanzo MR, Khayat R, Ponikowski P, Augostini R, Stellbrink C, Mianulli M, Abraham WT. Mechanisms and clinical consequences of untreated central sleep apnea in heart failure. J Am Coll Cardiol. 2015;65:72–84.
3. Ponikowski P, Anker SD, Chua TP, Francis D, Banasiak W, Poole-Wilson PA, Coats AJ, Piepoli M. Oscillatory breathing patterns during wakefulness in patients with chronic heart failure: clinical implications and role of augmented peripheral chemosensitivity. Circulation. 1999;100:2418–24.
4. Berry RB, Budhiraja R, Gottlieb DJ, Gozal D, Iber C, Kapur VK, Marcus CL, Mehra R, Parthasarathy S, Quan SF, Redline S, Strohl KP, Davidson Ward SL, Tangredi MM, American Academy of Sleep Medicine. Rules for scoring respiratory events in sleep: update of the 2007 AASM Manual for the scoring of sleep and associated events. Deliberations of the sleep apnea definitions task force of the American academy of sleep medicine. J Clin Sleep Med. 2012;8:597–619.
5. Sleep-related breathing disorders in adults: recommendations for syndrome definition and measurement techniques in clinical research. The Report of an American Academy of Sleep Medicine Task Force. Sleep. 1999;22:667–89.
6. Practice parameters for the use of portable recording in the assessment of obstructive sleep apnea. Standards of Practice Committee of the American Sleep Disorders Association. Sleep. 1994;17:372–377.
7. Vaughn BV, Giallanza P. Technical review of polysomnography. Chest. 2008;134:1310–9.
8. Deak M, Epstein LJ. The history of polysomnography. Sleep Med Clin. 2009;4:313–21.
9. Kushida CA, Littner MR, Morgenthaler T, Alessi CA, Bailey D, Coleman Jr J, Friedman L, Hirshkowitz M, Kapen S, Kramer M, Lee-Chiong T, Loube DL, Owens J, Pancer JP, Wise M. Practice parameters for the indications for polysomnography and related procedures: an update for 2005. Sleep. 2005;28:499–521.
10. Sériès F. Should all congestive heart failure patients have a routine sleep apnea screening? Proc Can J Cardiol. 2015;31:935–9.
11. Li Y, Daniels LB, Strollo Jr PJ, Malhotra A. Should all congestive heart failure patients have a routine sleep apnea screening? Con Can J Cardiol. 2015;31:940–4.
12. Fischer J, Dogas Z, Bassetti CL, Berg S, Grote L, Jennum P, Levy P, Mihaicuta S, Nobili L, Riemann D, Puertas Cuesta FJ, Raschke F, Skene DJ, Stanley N, Pevernagie D, Executive Committee (EC) of the Assembly of the National Sleep Societies (ANSS), Board of the European Sleep Research Society (ESRS), Regensburg, Germany. Standard procedures for adults in accredited sleep medicine centres in Europe. J Sleep Res. 2012;21:357–68.
13. Newell J, Mairesse O, Verbanck P, Neu D. Is a one-night stay in the lab really enough to conclude? First-night effect and night-to-night variability in polysomnographic recordings among different clinical population samples. Psychiatry Res. 2012;200:795–801.
14. Le Bon O, Staner L, Hoffmann G, Dramaix M, San Sebastian I, Murphy JR, Kentos M, Pelc I, Linkowski P. The first-night effect may last more than one night. J Psychiatr Res. 2001;35:165–72.

15. Bruyneel M, Libert W, Ameye L, Ninane V. Comparison between home and hospital set-up for unattended home-based polysomnography: a prospective randomized study. Sleep Med. 2015;16:1434–8.
16. Bruyneel M, Ninane V. Unattended home-based polysomnography for sleep disordered breathing: current concepts and perspectives. Sleep Med Rev. 2014;18:341–7.
17. Zheng H, Sowers M, Buysse DJ, Consens F, Kravitz HM, Matthews KA, Owens JF, Gold EB, Hall M. Sources of variability in epidemiological studies of sleep using repeated nights of in-home polysomnography: SWAN sleep study. J Clin Sleep Med. 2012;8:87–96.
18. Fry JM, DiPhillipo MA, Curran K, Goldberg R, Baran AS. Full polysomnography in the home. Sleep. 1998;21:635–42.
19. Collop NA, Anderson WM, Boehlecke B, Claman D, Goldberg R, Gottlieb DJ, Hudgel D, Sateia M, Schwab R, Portable Monitoring Task Force of the American Academy of Sleep Medicine. Clinical guidelines for the use of unattended portable monitors in the diagnosis of obstructive sleep apnea in adult patients. Portable Monitoring Task Force of the American Academy of Sleep Medicine. J Clin Sleep Med. 2007;3:737–47.
20. Flemmons WW, Littner MR, Rowley JA, Gay P, Anderson WM, Hudgel DW, McEvoy RD, Loube DI. Home diagnosis of sleep apnea: a systematica review of literature. Chest. 2003;124:1543–79.
21. Nakayama-Ashida Y, Takegami M, Chin K, Sumi K, Nakamura T, Takahashi K, Wakamura T, Horita S, Oka Y, Minami I, Fukuhara S, Kadotani H. Sleep-disordered breathing in the usual lifestyle setting as detected with home monitoring in a population of working men in Japan. Sleep. 2007;31:419–25.
22. Kapoor M, Greenough G. Home sleep tests for Obstructive Sleep Apnea (OSA). J Am Board Fam Med. 2015;28:504–9.
23. Krawczyk M, Flinta I, Garncarek M, Jankowska EA, Banasiak W, Germany R, Javaheri S, Ponikowski P. Sleep disordered breathing in patients with heart failure. Cardiol J. 2013;20:345–55.
24. Quintana-Gallego E, Villa-Gil M, Carmona-Bernal C, Botebol-Benhamou G, Martínez-Martínez A, Sánchez-Armengol A, Polo-Padillo J, Capote F. Home respiratory polygraphy for diagnosis of sleep-disordered breathing in heart failure. Eur Respir J. 2004;24:443–8.
25. Pinna GD, Robbi E, Pizza F, Taurino AE, Pronzato C, La Rovere MT, Maestri R. Can cardio-respiratory polygraphy replace portable polysomnography in the assessment of sleep-disordered breathing in heart failure patients? Sleep Breath. 2014;18:475–82.
26. Polese JF, Santos-Silva R, Kobayashi RF, Pinto IN, Tufik S, Bittencourt LR. Portable monitoring devices in the diagnosis of obstructive sleep apnea: current status, advantages, and limitations. J Bras Pneumol. 2010;36:498–505.
27. Brack T, Tüer I, Clarenbach F, Senn O, Noll G, Russi EW, Bloch KE. Daytime Cheyne-Stokes respiration in ambulatory patients with severe congestive heart failure is associated with increased mortality. Chest. 2007;132:1463–71.
28. Maestri R, La Rovere MT, Robbi E, Pinna GD. Night-to-night repeatability of measurements of nocturnal breathing disorders in clinically stable chronic heart failure patients. Sleep Breath. 2011;15:673–8.
29. Brown LK. Are we ready for "unisomnography"? Sleep. 2015;38:7–9.
30. Masa JF, Duran-Cantolla J, Capote F, Cabello M, Abad J, Garcia-Rio F, Ferrer A, Fortuna AM, Gonzalez-Mangado N, de la Peña M, Aizpuru F, Barbe F, Montserrat JM, Spanish Sleep Network. Efficacy of home single-channel nasal pressure for recommending continuous positive airway pressure treatment in sleep apnea. Sleep. 2015;38:13–21.
31. Series F, Marc I, Cormier Y, La Forge J. Utility of nocturnal home oximetry for case finding in patients with suspected sleep apnea hypopnea syndrome. Ann Intern Med. 1993;119:449–53.
32. Ayappa I, Norman RG, Suryadevara M, Rapoport DM. Comparison of limited monitoring using a nasal-cannula flow signal to full polysomnography in sleep-disordered breathing. Sleep. 2004;27:1171–9.
33. Bar A, Pillar G, Dvir I, Sheffy J, Schnall RP, Lavie P. Evaluation of a portable device based on peripheral arterial tone for unattended home sleep studies. Chest. 2003;123:695–703.

34. Patel NP, Ahmed M, Rosen I. Split-night polysomnography. Chest. 2007;132:1664–71.
35. Elshaug AG, Moss JR, Southcott AM. Implementation of a split-night protocol to improve efficiency in assessment and treatment of obstructive sleep apnoea. Intern Med J. 2005;35:251–4.
36. The impact of split-night polysomnography for diagnosis and positive pressure therapy titration on treatment acceptance and adherence in sleep apnea/hypopnea. Sleep. 2000;3:17–24.
37. Pietzsch JB, Garner A, Cipriano LE, Linehan JH. An integrated health-economic analysis of diagnostic and therapeutic strategies in the treatment of moderate-to-severe obstructive sleep apnea. Sleep. 2011;34:695–709.
38. Sergi M, Rizzi M, Greco M, Andreoli A, Bamberga M, Castronovo C, Ferini-Strambi L. Validity of diurnal sleep recording performed by an ambulatory device in the diagnosis of obstructive sleep apnoea. Respir Med. 1998;92:216–20.
39. Sériès F, Cormier Y, La Forge J. Validity of diurnal sleep recording in the diagnosis of sleep apnea syndrome. Am Rev Respir Dis. 1991;143:947–9.
40. Mortara A, Sleight P, Pinna GD, Maestri R, Prpa A, La Rovere MT, Cobelli F, Tavazzi L. Abnormal awake respiratory patterns are common in chronic heart failure and may prevent evaluation of autonomic tone by measures of heart rate variability. Circulation. 1997;96:246–52.
41. Poletti R, Passino C, Giannoni A, Zyw L, Prontera C, Bramanti F, Clerico A, Piepoli M, Emdin M. Risk factors and prognostic value of daytime Cheyne-Stokes respiration in chronic heart failure patients. Int J Cardiol. 2009;137:47–53.
42. Giannoni A, Emdin M, Poletti R, Bramanti F, Prontera C, Piepoli M, Passino C. Clinical significance of chemosensitivity in chronic heart failure: influence on neurohormonal derangement, Cheyne-Stokes respiration and arrhythmias. Clin Sci (Lond). 2008;114:489–97.

Diagnostic Tools: Messages from Implanted Devices (Pacemakers as Diagnostic Tools)

11

Margherita Padeletti, Fabrizio Bandini, Edoardo Gronda, and Luigi Padeletti

Abbreviations

AF	Atrial fibrillation
AHI	Apnea-hypopnea index
CPAP	Continuous positive airway pressure therapy
CRT	Cardiac resynchronization therapy
CSA	Central sleep apnea
HF	Heart failure
ICD	Implantable cardioverter defibrillator
LVEF	Left ventricular ejection fraction
OSA	Obstructive sleep apnea
PSG	Polysomnography
RDE	Respiratory disturbance event
SA	Sleep apnea

M. Padeletti, MD (✉) • F. Bandini, MD
Department of Internal Medicine, Cardiology Unit, Ospedale del Mugello,
Borgo San Lorenzo, Florence, Italy
e-mail: marghepadeletti@gmail.com; fabrband@gmail.com

E. Gronda, MD
Cardiovascular Department, IRCCS MultiMedica, Sesto San Giovanni, Milan, Italy
e-mail: edoardo.gronda@multimedica.it

L. Padeletti, MD
Cardiovascular Department, IRCCS MultiMedica, Sesto San Giovanni, Milan, Italy

Chair of Cardiology, University of Florence, Florence, Italy
e-mail: lpadeletti@ftgm.it

© Springer International Publishing Switzerland 2017
M. Emdin et al. (eds.), *The Breathless Heart*,
DOI 10.1007/978-3-319-26354-0_11

11.1   Introduction

Sleep apnea (SA) is extremely common in people with HF. Estimates of prevalence are as high as 47–76 % [1–4]. Furthermore, well-established risk factors for HF, such as hypertension, coronary artery disease, and diabetes, are all adversely impacted by SA.

Sleep-disordered breathing is broadly divided into obstructive sleep apnea (OSA) and central sleep apnea (CSA) and increasingly has been recognized as an important factor in the development of several cardiovascular conditions [4, 5]. OSA, the most common form in the general population, is characterized by collapse of the upper airways. CSA is thought to be the result of intermittent alteration of the respiratory drive and hyperventilation (Cheyne-Stokes respiration) and is frequently seen in HF patients, perhaps as a result of pulmonary edema. Sleep apnea is of concern in patients with HF because it leads to intermittent hypoxemia, hypercapnia, and sympathetic excitation, and it may participate in a pathophysiological vicious cycle that contributes to deterioration in cardiovascular function. CSA is a powerful independent predictor of poor prognosis in patients with congestive HF [6]. It is important to note that the classic symptoms of Cheyne-Stokes respiration, which are fragmented sleep, paroxysmal nocturnal dyspnea, orthopnea, and daytime fatigue, can easily be interpreted as worsening HF symptoms [7]. Management of CSA is less well defined compared to OSA, which is well established. CSA has been linked to worse prognosis in HF, but it is still debated whether this finding is a reflection of underlying cardiac pathology or whether the diagnosis carries independent adverse prognostic implications. Optimal specific treatment for CSA is being debated, but it is well established that treatment of HF with beta-blockers or cardiac resynchronization therapy [8] improves CSA and that worsening HF is associated with increased CSA. Thus, diagnosis and monitoring may help to assess treatments and allow identification of worsening HF.

The gold standard to diagnose sleep apnea is monitored polysomnography (PSG) in a sleep laboratory. This modality uses multiple biometric recording devices to accurately quantify the number of apnea (cessation of airflow for at least 10 s) and hypopnea (respiratory event with a ≥ 30 % reduction in thoracoabdominal movement or airflow as compared to baseline lasting at least 10 s and with a ≥ 4 % oxygen desaturation) episodes occurring during a night's sleep. The severity of SA is commonly quantified by the apnea-hypopnea index (AHI), which is the number of apneic and hypopneic events per hour. An AHI of 5–15 indicates mild disease, 15–30 indicates moderate disease, and >30 indicates severe disease [9]. Differently from patients referred for OSA diagnosis, who usually present with associated symptoms such as snoring, apneas, and/or excessive daytime sleepiness, patients with cardiovascular disorders are frequently nonsleepy and less symptomatic [10–12]. It has been demonstrated that symptoms and Sleepiness Scale score (Epworth) are less reliable in detecting SA in HF patients [11, 12]. Consequently in about 80 % of HF, SA remains undiagnosed [10, 13–16].

SA, especially in association with HF, has been linked to a host of other cardiac arrhythmias, including nocturnal paroxysmal asystole, bradyrhythmias, atrioventricular nodal block, supraventricular tachycardia, and non-sustained ventricular tachycardia [17]. People with OSA have dramatically increased risk of sudden cardiac death during sleep. This risk was clearly associated with the AHI [18]. In patients implanted with a cardioverter defibrillator (ICD), the AHI showed to be positively correlated to the number of appropriate ICD therapies [19]. Bitter et al. demonstrated among HF patients with an ICD that both CSA and OSA are independently associated with an increased risk for ventricular arrhythmias and appropriate cardioverter defibrillator therapies [20]. SA is also an independent predictor of new-onset atrial fibrillation (AF) [21] and may be a causative factor in the development of AF [22]. Moreover, SA increases likelihood for AF recurrence postcardioversion [23], and this recurrence decreases after CPAP therapy [24]. Overall, the prevalence of SA is nearly 60 % in patients implanted with devices for cardiac rhythm management, and the majority of them remain undiagnosed [10, 15, 16]. Particularly, SA is highly prevalent in patients indicated to cardiac resynchronization therapy (CRT) [25]. According to current ESC guidelines [26], CRT has a class I indication for patients with symptomatic HF, left ventricular ejection fraction (LVEF) $\leq 35\,\%$, and left bundle brunch block despite at least 3 months of optimal pharmacological therapy who are expected to survive at least 1 year with good functional status. It has been estimated that CRT candidates represent about 10 % of HF patients [27].

A high prevalence of SA in patients with cardiac implants requires a specific diagnosis strategy because diagnosing SA might represent a potential therapeutic target for reducing occurrence and recurrence of arrhythmia.

11.2 Automatic Detection of SA in Implantable Devices

Up to now, PSG remains the "gold standard" to diagnose SA, but a general screening extended to all patients with HF or rhythm disturbances is challenged by waiting lists of sleep laboratories and high-related costs [28]. Recently, automated detection of advanced breathing disorders [29, 30] has been developed in implantable cardiac devices. More than 750,000 new pacemakers and more than 250,000 new implantable cardioverter defibrillators (ICDs, including those providing CRT) are implanted annually worldwide [31].

Some commercially available cardiac devices use minute ventilation sensors to adjust heart rate (rate responsiveness) and have demonstrated the capability to detect breathing variations by using transthoracic impedance measurements. Impedance is a measure of opposition to the flow of electric current through a circuit. Impedance depends on the properties of the tissues between the electrodes. If biphasic current is introduced between the implanted lead and the pulse generator, variations in impedance can be measured. During the respiratory cycle, the thoracic cavity size and air content change. These changes correlate with impedance changes if correct filtering is applied. With this method, respiratory rate or relative changes in minute ventilation may be measured accurately [32]. On the basis of these principles, several manufacturers have developed thoracic impedance-based minute ventilation sensors for rate modulation. Several studies have suggested to use algorithms using implanted impedance-based minute ventilation sensors as a screening tool for detecting SA [29, 30, 33, 34].

11.2.1 Boston Scientific Technology

The latest pacemakers, ICDs and CRT devices from Boston Scientific include the AP Scan™ (or ApneaScan™) feature, which uses transthoracic impedance measurements to monitor breathing patterns.

Device-based algorithm automatically detects apnea/hypopnea events by measuring reductions in tidal volume using transthoracic impedance: the device automatically considers a respiratory disturbance event (RDE) when breathing amplitude is reduced by 27 % or more for at least 10 sec, including full breathing pauses (Fig. 11.1).

This is consistent with the clinical definition of apnea and hypopnea reported above. Similarly to the AHI, the number of occurred RDE defines the different grade of sleep-disordered breathing. AP Scan™ diagnostic feature displays a trend of the AHI: each value of AHI represents the nightly average number of RDE, calculated as the total number of RDE occurred during the programmed sleep time divided by the total sleep hours. Sleep time is determined by a clock and is programmed by the physician based on patient's habits; to increase the likelihood that the patient is asleep during the data acquisition, the algorithm begins to acquire the data 1 h after the programmed "sleep start time" and terminates data capture 1 h before the "wake-up time." The AP Scan™ was validated with simultaneous PSG

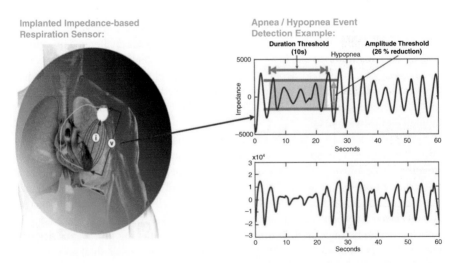

Fig. 11.1 An event of apnea/hypopnea is automatically detected by the device when the reduction in respiratory signal amplitude is greater than 26 % vs baseline. The respiratory signal is based on the transthoracic impedance measured by the sensor (Courtesy of Boston Scientific)

on pacemaker population, showing that AHI is correlated with clinic AHI (R=0.8), with 82% sensitivity and 88% specificity in identifying severe SA patients (AHI ≥ 30) [35]. During the follow-up visits post-implant, the AP Scan™ recordings can be checked by the physician over the course of 1 year. To facilitate the clinical interpretation of the respiratory disturbance trend, the graph shows a threshold at 32 events/hour, which approximately represent the clinical threshold for severe SA (AHI ≥ 30). Values above this threshold may suggest the need for further investigation to determine whether there is a severe breathing disorder during sleep (Fig. 11.2).

Figure 11.3 shows the screen of the device programmer where AP Scan™ is displayed in correlation with other two clinically relevant parameters: respiratory rate and activity level. All these trends can be checked with different granularity, selecting different viewing windows from 1 week up to 1 year; furthermore the physician, using the slider, can select and check specific days.

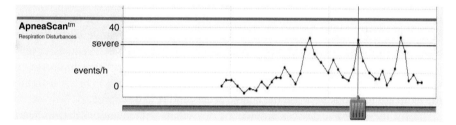

Fig. 11.2 Example of respiratory disturbance index (RDI) trend of Boston Scientific devices, showing the threshold of 32 events/hour as a threshold suggesting the possible need for further clinical investigation (Courtesy of Boston Scientific)

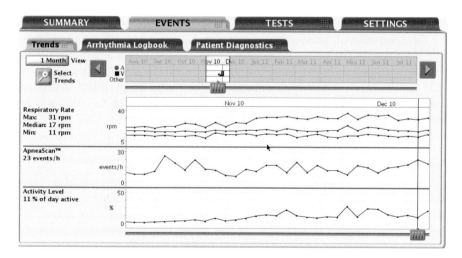

Fig. 11.3 Screenshot of the programmer showing respiratory rate, AP Scan™ and activity level automatically detected from the implanted device (Courtesy of Boston Scientific)

Transthoracic impedance measurements of ventilation are qualitative estimates of ventilation and do not allow a quantitative flow measurement, which constitutes a limitation for subtle hypopnea recognition. Also, this system does not assess directly the severity of nocturnal hypoxia, which is the landmark of SA. However, the duration of abnormal respiratory events is available and reflects the severity of intermittent hypoxia. Both sleep macrostructure and microarousals are not detected by the device. To address this limitation, the patient's sleep period can be adjusted in accordance with patient's sleep habits to ensure a high probability of sleep during the recording period.

In conclusion, although AP Scan™ is not intended to replace existing clinical tests and is not a surrogate for full PSG examination, it can help the physician to identify implanted patients at risk of severe SA, who may benefit from further investigation and potential better treatment.

Furthermore, an implanted cardiac device with a respiratory sensing function may provide not only clinically useful diagnostics for sleep-related breathing disorders but also the possibility to closely track the benefit of treatment and to have further insights into the pathophysiological mechanisms linking SA to HF. It has been well established by a meta-analysis [30] that the hemodynamic improvement induced by CRT is associated with a decrease in SA severity (AHI reduction, particularly in CSA), and it can be useful to analyze the temporal relationship between hemodynamic improvement and SA. Also the algorithm can help in better defining the temporal relations between the apneic events and ICD discharge.

Lastly, these cardiac devices provide the physicians with numerous data as heart rhythm (HR), heart rate variability (HRV), respiratory variables such as AHI, and device interventions that may be integrated with clinical variables to obtain a more complete score of prognostic stratification, through the use of appropriate statistical models. This is particularly true in the setting of patients on optimized pharmacological treatment, with left ventricular dysfunction (LVEF < 40 %), treated with ICD or CRT-D.

The observational, prospective, single-arm study DASAP-HF (ClinicalTrials. gov Identifier: NCT02620930) has been designed to validate the performance of AHI value calculated by AP Scan™ algorithm vs PSG in patients implanted with ICD or CRT-D. As a secondary objective of the study, the incidence of clinical events after 24 months of enrollment and its association with the AHI will be assessed.

11.2.2 LivaNova Technology

With the SA monitoring function, devices from LivaNova provide the physician with automatic screening of recipient patients for the risk of severe SA. SA monitoring has been designed to detect, count, and report abnormal breathing overnight events. These events are detected using the minute ventilation signal. This allows the calculation of AHI over the last 6 months, representing sleep-disordered breathing events. The SA monitoring feature provides information on the number of abnormal breathing patterns in the minute ventilation signal overnight, which could be used as an indicator of potential underlying breathing pathologies such as sleep apnea syndrome. Depending on patient profile and/or other symptoms, the physician may discuss with the patient and schedule a neurologist or a sleep specialist visit, as appropriate. The pacemaker determines ventilation by measuring transthoracic impedance (in single-chamber devices, a bipolar lead is required to operate the sensor). By emitting very low pulses of electrical current between the lead tip and the pacemaker can, the device is able to measure the transthoracic impedance as it changes with inspiration and expiration. (Fig. 11.4). Variations in lung volume during breathing cause the impedance to change (e.g., due to the tissue dilatation, air volume in the lungs, blood volume in vessels, etc.), resulting in a change in the measured voltage. By using Ohm's law, which states that the impedance (Z) is equal to the voltage (V) divided by the current (I) ($Z = V/I$), the device determines the transthoracic impedance over time ($dZ = dV/I$). This measurement is performed every 125 ms (8 Hz), in order to calculate the minute ventilation (MV), which corresponds to the amplitude (A) divided by the period (P) (Fig. 11.5) [30].

Fig. 11.4 Dual-chamber pacemaker – minute ventilation. Current is injected between the tip electrode and the pacemaker can. The voltage between the ring electrode and the pacemaker can is measured, and the resulting impedance (Z) is calculated (Courtesy of LivaNova)

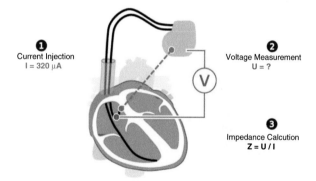

Fig. 11.5 Measure of MV in dynamic impedance: for each cycle (inspiration-expiration), the sensor measures a MIN (+) and a MAX (+) value, extracting an AMPLITUDE, and a PERIOD (Courtesy of LivaNova)

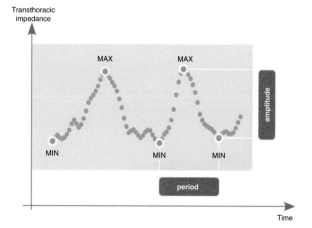

11.2.2.1 Abnormal Breathing Pattern Identification

The SA monitoring algorithm analyzes the transthoracic impedance signal during the night to detect, count, and store abnormal breathing patterns in the pacemaker memory, making them available in the programming screen during patients' follow-up.

At each identified breathing cycle, the ventilation sensor provides a period, an amplitude, and a marker (characteristic of the reliability of this cycle). Using these data, the software is able to validate/exclude the cycle (according to the reliability marker and/or to previous cycles) and check for ventilation pauses and/or for ventilation reductions.

11.2.2.2 Calculation of the AHI

At the end of the monitoring period, which is a 5-h programmable period between 22:00 and 06:00 (by default 00:00–05:00), the total number of ventilation pauses and reductions is divided by five to obtain an occurrence of events per hour, i.e., AHI. AHI is calculated every night and reported since the last follow-up (covering up to the last 6 months). The AHI trend is displayed on the programmer screen together with the trend of time spent in AF (on a daily basis) (Fig. 11.6a). For the night preceding the pacemaker interrogation, the hourly number of respiratory disturbances during the monitoring 5-h period is displayed together with the heart rate curve (Fig. 11.6b). A graph is also displayed to show the cumulative distribution of events (since last follow-up visit) by their duration (step of 10 sec) (Fig. 11.6c).

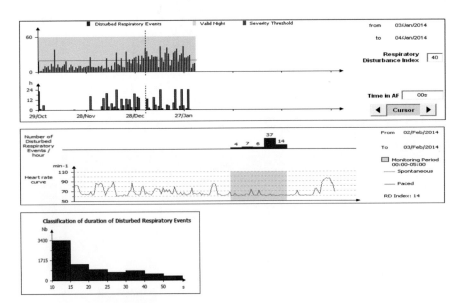

Fig. 11.6 (**a**) RDI and AF trends, (**b**) 5-h RDI and heart rate curve, and (**c**) classification of duration of disturbed respiratory events (Courtesy of LivaNova)

The DREAM pilot study was designed to assess the most recent version of this algorithm in terms of accuracy in identifying severe SA in pacemaker patients (Reply 200 pacemakers, LivaNova).

In a population of 40 unselected patients with a dual-chamber (75%) or a single-chamber (25%) Reply 200 pacemakers, a polysomnography (PSG) was carried out, roughly 2 months after implant. The aim of the study was to compare the AHI calculated by the device vs the AHI values determined by the PSG during the same night: the AHI from the device identified patients with severe SA with an 88.9% sensitivity and 84.6% specificity. By using a receiver operating characteristic (ROC) curve approach, the resulting optimal AHI cutoff to identify severe SA (best compromise between sensitivity and specificity) was 20 events/h. The authors concluded that this transthoracic impedance-derived method for severe SA screening/diagnosis and follow-up may improve the management of patients in routine cardiology practice [30].

Conclusion

In conclusion, SA is a common comorbidity in HF patients, with a worse prognostic outcome. Implantable devices with SA detection algorithm help physicians in screening diagnostic and follow-up therapy and monitoring efficacy of the therapeutic strategies.

Acknowledgments The authors thank Ilaria Vicini (Boston Scientific) and Chiara Angelone (LivaNova) for skillful technical assistance.

References

1. Sin DD, Fitzgerald F, Parker JD, Newton G, Floras JS, Bradley TD. Risk factors for central and obstructive sleep apnea in 450 men and women with congestive heart failure. Am J Respir Crit Care Med. 1999;160:1101–6.
2. Vazir A, Hastings PC, Dayer M, McIntyre HF, Henein MY, Poole-Wilson PA, Cowie MR, Morrell MJ, Simonds AK. A high prevalence of sleep disordered breathing in men with mild symptomatic chronic heart failure due to left ventricular systolic dysfunction. Eur J Heart Fail. 2007;9:243–50.
3. Javaheri S. Sleep disorders in systolic heart failure: a prospective study of 100 male patients. The final report. Int J Cardiol. 2006;106:21–8.
4. Javaheri S, Parker TJ, Liming JD, Corbett WS, Nishiyama H, Wexler L, Roselle GA. Sleep apnea in 81 ambulatory male patients with stable heart failure. Types and their prevalences, consequences and presentations. Circulation. 1998;97:2154–9.
5. Mooe T, Franklin KA, Holmstrom K, Rabben T, Wiklund U. Sleep-disordered breathing and coronary artery disease: long-term prognosis. Am J Respir Crit Care Med. 2001;164:1910–3.
6. Lanfranchi PA, Braghiroli A, Bosimini E, Mazzuero G, Colombo R, Donner CF, Giannuzzi P. Prognostic value of nocturnal cheyne-stokes respiration in chronic heart failure. Circulation. 1999;99:1435–40.
7. Naughton M, Benard D, Tam A, Rutherford R, Bradley TD. Role of hyperventilation in the pathogenesis of central sleep apneas in patients with congestive heart failure. Am Rev Respir Dis. 1993;148:330–8.
8. Gabor JY, Newman DA, Barnard-Roberts V, Korley V, Mangat I, Dorian P, Hanly PJ. Improvement in cheyne-stokes respiration following cardiac resynchronisation therapy. Eur Respir J. 2005;26:95–100.

9. Jaffe LM, Kjekshus J, Gottlieb SS. Importance and management of chronic sleep apnoea in cardiology. Eur Heart J. 2013;34(11):809–15.
10. Garrigue S, Pepin JL, Defaye P, Murgatroyd F, Poezevara Y, Clémenty J, Lévy P. High prevalence of sleep apnea syndrome in patients with long-term pacing: the European multicenter polysomnographic study. Circulation. 2007;115:1703–9.
11. Kasai T, Bradley TD. Obstructive sleep apnoea and heart failure. J Am Coll Cardiol. 2011;57:119–27.
12. Arzt M, Young T, Finn L, Skatrud JB, Ryan CM, Newton GE, Mak S, Parker JD, Floras JS, Bradley TD. Sleepiness and sleep in patients with both systolic heart failure and obstructive sleep apnea. Arch Intern Med. 2006;166:1716–22.
13. Bradley TD, Floras JS. Sleep apnea and heart failure: part I: obstructive sleep apnea. Circulation. 2003;107:1671–8.
14. Bradley TD, Floras JS. Sleep apnea and heart failure: part II: central sleep apnea. Circulation. 2003;107:1822–6.
15. Grimm W, Sharkova J, Heitmann J, Jerrentrup A, Koehler U, Maisch B. Sleep-disordered breathing in recipients of implantable defibrillators. PACE. 2009;32:S8–11.
16. Grimm W, Apelt S, Timmesfeld N, Koehler U. Sleep-disordered breathing in patients with implantable cardioverter-defibrillator. Europace. 2013;15(4):515–22.
17. Roche F, Xuong AN, Court-Fortune I, Costes F, Pichot V, Duverney D, Vergnon JM, Gaspoz JM, Barthélémy JC. Relationship among the severity of sleep apnea syndrome, cardiac arrhythmias, and autonomic imbalance. Pacing Clin Electrophysiol. 2003;26:669–77.
18. Gami AS, Howard DE, Olson EJ, Somers VK. Day-night pattern of sudden death in obstructive sleep apnea. N Engl J Med. 2005;352:1206–14.
19. Tomaello L, Zanolla L, Vassanelli C, LoCascio V, Ferrari M. Sleep disordered breathing is associated with appropriate implantable cardioverter defibrillator therapy in congestive heart failure patients. Clin Cardiol. 2010;33:E27–30.
20. Bitter T, Westerheide N, Prinz C, Hossain MS, Vogt J, Langer C, Horstkotte D, Oldenburg O. Cheyne-stokes respiration and obstructive sleep apnoea are independent risk factors for malignant ventricular arrhythmias requiring appropriate cardioverter-defibrillator therapies in patients with congestive heart failure. Eur Heart J. 2011;32:61–74.
21. Gami AS, Hodge DO, Herges RM, Olson EJ, Nykodym J, Kara T, Somers VK. Obstructive sleep apnea, obesity, and the risk of incident atrial fibrillation. J Am Coll Cardiol. 2007;49:565–71.
22. Mehra R, Benjamin EJ, Shahar E, Gottlieb DJ, Nawabit R, Kirchner HL, Sahadevan J, Redline S. Association of nocturnal arrhythmias with sleep-disordered breathing: the sleep heart health study. Am J Respir Crit Care Med. 2006;173(8):910–6.
23. Gami AS, Pressman G, Caples SM, Kanagala R, Gard JJ, Davison DE, Malouf JF, Ammash NM, Friedman PA, Somers VK. Association of atrial fibrillation and obstructive sleep apnea. Circulation. 2004;110:364–7.
24. Kanagala R, Murali NS, Friedman PA, et al. Obstructive sleep apnea and the recurrence of atrial fibrillation. Circulation. 2003;107:2589–94.
25. European Heart Rhythm Association (EHRA), European Society of Cardiology (ESC), Heart Rhythm Society, Heart Failure Society of America (HFSA), American Society of Echocardiography (ASE), American Heart Association (AHA), European Association of Echocardiography (EAE) of ESC, Heart Failure Association of ESC (HFA), Daubert JC, Saxon L, Adamson PB, Auricchio A, Berger RD, Beshai JF, Breithard O, Brignole M, Cleland J, DeLurgio DB, Dickstein K, Exner DV, Gold M, Grimm RA, Hayes DL, Israel C, Leclercq C, Linde C, Lindenfeld J, Merkely B, Mont L, Murgatroyd F, Prinzen F, Saba SF, Shinbane JS, Singh J, Tang AS, Vardas PE, Wilkoff BL, Zamorano JL, Anand I, Blomström-Lundqvist C, Boehmer JP, Calkins H, Cazeau S, Delgado V, Estes NA, Haines D, Kusumoto F, Leyva P, Ruschitzka F, Stevenson LW, Torp-Pedersen CT. EHRA/HRS expert consensus statement on cardiac resynchronization therapy in heart failure: implant and follow-up recommendations and management. Europace. 2012;14:1236–86.

26. Authors/Task Force Members, Priori SG, Blomström-Lundqvist C, Mazzanti A, Blom N, Borggrefe M, Camm J, Elliott PM, Fitzsimons D, Hatala R, Hindricks G, Kirchhof P, Kjeldsen K, Kuck KH, Hernandez-Madrid A, Nikolaou N, Norekvål TM, Spaulding C, Van Veldhuisen DJ. 2015 ESC Guidelines for the management of patients with ventricular arrhythmias and the prevention of sudden cardiac death: the Task Force for the Management of Patients with Ventricular Arrhythmias and the Prevention of Sudden Cardiac Death of the European Society of Cardiology (ESC) Endorsed by: Association for European Paediatric and Congenital Cardiology (AEPC). Eur Heart J. 2015;36(41):2793–867.
27. Hatala R, Lunati M, Calvi V, Favale S, Goncalvesová E, Haim M, Jovanovic V, Kaczmarek K, Kautzner J, Merkely B, Pokushalov E, Revishvili A, Theodorakis G, Vatasescu R, Zalevsky V, Zupan I, Vicini I, Corbucci G. Clinical implementation of cardiac resynchronization therapy-regional disparities across selected ESC member countries. Ann Noninvasive Electrocardiol. 2015;20(1):43–52.
28. Agusti A, Hedner J, Marin JM, Barbé F, Cazzola M, Rennard S. Night-time symptoms: a forgotten dimension of COPD. Eur Respir Rev. 2011;20:183–94.
29. Shalaby A, Atwood C, Hansen C, Konermann M, Jamnadas P, Lee K, Willems R, Hartley J, Stahmann J, Kwok J, Ni Q, Neuzner J. Feasibility of automated detection of advanced sleep disordered breathing utilizing an implantable pacemaker ventilation sensor. Pacing Clin Electrophysiol. 2006;29:1036–43.
30. Defaye P, de la Cruz I, Martí-Almor J, Villuendas R, Bru P, Sénéchal J, Tamisier R, Pépin JL. A pacemaker transthoracic impedance sensor with an advanced algorithm to identify severe sleep apnea: the DREAM European study. Heart Rhythm. 2014;11(5):842–8.
31. Mond HG, Proclemer A. The 11th world survey of cardiac pacing and implantable cardioverter-defibrillators: calendar year 2009 – a World Society of Arrhythmia's project. Pacing Clin Electrophysiol. 2011;34(8):1013–27.
32. Simon R, Ni Q, Willems R, Hartley JW, Daum DR, Lang D, Ward K, Gill J. Comparison of impedance minute ventilation and direct measured minute ventilation in a rate adaptive pacemaker. Pacing Clin Electrophysiol. 2003;26(11):2127–33.
33. Scharf C, Cho YK, Bloch KE, Brunckhorst C, Duru F, Balaban K, Foldvary N, Liu L, Burgess RC, Candinas R, Wilkoff BL. Diagnosis of sleep-related breathing disorders by visual analysis of transthoracic impedance signals in pacemakers. Circulation. 2004;110:2562–7.
34. Defaye P, Pepin JL, Poezevara Y, Mabo P, Murgatroyd F, Lévy P, Garrigue S. Automatic recognition of abnormal respiratory events during sleep by a pace-maker transthoracic impedance sensor. J Cardiovasc Electrophysiol. 2004;15:1034–40.
35. Lamba J, Simpson CS, Redfearn DP, Michael KA, Fitzpatrick M, Baranchuk A. Cardiac resynchronization therapy for the treatment of sleep apnoea: a meta-analysis. Europace. 2011;13(8):1174–9.

Targeting and Treating Apneas

12

Claudio Passino, Alberto Giannoni, Alberto Aimo,
Gianluca Mirizzi, and Michele Emdin

Abbreviations

AHI	Apnea/hypopnea index
ASV	Adaptive servo-assisted ventilation
BZP	Benzodiazepines
BIPAP	Bi-level positive airway pressure
CB	Carotid body
CBD	Carotid body denervation
CPAP	Continuous positive airway pressure
CSA	Central sleep apnea
CSR	Cheyne-Stokes respiration
EPAP	Expiratory positive airway pressure
$FetCO_2$-$FiCO_2$	Difference in end-tidal CO_2 and inspired CO_2
HCVR	Hypercapnic ventilator response
HF	Heart failure
HFrEF	Heart failure with reduced ejection fraction
HVR	Hypoxic ventilatory response
ICD	Implantable cardioverter-defibrillator

How should we treat apneas? Treating downstream: CPAP vs. servo-ventilation
Treating upstream: which target? (hemodynamics, chemoreflex, others)
When should we treat apneas? When should we not?

C. Passino (✉) • A. Aimo • M. Emdin
Life Science Institute, Scuola Superiore Sant'Anna, Pisa, Italy

Division of Cardiology and Cardiovascular Medicine, Fondazione Toscana G. Monasterio,
Pisa, Italy
e-mail: passino@ftgm.it; a.aimo@sssup.it; emdin@ftgm.it

A. Giannoni • G. Mirizzi
Division of Cardiology and Cardiovascular Medicine, Fondazione Toscana G. Monasterio,
Pisa, Italy
e-mail: alberto.giannoni@ftgm.it; gianluca.mirizzi@ftgm.it

© Springer International Publishing Switzerland 2017
M. Emdin et al. (eds.), *The Breathless Heart*,
DOI 10.1007/978-3-319-26354-0_12

IPAP	Inspiratory positive airway pressure
LV	Left ventricular
LVEF	Left ventricular ejection fraction
NYHA	New York Heart Association
OMT	Optimal medical treatment
OSA	Obstructive sleep apnea
$PaCO_2$	Partial pressure of carbon dioxide in the arterial blood
PB	Periodic breathing
NIV	Noninvasive mechanical ventilation
PCWP	Pulmonary capillary wedge pressure
PSQI	Pittsburgh Sleep Quality Index
R-BNP	Recombinant form of the natural human B-type natriuretic peptide
RSNA	Renal sympathetic nerve activity
VA	Alveolar ventilation
VCO_2	Constant volume of body production of CO_2

12.1 Introduction

How should we treat apneas? Should we choose treatments acting downstream the pathophysiological cascade and applicable only to sleep apneas, such as mechanical ventilation techniques or phrenic nerve stimulation (as discussed in Chap. 13), or should we favor pathophysiological triggers, as improvement of hemodynamics and/or modulation of the apneic threshold? Would it be possible, as a future perspective, to act on chemoreceptors by specific interventions? Is it really necessary to treat all patients with evidence of periodic breathing/Cheyne-Stokes respiration (CSR) phenomenon? Or should we better identify those patients in whom PB/CSR is truly a risky condition? These questions will all be addressed here below.

12.2 How Should We Treat Apneas? Treating Downstream: CPAP Versus Servo-ventilation

12.2.1 Noninvasive Mechanical Ventilation

The use of noninvasive mechanical ventilation (NIV) for the treatment of sleep-related breathing disorders was originally proposed for obstructive sleep apnea (OSA) syndrome. In this setting, several studies confirmed the utility of NIV in symptom relief and in improvement of quality of sleep. In the most recent years, the possibility to use NIV also for treatment of central apneas (central sleep apnea, CSA; Cheyne-Stokes respiration, CSR) in patients with chronic heart failure (HF) has been explored with conflicting results.

12.2.2 Types of Noninvasive Ventilation

12.2.2.1 Continuous Positive Airway Pressure (CPAP)

CPAP is currently the most widely used type of noninvasive ventilation. Its use has been proposed, besides in the emergency room setting, for the treatment of OSA and breathing pattern abnormalities observed in patients with HF. A constant level of positive pressure is delivered to the patient during spontaneous breathing, preventing intermittent collapses of the upper airways; this results in a significant reduction of the number of apnea episodes. In addition, CPAP treatment is able to induce an improvement in functional residual capacity, in daytime gas exchange, and in systolic left ventricular function in HF patients with OSA [1].

12.2.2.2 Auto-CPAP

Auto-CPAP is delivered via a self-titrating CPAP device, which uses different algorithms to detect variations in the degree of obstruction and changes the pressure level to restore normal breathing. Auto-CPAP is able to compensate for body posture during sleep, stage of sleep, and other factors that affect upper airway collapsibility. The auto-CPAP can be used for those patients with OSA related to position, in whom positional maneuvers are not tolerated [2]; it can also be used during cardiorespiratory monitoring to detect the best pressure value to be used later with fixed CPAP for treatment of OSA.

12.2.2.3 Bi-level Positive Airway Pressure (BIPAP)

Bi-level positive airway pressure (BIPAP) is also used for sleep-related disorders (including those associated with chronic heart failure), but its main indication is in pathological conditions associated with hypoventilation. The BIPAP devices deliver a higher pressure during inspiration (inspiratory positive airway pressure, IPAP) and a lower pressure during expiration (expiratory positive airway pressure, EPAP). The gradient between IPAP and EPAP (pressure support ventilation) is crucial in maintaining adequate alveolar ventilation and reducing $PaCO_2$. The IPAP acts also in reducing the work of breathing and fatigue, by reducing the workload of respiratory muscles; EPAP has the function of maintaining the patency of the upper airway, to control obstructive apnea and to improve the functional residual capacity. Main indications for BIPAP include patients with OSA who cannot tolerate exhaling against a high-fixed CPAP pressure, neuromuscular disorders, complex sleep apnea, central apnea in chronic heart failure, and obesity hypoventilation syndrome [3, 4].

12.2.2.4 Adaptive Servo-assisted Ventilation

The adaptive servo-assisted ventilation (ASV) has been developed for the treatment of central apnea syndrome in patients with chronic heart failure. These devices, which are more complex than CPAP and BIPAP, provide expiratory and inspiratory support and are able to automatically adjust the inspiratory pressure support for each inspiration within a prespecified range. To determine the degree of pressure support needed, the ASV algorithm continuously calculates target ventilation. Based on respiratory rate and tidal volume, the target is usually 90 % of the patient's recent average ventilation. Different algorithms have been used to achieve synchronization between pressure support and patient's breathing pattern. These algorithms based on patient's recent average respiratory rate and amplitude and instantaneous direction, magnitude, and rate of change of the patient's airflow deliver different degrees and rates of ventilatory support. In practice, when a central apnea or hypopnea occurs, support initially continues to reflect the patient's recent breathing pattern: if the apnea persists, the device increasingly uses the backup respiratory rate. The advantage of such devices relies on the fact that minimal support is delivered during stable breathing, in theory reducing the adverse hemodynamic effects of NIV. The aim is the stabilization of breathing pattern and to reduce the respiratory alkalosis and hypocapnia occurring during hyperpneas that can trigger apnea reentry cycles [5].

12.2.3 NIV in OSA Syndrome

OSA, differently from central apneas, is characterized by intermittent complete or partial collapse of the upper airway. This pattern of breathing has been associated with several cardiovascular diseases, including systemic hypertension, heart failure, arrhythmias, coronary artery disease, and pulmonary hypertension. Several studies have demonstrated the benefit of NIV in the treatment of OSA. In hypertensive patients, CPAP therapy drops blood pressure by 10 mmHg on average in patients with moderate-to-severe sleep apnea [6, 7]. In patients affected by coronary artery disease and comorbid for OSA, treatment with CPAP reduces angina and nocturnal myocardial ischemia [8] and decreases the incidence of both fatal and nonfatal cardiovascular events approaching the risk observed in simple snorers [9].

In addition to central apneas, patients with heart failure may experience OSA: a number of studies reported a high prevalence of OSA among patients with heart failure (11–38 %) [10]. Patients with heart failure, both with preserved and reduced ejection fraction, and OSA are usually overweight and snore habitually; the association between the severity of heart failure and the occurrence of OSA is weaker than for central apneas, with a 15 % incidence of OSA in patients with mild systolic left ventricular dysfunction [11]. In such patients, CPAP abolishes acute OSA and related hypoxia; reduces nocturnal heart rate, blood pressure, and left ventricular afterload; and improves the neural control of blood pressure and heart rate by increasing baroreflex sensitivity [12, 13]. One mechanism of benefit is likely related to the reduction of the sympathetically mediated vasoconstriction exerted by CPAP in patients with heart failure and OSA [14].

In the setting of heart failure, CPAP therapy has been shown to improve both systolic [15] and diastolic function [16]. The improvement was more marked in patients with a LVEF above 30 % [17]. However, these data have not been confirmed in a randomized, double-blind, crossover study [18]. OSA has been associated with higher mortality in patients with heart failure [19]; however, the impact of CPAP therapy on mortality in patients with heart failure and OSA has not been shown yet.

Based on the abovementioned data, current clinical indications for NIV treatment in OSA rely on the presence of symptoms and of markers of hypoventilation, in the presence of an apnea/hypopnea index (AHI) higher than 15 events/h [20].

12.2.4 NIV in Central Apneas

In patients with HF, CPAP reduces LV transmural pressure and afterload, by increasing intrathoracic pressure [21], and LV preload by reducing end-diastolic volume and pressure [22]. The acute effects in awake patients of CPAP treatment between 5 and 10 cm H_2O on cardiac output are dependent on cardiac preload and rhythm; an increase is observed in patients with high LV filling pressure (i.e., >12 mmHg) and a decrease in those with low LV filling pressure (i.e., <12 mmHg) [23] or atrial fibrillation [24]. However, long-term adverse hemodynamic effects are not known. First studies on the effects of CPAP on central apneas in patients with HF did not demonstrate a significant effect on CSA relief, probably because of differences in how CPAP was applied (short periods, fixed pressure support, with limited patient familiarization with the device). Conversely, following studies in which patients were acclimatized to CPAP with a gradual titration to higher pressures, a positive effect was described, with reduction in AHI up to 67 % [25–28]. In these studies, the reduction in the incidence of apneas was paralleled by an increase in resting $PaCO_2$, an improvement in LVEF [25], and an increased inspiratory muscle strength [26]; in addition, positive effects were also observed on the degree of functional mitral regurgitation [27], sympathetic activation [25], and plasma levels of natriuretic peptides [27]. As concerns the prognostic value of CPAP in HF patients with CSA, a pivotal, short-term single-center study [29] suggested that CPAP, besides improving cardiac function in HF patients with CSA, had an impact on outcome, with a trend toward a reduced combined mortality plus cardiac transplantation. Already from this early study, compliance to treatment emerged as a central issue: in fact, among patients who were compliant with CPAP, the reduction in the combined rate of death and cardiac transplantation was significant. The multicenter CANPAP trial was published in 2005 and was aimed to establish whether CPAP on top of optimized HF therapy would improve CSA, morbidity, and mortality in HF patients with CSA [30]. The CANPAP randomized trial included 258 patients with HF and CSA (AHI > 15/h). Analysis was performed according to the intention-to-treat principle. In this trial CPAP attenuated central sleep apnea, improved nocturnal oxygenation, increased LVEF, lowered norepinephrine levels, and increased the distance at the 6-min walking test, but failed to demonstrate an increase in survival. The study suffered of several restraints: the main one was related to the fact that CPAP therapy, which was used by 85 % of treated subjects for approximately four hours per night, reduced the number of episodes of central apnea by 50 %, with an overall reduction of sleep-breathing disorder by only 25 %, resulting in a substantial under-treatment effect and a potential confounder of the study conclusions. A post hoc analysis of this trial revealed that when patients whose apnea-hypopnea index was not reduced below 15 by CPAP (n=43/110) were excluded from analysis, CPAP resulted in a greater increase in left ventricular ejection fraction at 3 months and significantly better transplant-free survival than control [31]. Survival analysis revealed a divergence of event rates in the first 18 months favoring the control group ($p < 0.02$), which reversed after 18 months to favor CPAP ($p < 0.06$). This suggests that CPAP had an early adverse effect in some subjects, but a late beneficial effect in others. Ultimately, the CANPAP trial lacked power to conclude that CPAP has an impact on survival in HF patients; indeed, the data do not support its routine use in HF patients with CSA.

Two other types of NIV have been evaluated in patients with HF: BIPAP support with a backup rate and ASV. The introduction in the clinical use of ASV devices for treatment of CSA was awaited with high expectations: from small studies, one night of ASV showed a higher improvement on the nocturnal breathing pattern and sleep quality in patients with HF, when compared with CPAP [5]. Furthermore, patients seemed to prefer ASV over CPAP, even during 6 months of treatment [32] with the consequent goal of improving compliance to treatment, which was one of the reasons of the failure of the CANPAP trial.

The SERVE-HF trial [33] was designed to evaluate the effect of treating CSA with an adaptive servo-ventilation (ASV) device in patients with heart failure and reduced ejection fraction. The trial randomly assigned 1325 patients with a left ventricular ejection fraction $\leq 45\%$, an AHI ≥ 15 events/h with a predominance of central events to optimal medical treatment with ASV or optimal medical treatment alone (control). The primary composite end point was death, lifesaving cardiovascular intervention, or unplanned hospitalization for worsening heart failure. As the CANPAP, the SERVE-HF suffered from poor compliance to treatment with the average time of ASV reported by authors equal to 3.4 h per night. Not only ASV had no significant effect on the primary end point, but all-cause and cardiovascular mortality were both increased with this therapy. The authors of the trial speculated that CSA might represent a compensatory mechanism with protective effects in heart failure with reduced ejection fraction (HFrEF) patients and that excess positive intrathoracic pressure caused by ASV might have had adverse cardiovascular consequences.

The CAT-HF study was a prospective, randomized, controlled, multicenter clinical trial in HF patients with either reduced or preserved ejection fraction and an AHI ≥ 15 events/h, designed to evaluate the safety and efficacy of minute ventilation-targeted adaptive servo-ventilation. It was stopped early due to safety concerns [34]. These two latter trials have raised serious concerns about the safety of ASV in HF patients.

The introduction of new generation ASV devices, claiming to be more effective and tolerated, has driven the design of a new trial, the ADVENT-HF, with a planned enrolment of about 850 patients with HFrEF and either obstructive sleep apnea or CSA using an advanced technology ASV device with automatic end-expiratory titration [35].

As conclusive remarks, the disappointing result of applying airway positive pressure to treat CSA in HF patients should not stop the research of treatments for this respiratory disorder. However, a deeper and rational approach, based on the pathophysiology of CSA, is required to positively treat a negative disorder in the complex scenario of heart failure, where pathophysiological mechanisms are strongly interlinked and interdependent.

12.3 How Should We Treat Apneas? Treating Upstream: Which Target? (Chemoreflex, Hemodynamics, Others)

12.3.1 Drugs

12.3.1.1 HF Therapies and Inotropes

Optimal medical treatment (OMT) should be the first step to pursue in patients presenting with HF and CSA/CSR. OMT should improve CSR/CSA by several mechanisms, such as improving cardiac output and thus decreasing circulatory delay and chemoreflex overactivation (see Chap. 5), reducing filling pressure and J receptor-related ventilatory stimulation, and increasing functional residual capacity by decreasing cardiac size and pleural effusion. All these positive effects of OMT may reduce both the chemoreflex and the plant gain, lowering the global loop gain and leading to ventilatory stability [36].

In fact, in a study from Solin et al., a subgroup of seven severe HF patients, awaiting heart transplantation, with initially high pulmonary capillary wedge pressure (PCWP) and central apneas underwent intensive medical treatment with various drugs (diuretics, nitrates, ACE inhibitors, or beta-blockers) including CPAP (but notably not during the night of CSR reassessment). Following this heterogeneous treatments, both PCWP (29.0 ± 2.6–22.0 ± 1.8 mmHg; $p < 0.001$) and AHI (38.5 ± 7.7–18.5 ± 5.3 events/h; $p = 0.005$) were reduced, independently of the drug used. Notably, respiratory instability was not completely abolished, but a certain degree of CSR was still persistent after OMT [37].

In a retrospective analysis of 50 consecutive patients with dilated cardiomyopathy (New York Heart Association, NYHA, classes II–IV and left ventricular ejection fraction $\leq 35\%$), a full-night polysomnography showed that patients in beta-blocker therapy (metoprolol or carvedilol) had lower prevalence of CSR (40 % versus 69 % using an AHI cutoff = 15 events/h) and lower AHI as compared to beta-blocker-free patients (8.7 ± 8.1 versus 19.8 ± 14.2 events/h, $p < 0.05$). Also lower Epworth sleepiness scores were found in patients receiving beta-blockers [38]. These data were confirmed also by the work of Tamura et al., in which a 57 % lower AHI was found in patients taking beta-blockers [39].

Similar data were found with captopril and spironolactone, although the entity of reduction in AHI was lower. On the contrary, ramipril and losartan showed a neutral and negative effect on sleep, respectively [40].

Although the vast majority of studies exploring the effect of neurohormonal antagonists on CSA/CSR are retrospective and some bias is inevitable, a specific effect of these drugs on CSA/CSR triggers, beyond reverse remodeling and improved hemodynamics, is biologically likely, considering that, on the one hand, chemoreceptors are influenced by both sympathetic activation and angiotensin II levels and on the other the chemoreflex system has an adrenergic output (see also Chap. 5, Sect. 5.2.2).

There is currently no information about the effect of inotropes on CSA/CSR, with the only exception of a trial on milrinone, which makes exertional ventilatory oscillation disappear in three patients with severe HF [41].

There are however some studies on the effect of inotropes on the chemoreflex, showing that low-dose dopamine reduces the ventilatory response to hypoxia [42], while dobutamine increases the ventilatory and sympathetic response to hypoxia and has a neutral effect to hyperoxic/hypercapnic response [43, 44].

In a prospective three-way crossover double-blind randomized study performed in seven chronic HF patients, the effects on chemoreflex sensitivity of the recombinant form of the natural human B-type natriuretic peptide (R-BNP) levosimendan were compared with placebo. While levosimendan seems to have a neutral effect on both peripheral and central chemoreceptors, R-BNP seems to increase peripheral chemosensitivity to hypoxia [45].

12.3.1.2 Acetazolamide

Acetazolamide is a mild diuretic agent causing metabolic acidosis [46]. It also acts as a respiratory stimulant, used for the prevention and treatment of PB/CSR related to high altitude or idiopathy. In 2006, the first evidence of efficacy of acetazolamide in the treatment of PB/CSR related to HF has been provided by Javaheri et al. [47]. In this double-blind, crossover study, 12 patients with systolic HF and PB/CSR were randomized to acetazolamide or placebo [47]. The two study arms were comparable at baseline, but after only 5 days, the number of central apneas per hour and the percentage of total sleep time spent below 90 % arterial oxygen saturation were significantly lower in patients treated with acetazolamide than in those receiving placebo [47]. Furthermore, patients receiving acetazolamide reported to sleep better and to feel more rested in the morning and less sleepy during the day [47]. In this study, acetazolamide was administered as a single dose of 3 mg/kg 30 min before bedtime in order to reduce the side effects of frequent administration of acetazolamide, most notably paresthesias and dyspnea [48]. Other studies, using different dosages (250 or 1000 mg o.p.d. or 250 mg b.i.d.), found significant reductions in the AHI [49–51].

The effect of acetazolamide has been ascribed mostly to mild metabolic acidosis, stimulating central chemoreceptors (as demonstrated by an increase in the hypercapnic ventilatory response – HCVR) [49, 52]. On the one hand, this effect would be beneficial, as the enhanced sensitivity to arterial CO_2 would result in a reduced apneic threshold, i.e., the partial pressure of carbon dioxide in the arterial blood ($PaCO_2$) below which ventilation is suppressed; acetazolamide would then reduce the probability of apnea at each given $PaCO_2$ level [53]. On the other hand, the increase in HCVR could represent an intrinsic limitation in acetazolamide efficacy, as enhanced HCVR promotes PB/CSR [54].

Another potential mechanism of action of acetazolamide is represented by its diuretic effect, leading to reduced pulmonary congestion, and improved gas exchanges in the lungs [47]. A potential drawback of acetazolamide therapy is the increased risk for hypokalemia, and then for arrhythmias [46]. At present, there are no large, long-term trials assessing its safety and efficacy in HF patients [48, 53].

12.3.1.3 Theophylline

After the demonstration that theophylline reduces the incidence of central apneas in premature infants (see also Chap. 3) [53], this drug has been considered for the treatment of PB/CSR in patients with HF. After the promising results of some small studies [55, 56], a double-blind, randomized, placebo-controlled, crossover study was performed by Javaheri et al., enrolling 15 patients with stable systolic HF. Oral theophylline, administered in order to reach therapeutic plasma concentrations (11 μg/mL; range, 7–15 μg/mL), reduced the AHI by around 50%, and improved arterial oxyhemoglobin saturation [57].

It has been demonstrated that, in the central nervous system, adenosine depresses ventilation, and at therapeutic serum concentrations, theophylline competes with adenosine for receptor binding [53]. This mechanism could explain the efficacy of theophylline in the reduction of central apneas and hypopneas. Of note, theophylline increases ventilation without affecting the HCVR [58], contrary to acetazolamide (see above).

A strict monitoring of serum theophylline levels must be performed in order to avoid side effects, most notably tachyarrhythmias and seizures, but also other symptoms of central nervous system excitation (headaches, insomnia, irritability, dizziness), and gastrointestinal symptoms (nausea, diarrhea) [59]. In addition, theophylline interacts with many drugs, such as antiepileptics (which reduce theophylline levels), antidepressants, antifungals, and some antiarrhythmics (which increase plasma theophylline), also diuretics (as the concomitant administration increases the risk for hypokalemia) [60]. Furthermore, there are controversial data about the possibility that long-term administration of theophylline could increase sympathetic tone [53], which would be deleterious for patients with HF. On the whole, the safety of theophylline administration to treat PB/CSR has never been assessed in dedicated studies [48, 53].

12.3.1.4 Benzodiazepines

Another potential approach was the administration of benzodiazepines (BZP). In fact, being PB/CSR an oscillatory and (partially) self-maintaining breathing pattern, the respiratory depression by BZP could block the hyperpneic phase, thus possibly stabilizing ventilation [61]. Nonetheless, two studies [61], one of which being a placebo-controlled, double-blind study [62], failed to detect any effect of BZP on PB/CSR in patients with HF. Of note, other respiratory depressants, namely, opioids, can exacerbate central apneas and should be avoided in patients with PB/CSR [48].

Progesterone agonists have been shown to facilitate gas exchanges in obese patients with obstructive apneas, resulting in fewer fluctuations in blood gas values; [63] an efficacy in PB/CSR has been postulated, but never demonstrated so far [64]. Finally, a beneficial effect of the antagonism of serotonin receptor 5-HT1A has also been reported in animals [65] and in single human patients with PB/CSR of neurological origin [66, 67], but no data are currently available in the setting of HF.

12.3.2 Gas Administration

12.3.2.1 Oxygen

Supplemental nasal oxygen administration during sleep is still a promising option for central apneas in patients with HF, as recently reviewed in [68]. Several studies recruiting a small number of patients with HF (from 7 to 36 patients) and supplementing O_2 (1–5 L/min) for a minimum of 1 night up to a maximum of 12 months administration have invariably shown a beneficial decrease of the AHI (from −28 up to −84%) and an amelioration of arterial oxyhemoglobin desaturation [68]. A high degree of heterogeneity in the study populations should be underlined: The majority of the study included patients with systolic HF (EF often below 45%) and with New York Heart Association functional classes II–IV, with different AHI cutoffs as entry criteria (AHI ≥ 5 or 15 events/h) and some studies also enrolling patients with OSA or mixed apneas. In a randomized, placebo-controlled, double-blind study, 1 week nocturnal administration of O_2 improves maximum exercise capacity [69], presumably mediated by a reduction in ventilatory response to CO_2. Moreover, oxygen therapy decreases sympathetic activity as evidenced by both microneurography and urinary norepinephrine excretion (50% reduction) [70, 71]. On the contrary, no effect on natriuretic peptides was observed after O_2 administration. In the three longest-term trials (3–12 months in duration, two randomized control trials and one nonrandomized trial), an average improvement in left ventricular ejection fraction of 5% (95% CI 0.3–98) was observed [72].

Two studies also compared the effect of nocturnal O_2 administration versus CPAP, while two other studies made a comparison with ASV. On the whole, nocturnal O_2 showed similar results as compared to CPAP in terms of AHI reduction, but resulted less effective than ASV, at least on the respiratory data [68]. Differently from CPAP/ASV, in the studies in which nocturnal O_2 was administered over several months, the compliance and tolerance were excellent. Further, with an estimated cost of around 200 dollars per month, oxygen therapy also resulted cost-effective, with an estimated total cost saving for the health care of around 10,000 dollars per year per patient [73]. Finally, again differently from CPAP/ASV, no case of death apparently related to nocturnal O_2 administration was reported; nevertheless, the effect of long-term O_2 in patients with HF remains unknown.

A small rise in $PaCO_2$ and thus an increase in the difference between prevailing partial pressure of carbon dioxide ($PaCO_2$) and the apneic $PaCO_2$ threshold, together with a reduction in ventilatory response to CO_2, and increasing body stores (e.g., lung contents) of O2 with underdamping effects are the most likely mechanisms through which O_2 administration may cause reduction of central apneas and lead to higher ventilatory stability [36].

Despite the several studies showing the beneficial effects of oxygen on central apnea, exercise capacity, and sympathetic activation, no prospective randomized placebo-controlled long-term study specifically designed to determine if O_2 therapy has the potential to decrease morbidity and mortality has been realized in HF so far [74].

12.3.2.2 Carbon Dioxide

Although oscillations in the $PaCO_2$ are known to drive the characteristic ventilatory fluctuations of CSR/CSA in heart failure (see Chaps. 4 and 5), the wide range of therapies so far investigated in patients with HF and CSR do not specifically target these oscillations. Based on the rationale that patients with CSR/CSA experience apneas when the $PaCO_2$ levels drop below the apneic threshold, the effect of inhaled CO_2 on CSR/CSA has also been investigated.

Previous attempts to treat CSA/CSR by administering CO_2 have either used a constant concentration or flow rate of CO_2 throughout the CSA/CSR cycle (static administration pattern) [75–78].

The administration of CO_2 was actually really effective in suppressing CSA/CSR, with a stabilizing effect superior than O_2 administration, as may be predicted by the physiology of breathing and the pathophysiology of CSA/CSR, where CO_2 plays a key role (see also Chaps. 2, 4, and 5). Indeed in the study of Steens et al [75], inhaled CO_2 (3 % constant flow) virtually eradicates CSA/CSR in patients; however, it was found that this therapy negatively affected some features of sleep structure such as sleep latency. The same remarkable effect on CSA/CSR was shown by Andreas, who added CO_2 to O_2 administration, again completely abolishing CSA/CSR [78]. However, an undesirable increase in sympathetic outflow was observed [78] and later confirmed by Lorenzi-Filho and coworkers [77], deflating any enthusiasm about CO_2 administration in HF patients, where sympathetic activation is usually detrimental. Furthermore, a fixed increase in inspired CO_2 concentration mandates an increase in ventilation and therefore increases the work of breathing. This has often been commented on in previous studies but not always quantified. However, it may be easily calculated by the following equation:

$$VA = \frac{VCO_2}{\left(FetCO_2 - FiCO_2\right)}$$ where VA is the alveolar ventilation, VCO_2 is a constant

volume of body production of CO_2, and $FetCO_2$-$FiCO_2$ is the difference in end-tidal CO_2 and inspired CO_2. Using this calculation, which provides only a lower limit on the increment in ventilation, ventilation with constant CO_2 is increased by up to 96 % (24–96 %). Adding dead space is an alternative way to elevate end-tidal CO_2 with potential effect on breathing stability. Sommer [79] and Banzett [80] developed devices that give added inspired CO_2 during the patient's hyperventilation phase to increase end-tidal CO_2, effectively minimizing changes in alveolar gases during hyperpnea. However, this was achieved at the cost of increased ventilation, similar to static supplementary CO_2 administration.

By carefully targeting therapy to a certain proportion of the CSA/CSR cycle, it would be possible to fill in the troughs of CO_2 producing the hypopneic phase of ventilation while minimizing the overall dose of CO_2 delivered so that there is not a substantial increase in mean CO_2 and ventilation. Using mathematical modeling, Mebrate et al. explored the consequences of dynamic CO_2 administration, with different timing and dosing algorithms [81].

The optimal time window identified by mathematical simulation and corresponding to peak hyperventilation was then tested using an automated system and a rotatory valve mixing air with CO_2 in both healthy subjects reproducing voluntary periodic breathing and a small group of HF patients with spontaneous daytime CSR. Dynamic CO_2 was actually able to stabilize both CO_2 and ventilatory oscillations (43 and 68 % in HF patients, respectively), minimizing the dose delivered (only 0.5 % CO_2) and thus the increase in both end-tidal CO_2 and ventilation, compared with static CO_2 [82].

This may be of potential clinical interest, but further studies in larger cohort, with some specific information about the effect of dynamic CO_2 on the sympathetic system are mandatory, before challenging this kind of intervention in randomized control trials.

12.3.3 Devices and Surgery

12.3.3.1 Overdrive Pacing, Cardiac Resynchronization Therapy, and Dynamic Pacing

In 15 subjects, some of whom had mild left ventricular systolic dysfunction (n=4%, 27%), atrial overdrive pacing was shown to improve central and obstructive sleep apnea. These subjects had permanent atrial-synchronized ventricular pacemakers placed for symptomatic sinus bradycardia. Nocturnal atrial overdrive (from 51 ± 8 to 72 ± 4 beats per minute) moderately decreased AHI (from 28 ± 22 to 11 ± 14 events/h), improved arterial oxyhemoglobin desaturation, and decreased arousals. It should be emphasized that in these patients, central apneas accounted for most of the disordered breathing events and drive the reduction after pacing. The mechanisms of action remain unclear [83]. In a second randomized, crossover study, 12 patients (LVEF $38.3 \pm 13.6\%$) with indications for a dual-chamber pacemaker or defibrillator (ICD) were randomized to algorithm ON-OFF (group A) or OFF-ON (group B). Patients had this time mainly OSA and mixed apneas (9 and 3 patients, respectively). In these patients, long-term dynamic atrial overdrive pacing did not improve AHI and Pittsburgh Sleep Quality Index (PSQI) questionnaire [84].

In another study from the same group, Sinha et al demonstrated that cardiac resynchronization therapy (CRT) leads to a reduction of central apneas and to increased sleep quality in patients with HF and CSA/CSR [85]. Twenty-four patients with HF (LVEF $24 \pm 6\%$), and left bundle branch block (QRS duration 173 ± 22 ms), underwent CRT: 14 patients showed CSA/CSR (AHI>5 events/h), and 10 patients did not. After 17 ± 7 weeks of CRT, there is a significant decrease in AHI (19.2 ± 10.3– 4.6 ± 4.4, $p<0.001$) and PSQI (10.4 ± 1.6–3.9 ± 2.4, $p<0.001$) and a significant increase in SaO_2min (84 ± 5–$89 \pm 2\%$, $p<0.001$), in HF patients with CSA/CSR, while no change was observed in patients without CSR/CSA. Authors discussed that this finding may partly justify the prognostic improvement observed in HF patients undergoing CRT.

Dynamic manipulation of cardiac output via pacemaker fluctuations obtained by adjusting heart rate (by 30 beats/min) or atrioventricular delay (between optimal and non optimal values) or both, with period of 60 s in 19 heart failure patients (age 73+/−11, EF 29+/−12%), was able to engender both oscillation in end-tidal CO_2

and ventilation, by likely recruiting the CO_2 reserve stored in the peripheral venous system [86]. While this pacemaker manipulation has so far been developed for inducing experimental periodic breathing, this may potentially be applied for stabilizing breathing as dynamic CO_2, but with the great advantage of using intracorporeal CO_2, without any need of face mask and nasal *cannulae* and no risk of CO_2 toxicity [87].

12.3.3.2 Heart Transplantation, Valve Surgery, and Ventricular Assist Devices

Cardiac transplantation usually eliminates CSA/CSR, due to the reversal of the hemodynamic features of HF that mediate CSR/CSA onset and maintenance [88–90]. However, OSA may develop after cardiac transplantation [91]. Indeed, weight gain is common in transplant recipients, due to both the use of steroids and improved quality of life, and obesity is known to increase the risk of OSA. A relatively large study number in cardiac transplant recipients showed a 36 % prevalence of OSA, using an AHI cutoff of 15 events/h and an average index of 50 events/h, with OSA indeed related with the weight gain after cardiac transplantation [92].

Similarly, some case reports have pointed out that CSA/CSR is ameliorated after either mitral valve repair [93] or replacement [94].

In other case reports, the effect of ventricular assist device implantation on apneas was evaluated, showing conflicting results. A patient with end-stage HF first underwent biventricular assist device implantation, obtaining CSA and OSA resolution, and then heart transplantation, with recurrence of OSA, probably due to weight gain [95]. In the study of Padeletti et al., three patients with acute decompensation of end-stage congestive HF were evaluated before and after the implantation of a monoventricular assist device; CSA/CSR was slightly reduced in two patients and actually worsened in one patient, despite hemodynamic improvement [96].

12.3.3.3 Chemoreflex Modulation or Demolition?

As already reviewed in Chap. 5, the role played by increased chemosensitivity on the HF progression has recently received attention, since it is thought to contribute to sympathetic overactivation, to CSA/CSR genesis, [97], and finally to increased mortality in HF [98, 99].

Therefore, therapeutic intervention targeting either peripheral or central chemoreceptor can have the potential to simultaneously improve breathing stability, the adrenergic outflow, and eventually quality of life and mortality in HF. While there are some promising data collected in the animal setting concerning the treatment of peripheral chemoreceptors, currently there are no data about the possibility of treating central chemoreceptors.

In experimentally induced HF, an enhancement of peripheral chemosensitivity associated with elevated sympathetic outflow and desensitization of the baroreflex, as well as with increased ventilatory instability, has been thoroughly demonstrated by the group of Shultz [100].

Notably, selective bilateral surgical elimination of the carotid bodies reduced central presympathetic neuronal activation, normalized sympathetic outflow and baroreflex sensitivity, and stabilized breathing function in animal with HF. In pacing-induced HF rabbits (CHF-sham), ventilatory responses to hypoxia were augmented compared to healthy animals (sham-sham) and reduced after bilateral carotid body denervation (CBD). Bilateral CBD also reduced resting renal sympathetic nerve activity (RSNA: $43\pm5\%$ CHF-sham versus $25\pm1\%$ CHF-CBD max, $p<0.05$) to values comparable to healthy rabbits ($23\pm2\%$ in sham-sham). Low-frequency/high-frequency heart rate variability ratio was similarly increased in CHF and reduced by CBD ($p<0.05$). Finally, respiratory rate variability index and apnea-hypopnea index were increased in CHF-sham animals and reduced in CHF-CBD animals ($p<0.05$). Finally, arrhythmia incidence was increased in CHF-sham and reduced in CHF-CBD animals (213 ± 58 events/h versus 108 ± 48 events/h, $p<0.05$). Furthermore, ventricular systolic and diastolic volumes were reduced, and ejection fraction increased ($41\pm5\%$ versus $54\pm2\%$, $p<0.05$) [101].

Similar findings were obtained also in rats with HF induced by coronary ligation. In this case, a selective unilateral CBD reduced the central presympathetic neuronal activation by 40%, normalized indexes of sympathetic outflow and baroreflex sensitivity, and reduced the incidence of apneas in HF animals from 16.8 ± 1.8–8.0 ± 1.4 events/h. Remarkably, when CB ablation was performed early, a positive effect on both cardiac remodeling and arrhythmias was obtained. Moreover, early CB ablation improved survival at 3 months follow-up from 45% to 85% [102].

Interestingly, a case report from a heart failure patient in which unilateral CB ablation was performed showed again promising results with significant improvement in autonomic balance and breathing variability. Taken together, these data support the idea that CB ablation could represent a novel therapeutic strategy to reduce cardiorespiratory and autonomic dysfunction in HF potentially improving survival.

Some safety concerns have however been raised [103]. Indeed, CBs are the main sensors of hypoxia, with only a minor contribution of aortic bodies in humans [104]. Therefore, an irreversible bilateral surgical CB demolition seems far from desirable in HF patients, in whom a quick response to hypoxia as in acute life-threatening conditions is indeed necessary. Monolateral CB surgery, as already tested in rats [102], or, alternatively, a reversible pharmacological/non-pharmacological CB modulation could succeed in blunting the negative effects of PC overactivity, without affecting its physiological function [105].

Another possibility is to indirectly interfere with chemoreflex activity, primarily acting on the baroreflex and the ergoreflex, since the peripheral feedbacks are all integrated at brainstem level (see also Chap. 5). While, no data about the baroreflex modulation of chemosensitivity and CSA/CSR are currently available, preliminary results in animals make exercise training (EXT) a fascinating option. Indeed, it has long been known that EXT has a positive effect on a reflex originating from the peripheral muscles as the ergoreflex [106]. Likewise, the positive effect of EXT on sympathovagal balance are widely acknowledged and partly attributed to restoration of the baroreflex [107]. In the experimental setting, it was shown that EXT decreases hypoxia-evoked afferent activity from CB and hypoxia-evoked increases in RSNA [108]. While the effect of EXT on OSA is also well known and mainly linked to weight loss, no data are currently available about the effect of this therapy on CSA/CSR. However, Zurek M et al. demonstrated that EXT leads to the disappearance of exertional oscillatory ventilation (conceptually linked with CSA/CSR) in about 70 % of the HF patient subgroup after training (versus 2.3 % in the control group) [109].

A specific kind of training acting on inspiratory muscle may add further benefits in HF patients. Indeed, 32 HF patients were randomized to inspiratory muscle training (IMT) or placebo for 12 weeks using a specific device and instructed to maintain diaphragmatic breathing with a breathing rate of 15–20 breaths/min. For the IMT group, inspiratory load was set at 30 % of maximal static inspiratory pressure, and weekly training loads were adjusted to maintain 30 % of the maximal inspiratory pressure. IMT resulted in marked improvement in inspiratory muscle strength and improvement in functional capacity and quality of life. Remarkably a reduction in exertional ventilatory oscillation was observed. A potential beneficial effect of ergo-receptors on chemoreceptors may be hypothesized [110]. Finally, a completely different kind of respiration, with the slow and deep breathing (6 breaths/min) typical of Yoga mantra and rosary prayer, is known not only to reduce dyspnea and improve exercise performance in HF [111, 112] but also to decrease the chemoreflex sensitivity to hypoxia and hypercapnia [113], with thus potential beneficial effects on HF-related CSR.

12.4   When Should We Treat Apneas? When Should We Not? Conclusive Remarks

CANPAP and SERVE-HF, two multicenter, randomized controlled phase III trials on noninvasive mechanical ventilation to cure sleep CSR in systolic HF, have failed to show any improvement in survival and rather evidenced poor compliance and an incremental risk of mortality in the treated population. This reproducible negative result raises doubt about whether treating CSR is advisable or not [114]. However, PB/CSR occurs often at daytime in awake patients, and even during effort, its presence holding an independent, additive prognostic value, as compared with central sleep apnea [115–117]. Noninvasive mechanical ventilation acts on apneas "downstream" and only in asleep patients, with a poor compliance, and has no recognized favorable effect "upstream" on pathophysiological triggers, being, therefore, not able to treat daytime apnea. Several diverse attempts have been made to cure PB/CSR acting on altered chemoreflex sensitivity to hypoxia and/or hypercapnia or alternatively on circulatory delay, which both represent the main pathways to PB/CSR initiation and maintenance. Regarding the latter target, as shown throughout the present chapter, guideline-recommended pharmacologic therapy and cardiac resynchronization therapy are effective in decreasing periodic breathing by improving hemodynamics. On the other hand, inhalation of pure oxygen, of carbon dioxide, or of oxygen/carbon dioxide mixtures and the administration of acetazolamide differently play with chemoreceptors (either decreasing or further increasing chemosensitivity) and with apnea threshold, globally decreasing periodic breathing incidence. The observation of reduced exercise tolerance as undesirable "collateral effect" of acetazolamide treatment by Fontana et al. [49] and Apostolo et al. [118] raises a question, together with the negative effects on outcome of noninvasive mechanical ventilation [119]: Is PB/CSR always detrimental or only in a subset of patients? Future studies are warranted, which should investigate how to identify patients, in whom PB/CSR is no more compensatory, as in Naughton's hypothesis, but promoting the evolution of heart failure disease and life-threatening events, in order to consider only this subset for treatment. It seems reasonable to propose that the diagnostic workup for PB/CSR/central apneas would not aim only to detect the presence/absence of the phenomenon, but better to consider, as a guide to decision-making for treatment possible predictors of efficacy. A list of potential predictors of therapy effectiveness could be the following: (a) PB/CSR severity, as identified by polygraphy (e.g., daytime occurrence and/or apnea/hypopnea index >30); (b) the quantification of chemoreflex activation (notably another predictor of poor outcome in HF), circulatory delay, and plant gain (still often overlooked in HF) for a tailored approach; (c) the level of neurohormonal activation (plasma concentration of nor-epinephrine or B-type natriuretic peptides); and (d) the severity of underlying cardiac function or a combination of all these predictors. Therefore treatment success should be based on three prerequisites/goals: the proof that the underlying disease is treated, the expected benefit on symptoms, and the evidence that further pathological consequences are prevented. These benefits should be accompanied by treatment safety profile and patients' compliance to therapy (Fig. 12.1).

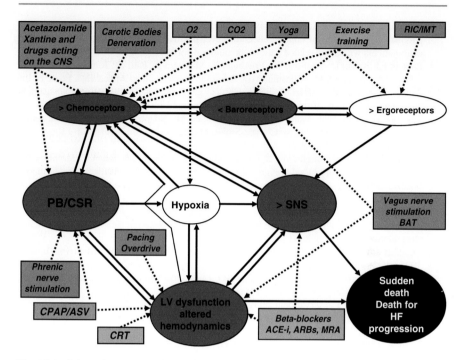

Fig. 12.1 Schematic representation of the pathophysiological contribution of Cheyne-Stokes respiration to disease progression and of therapies currently targeting ventilatory instability in heart failure

Solid arrows indicate direct pathophysiological effects/influences. *Dotted arrows* link established or potential therapeutic interventions with HF-related targets

In *red*, factors with detrimental prognostic significance in HF; in *green*, therapies with proven positive prognostic impact in HF; in *blue*, therapies with unknown effect on survival; and, in *violet*, therapies with neutral or potentially negative impact on survival

ACE-i angiotensin-converting enzyme inhibitors, *ARB* angiotensin receptor blockers, *ASV* assisted servo-ventilation, *BAT* baroreceptor activation therapy, *CPAP* continuous positive airway pressure, *CNS* central nervous system, *CRT* cardiac resynchronization therapy, *CSR* Cheyne-Stokes respiration, *HF* heart failure, *IMT* inspiratory muscle training, *MRA* mineralocorticoid receptor antagonist, *LV* left ventricular, *HF* heart failure, *PB* periodic breathing, *RIC* remote ischemic conditioning

Gently taken and adapted with permission from Giannoni A, Mirizzi G, Aimo A, Emdin M, Passino C. Peripheral reflex feedbacks in chronic heart failure: Is it time for a direct treatment? World J Cardiol. 2015;7:824–8

References

1. Theerakittikul T, Ricaurte B, Aboussouan LS. Noninvasive positive pressure ventilation for stable outpatients: CPAP and beyond. Cleve Clin J Med. 2010;77:705–14.
2. Meurice JC, Cornette A, Philip-Joet F, Pepin JL, Escourrou P, et al. Evaluation of autoCPAP devices in home treatment of sleep apnea/hypopnea syndrome. Sleep Med. 2007;8: 695–703.

3. Kushida CA, Littner MR, Hirshkowitz M, American Academy of Sleep Medicine. Practice parameters for the use of continuous and bilevel positive airway pressure devices to treat adult patients with sleep related patients breathing disorders. Sleep. 2006;29:375–80.
4. Epstein LJ, Kristo D, Strollo Jr PJ, Friedman N, Malhotra A, Patil SP, Ramar K, Rogers R, Schwab RJ, Weaver EM, Weinstein MD, Adult Obstructive Sleep Apnea Task Force of the American Academy of Sleep Medicine. Clinical guideline for the evaluation, management and long-term care of obstructive sleep apnea in adults. J Clin Sleep Disord. 2009;5:263–76.
5. Teschler H, Döhring J, Wang YM, Berthon-Jones M. Adaptive pressure support servo-ventilation: a novel treatment for Cheyne-Stokes respiration in heart failure. Am J Respir Crit Care Med. 2001;164:614–9.
6. Pepperell JC, Ramdassingh-Dow S, Crosthwaite N, Mullins R, Jenkinson C, Stradling JR, Davies RJ. Ambulatory blood pressure after therapeutic and subtherapeutic nasal continuous positive airway pressure for obstructive sleep apnoea: a randomised parallel trial. Lancet. 2002;359:204–10.
7. Becker HF, Jerrentrup A, Ploch T, Grote L, Penzel T, Sullivan CE, Peter JH. Effect of nasal continuous positive airway pressure treatment on blood pressure in patients with obstructive sleep apnea. Circulation. 2003;107:68–73.
8. Franklin KA, Nilsson JB, Sahlin C, Naslund U. Sleep apnoea and nocturnal angina. Lancet. 1995;345:1085–7.
9. Marin JM, Carrizo SJ, Vicente E, Agusti AG. Long-term cardiovascular outcomes in men with obstructive sleep apnoea-hypopnoea with or without treatment with continuous positive airway pressure: an observational study. Lancet. 2005;365:1046–53.
10. Bradley TD, Floras JS. Sleep apnea and heart failure: part I: obstructive sleep apnea. Circulation. 2003;107:1671–8.
11. Vazir A, Hastings PC, Dayer M, McIntyre HF, Henein MY, Poole-Wilson PA, Cowie MR, Morrell MJ, Simonds AK. A high prevalence of sleep disordered breathing in men with mild symptomatic chronic heart failure due to left ventricular systolic dysfunction. Eur J Heart Fail. 2007;9:243–50.
12. Tkacova R, Rankin F, Fitzgerald FS, Floras JS, Bradley TD. Effects of continuous positive airway pressure on obstructive sleep apnea and left ventricular afterload in patients with heart failure. Circulation. 1998;98:2269–75.
13. Tkacova R, Dajani HR, Rankin F, Fitzgerald FS, Floras JS, Bradley TD. Continuous positive airway pressure improves nocturnal baroreflex sensitivity of patients with heart failure and obstructive sleep apnea. J Hypertens. 2000;18:1257–62.
14. Usui K, Bradley TD, Spaak J, Ryan CM, Kubo T, Kaneko Y, Floras JS. Inhibition of awake sympathetic nerve activity of heart failure patients with obstructive sleep apnea by nocturnal continuous positive airway pressure. J Am Coll Cardiol. 2005;45:2008–11.
15. Mansfield DR, Gollogly NC, Kaye DM, Richardson M, Bergin P, Naughton MT. Controlled trial of continuous positive airway pressure in obstructive sleep apnea and heart failure. Am J Respir Crit Care Med. 2004;169:361–6.
16. Arias MA, Garcia-Rio F, Alonso-Fernandez A, Mediano O, Martinez I, Villamor J. Obstructive sleep apnea syndrome affects left ventricular diastolic function: effects of nasal continuous positive airway pressure in men. Circulation. 2005;112:375–83.
17. Egea CJ, Aizpuru F, Pinto JA, Ayuela JM, Ballester E, Zamarron C, Montserrat JM, Barbe F, Alonso-Gomez AM, Rubio R, Lobo JL, Duran-Cantolla J, Zorrilla V, Nuñez R, Cortés J, Jiménez A, Cifrián J, Ortega M, Carpizo R, Sánchez A, Terán J, Iglesias L, Fernández C, Alonso ML, Cordero J, Roig E, Pérez F, Muxi A, Gude F, Amaro A, Calvo U, Masa JF, Utrabo I, Porras Y, Lanchas I, Sánchez E. Cardiac function after CPAP therapy in patients with chronic heart failure and sleep apnea: a multicenter study. Sleep Med. 2008;9:660–6.
18. Smith LA, Vennelle M, Gardner RS, McDonagh TA, Denvir MA, Douglas NJ, Newby DE. Auto-titrating continuous positive airway pressure therapy in patients with chronic heart failure and obstructive sleep apnoea: a randomized placebo-controlled trial. Eur Heart J. 2007;28:1221–7.

19. Wang H, Parker JD, Newton GE, Floras JS, Mak S, Chiu KL, Ruttanaumpawan P, Tomlinson G, Bradley TD. Influence of obstructive sleep apnea on mortality in patients with heart failure. J Am Coll Cardiol. 2007;49:1625–31.

20. Robert D, Argaud L. Non-invasive positive ventilation in the treatment of sleep-related breathing disorders. Sleep Med. 2007;8:441–52.

21. Naughton MT, Rahman MA, Hara K, Floras JS, Bradley TD. Effect of continuous positive airway pressure on intrathoracic and left ventricular transmural pressures in patients with congestive heart failure. Circulation. 1995;91:1725–31.

22. Mehta S, Liu PP, Fitzgerald FS, Allidina YK, Bradley TD. Effects of continuous positive airway pressure on cardiac volumes in patients with ischemic and dilated cardiomyopathy. Am J Respir Crit Care Med. 2000;161:128–34.

23. De Hoyos A, Liu PP, Benard DC, Bradley TD. Haemodynamic effects of continuous positive airway pressure in humans with normal and impaired left ventricular function. Clin Sci (Lond). 1995;88:173–8.

24. Kiely JL, Deegan P, Buckley A, Shiels P, Maurer B, McNicholas WT. Efficacy of nasal continuous positive airway pressure therapy in chronic heart failure: importance of underlying cardiac rhythm. Thorax. 1998;53:957–62.

25. Naughton MT, Benard DC, Liu PP, Rutherford R, Rankin F, Bradley TD. Effects of nasal CPAP on sympathetic activity in patients with heart failure and central sleep apnea. Am J Respir Crit Care Med. 1995;152:473–9.

26. Granton JT, Naughton MT, Benard DC, Liu PP, Goldstein RS, Bradley TD. CPAP improves inspiratory muscle strength in patients with heart failure and central sleep apnea. Am J Respir Crit Care Med. 1996;153:277–82.

27. Tkacova R, Liu PP, Naughton MT, Bradley TD. Effect of continuous positive airway pressure on mitral regurgitant fraction and atrial natriuretic peptide in patients with heart failure. J Am Coll Cardiol. 1997;30:739–45.

28. Arzt M, Schulz M, Wensel R, Montalvan S, Blumberg FC, Riegger GA, Pfeifer M. Nocturnal continuous positive airway pressure improves ventilatory efficiency during exercise in patients with chronic heart failure. Chest. 2005;127:794–802.

29. Sin DD, Logan AG, Fitzgerald FS, Liu PP, Bradley TD. Effects of continuous positive airway pressure on cardiovascular outcomes in heart failure patients with and without Cheyne-Stokes respiration. Circulation. 2000;102:61–6.

30. Bradley TD, Logan AG, Kimoff RJ, Series F, Morrison D, Ferguson K, Belenkie I, Pfeifer M, Fleetham J, Hanly P, et al. Continuous positive pulmonary airway pressure for central sleep apnea and heart failure. N Engl J Med. 2005;353:2025–33.

31. Arzt M, Floras JS, Logan AG, Kimoff RJ, Series F, Morrison D, Ferguson K, Belenkie I, Pfeifer M, Fleetham J, Hanly P, Smilovitch M, Ryan C, Tomlinson G, Bradley TD, CANPAP Investigators. Suppression of central sleep apnea by continuous positive airway pressure and transplant-free survival in heart failure: a post hoc analysis of the Canadian Continuous Positive Airway Pressure for Patients with Central Sleep Apnea and Heart Failure Trial (CANPAP). Circulation. 2007;115:3173–80.

32. Philippe C, Stoica-Herman M, Drouot X, Raffestin B, Escourrou P, Hittinger L, Michel PL, Rouault S, d'Ortho MP. Compliance with and efficacy of adaptive servo-ventilation (ASV) versus continuous positive airway pressure (CPAP) in the treatment of Cheyne-Stokes respiration in heart failure over a six month period. Heart. 2005;92:337–42.

33. Cowie MR, Woehrle H, Wegscheider K, Angermann C, d'Ortho MP, Erdmann E, Levy P, Simonds AK, Somers VK, Zannad F, Teschler H. Adaptive servo-ventilation for central sleep apnea in systolic heart failure. N Engl J Med. 2015;373:1095–105.

34. Fiuzat M, Oldenberg O, Whellan DJ, Woehrle H, Punjabi NM, Anstrom KJ, Blase AB, Benjafield AV, Lindenfeld J, O'Connor CM. Lessons learned from a clinical trial: design, rationale, and insights from the cardiovascular improvements with minute ventilation-targeted Adaptive Servo-Ventilation (ASV) therapy in Heart Failure (CAT-HF) study. Contemp Clin Trials. 2016;47:158–64.

35. National Institutes of Health. Effect of Adaptive Servo Ventilation (ASV) on survival and hospital admissions in heart failure (ADVENT-HF). https://clinicaltrials.gov/ct2/show/NCT01128816

36. Javaheri S. Central sleep apnea in congestive heart failure: prevalence, mechanisms, impact, and therapeutic options. Semin Respir Crit Care Med. 2005;26:44–55.

37. Solin P, Bergin P, Richardson M, Kaye DM, Walters EH, Naughton MT. Influence of pulmonary capillary wedge pressure on central apnea in heart failure. Circulation. 1999;99:1574–9.

38. Köhnlein T, Welte T. Does beta-blocker treatment influence central sleep apnoea? Respir Med. 2007;101:850–3.

39. Tamura A, Kawano Y, Naono S, Kotoku M, Kadota J. Relationship between beta-blocker treatment and the severity of central sleep apnea in chronic heart failure. Chest. 2007;131:130–5.

40. Jiménez JA, Greenberg BH, Mills PJ. Effects of heart failure and its pharmacological management on sleep. Drug Discov Today Dis Model. 2011;8:161–6.

41. Ribeiro JP, Knutzen A, Rocco MB, Hartley LH, Colucci WS. Periodic breathing during exercise in severe heart failure. Reversal with milrinone or cardiac transplantation. Chest. 1987;92:555–6.

42. Niewinski P, Tubek S, Banasiak W, Paton JF, Ponikowski P. Consequences of peripheral chemoreflex inhibition with low-dose dopamine in humans. J Physiol. 2014;592:1295–308.

43. Velez-Roa S, Kojonazarov B, Ciarka A, Godart P, Naeije R, Somers VK, van de Borne P. Dobutamine potentiates arterial chemoreflex sensitivity in healthy normal humans. Am J Physiol Heart Circ Physiol. 2003;285:H1356–61.

44. Velez-Roa S, van de Borne P, Somers VK. Dobutamine potentiates the peripheral chemoreflex in patients with congestive heart failure. J Card Fail. 2003;9:380–3.

45. Bocchi EA, Moura LZ, Issa VS, Cruz F, Carvalho VO, Guimarães GV. Effects of the recombinant form of the natural human B-type natriuretic peptide and levosimendan on pulmonary hyperventilation and chemosensivity in heart failure. Cardiovasc Ther. 2013;31:100–7.

46. Brunton L, Chabner B, Knollman B. Goodman and Gilman's The pharmacological basis of therapeutics. 12th edn, New York, The McGraw-Hill Companies Inc.; 2011.

47. Javaheri S. Acetazolamide improves central sleep apnea in heart failure: a double-blind, prospective study. Am J Respir Crit Care Med. 2006;173:234–7.

48. Grayburn RL, Kaka Y, Tang WH. Contemporary insights and novel treatment approaches to central sleep apnea syndrome in heart failure. Curr Treat Options Cardiovasc Med. 2014;16:322.

49. Fontana M, Emdin M, Giannoni A, Iudice G, Baruah R, Passino C. Effect of acetazolamide on chemosensitivity, Cheyne-Stokes respiration, and response to effort in patients with heart failure. Am J Cardiol. 2011;107:1675–80.

50. DeBacker WA, Verbraecken J, Willemen M, Wittesaele W, DeCock W, Van deHeyning P. Central apnea index decreases after prolonged treatment with acetazolamide. Am J Respir Crit Care Med. 1995;151:87–91.

51. White DP, Zwillich CW, Pickett CK, Douglas NJ, Findley LJ, Weil JV. Central sleep apnea. Improvement with acetazolamide therapy. Arch Intern Med. 1982;142:1816–9.

52. Javaheri S, Sands SA, Edwards BA. Acetazolamide attenuates Hunter-Cheyne-Stokes breathing but augments the hypercapnic ventilatory response in patients with heart failure. Ann Am Thorac Soc. 2014;11:80–6.

53. Javaheri S. Sleep-related breathing disorders in heart failure. In: Mann DL, editor. Heart failure. A companion to Braunwald's heart disease. Philadelphia: Elsevier Saunders; 2004.

54. Dempsey JA, Smith CA, Blain GM, Xie A, Gong Y, Teodorescu M. Role of central/peripheral chemoreceptors and their interdependence in the pathophysiology of sleep apnea. Adv Exp Med Biol. 2012;758:343–9.

55. Dowell AR, Heyman A, Sieker HO, Tripathy K. Effect of aminophylline on respiratory-center sensitivity in Cheyne-Stokes respiration and in pulmonary emphysema. N Engl J Med. 1965;273:1447–53.

56. Tomcsányi J, Karlócai K. Effect of theophylline on periodic breathing in congestive heart failure measured by transcutaneous oxygen monitoring. Eur J Clin Pharmacol. 1994;46:173–4.
57. Javaheri S, Parker TJ, Wexler L, Liming JD, Lindower P, Roselle GA. Effect of theophylline on sleep-disordered breathing in heart failure. N Engl J Med. 1996;335:562–7.
58. Javaheri S, Guerra L. Lung function, hypoxic and hypercapnic ventilatory responses, and respiratory muscle strength in normal subjects taking oral theophylline. Thorax. 1990;45: 743–7.
59. Barnes PJ. Theophylline. Am J Respir Crit Care Med. 2013;188:901–6.
60. Karalliedde LD, Clarke S, Gotel U, Karalliedde J. Adverse drug interactions: a handbook for prescribers. Boca Raton: CRC Press; 2010.
61. Guilleminault C, Clerk A, Labanowski M, Simmons J, Stoohs R. Cardiac failure and benzodiazepines. Sleep. 1993;16:524–8.
62. Biberdorf DJ, Steens R, Millar TW, Kryger MH. Benzodiazepines in congestive heart failure: effects of temazepam on arousability and Cheyne-Stokes respiration. Sleep. 1993;16: 529–38.
63. Kimura H, Tatsumi K, Kunitomo F, Okita S, Tojima H, Kouchiyama S, Masuyama S, Shinozaki T, Mikami M, Watanabe S. Obese patients with sleep apnea syndrome treated by progesterone. Tohoku J Exp Med. 1988;156:151–7.
64. Eckert DJ, Jordan AS, Merchia P, Malhotra A. Central sleep apnea: pathophysiology and treatment. Chest. 2007;131:595–607.
65. Moore MW, Chai S, Gillombardo CB, Carlo A, Donovan LM, Netzer N, Strohl KP. Two weeks of buspirone protects against posthypoxic ventilatory pauses in the C57BL/6J mouse strain. Respir Physiol Neurobiol. 2012;183(1):35–40.
66. Wilken B, Lalley P, Bischoff AM, Christen HJ, Behnke J, Hanefeld F, Richter DW. Treatment of apneustic respiratory disturbance with a serotonin-receptor agonist. J Paediatr. 1994;130:89–94.
67. El-Khatib MF, Kiwan RA, Jamaleddine GW. Buspirone treatment for apneustic breathing in brain stem infarct. Respir Care. 2003;48:956–8.
68. Bordier P, Lataste A, Hofmann P, Robert F, Bourenane G. Nocturnal oxygen therapy in patients with chronic heart failure and sleep apnea: a systematic review. Sleep Med. 2016;17:149–57.
69. Andreas S, Clemens C, Sandholzer H, Figulla HR, Kreuzer H. Improvement of exercise capacity with treatment of Cheyne-Stokes respiration in patients with congestive heart failure. J Am Coll Cardiol. 1996;27:1486–90.
70. Andreas S, Bingeli C, Mohacsi P, Lischer TF, Noll G. Nasal oxygen and muscle sympathetic nerve activity in heart failure. Chest. 2003;123:366–71.
71. Staniforth AD, Kinneart WJM, Hetmanski DJ, Hetmanski DJ, Cowley AJ. Effect of oxygen on sleep quality, cognitive function and sympathetic activity in patients with chronic heart failure and Cheyne-Stokes respiration. Eur Heart J. 1998;19:922–8.
72. Aurora RN, Chowdhuri S, Ramar K, Bista SR, Casey KR, Lamm CI, Kristo DA, Mallea JM, Rowley JA, Zak RS, Tracy SL. The treatment of central sleep apnea syndromes in adults: practice parameters with an evidence-based literature review and meta-analyses. Sleep. 2012;35:17–40.
73. Seino Y, Imai H, Nakamoto T, Araki Y, Sasayama S, CHF-HOT. Clinical efficacy and cost-benefit analysis of nocturnal home oxygen therapy in patients with central sleep apnea caused by chronic heart failure. Circ J. 2007;71:1738–43.
74. Javaheri S. Pembrey's dream: the time has come for a long-term trial of nocturnal supplemental nasal oxygen to treat central sleep apnea in congestive heart failure. Chest. 2003;123:322–5.
75. Steens RD, Millar TW, Su X, et al. Effect of inhaled 3 % CO_2 on Cheyne-Stokes respiration in congestive heart failure. Sleep. 1994;17:61–8.
76. Szollosi I, Jones M, Morrell MJ, Helfet K, Coats AJ, Simonds AK. Effect of CO_2 inhalation on central sleep apnea and arousals from sleep. Respiration. 2004;71:493–8.

77. Lorenzi-Filho G, Rankin F, Bies I, Douglas Bradley TD. Effects of inhaled carbon dioxide and oxygen on Cheyne-Stokes respiration in patients with heart failure. Am J Respir Crit Care Med. 1999;159:1490–8.
78. Andreas S, Weidel K, Hagenah G, Heindl S. Treatment of Cheyne-Stokes respiration with nasal oxygen and carbon dioxide. Eur Respir J. 1998;12:414–9.
79. Sommer LZ, Iscoe S, Robicsek A, Kruger J, Silverman J, Rucker J, Dickstein J, Volgyesi GA, Fisher JA. A simple breathing circuit minimizing changes in alveolar ventilation during hyperpnoea. Eur Respir J. 1998;12:698–701.
80. Banzett RB, Garcia RT, Moosair SH. Simple contrivance "clamps" and tidal PCO_2 and PO_2 despite rapid changes in ventilation. J Appl Physiol. 2000;88:1597–600.
81. Mebrate Y, Willson K, Manisty CH, Baruah R, Mayet J, Hughes AD, Parker KH. Francis DP (2009) Dynamic CO_2 therapy in periodic breathing: a modeling study to determine optimal timing and dosage regimes. J Appl Physiol. 2009;107:696–706.
82. Giannoni A, Baruah R, Willson K, Mebrate Y, Mayet J, Emdin M, Hughes AD, Manisty CH, Francis DP. Real-time dynamic carbon dioxide administration: a novel treatment strategy for stabilization of periodic breathing with potential application to central sleep apnea. J Am Coll Cardiol. 2010;56(22):1832–7.
83. Garrigue S, Bordier P, Jaïs P, Shah DC, Hocini M, Raherison C, Tunon De Lara M, Haïssaguerre M, Clementy J. Benefit of atrial pacing in sleep apnea syndrome. N Engl J Med. 2002;346:404–12.
84. Sinha AM, Bauer A, Skobel EC, Markus KU, Ritscher G, Noelker G, Breithardt OA, Brachmann J, Stellbrink C. Long-term effects of dynamic atrial overdrive pacing on sleep-related breathing disorders in pacemaker or cardioverter defibrillator recipients. Pacing Clin Electrophysiol. 2009;32:S219–22.
85. Sinha AM, Skobel EC, Breithardt OA, Norra C, Markus KU, Breuer C, Hanrath P, Stellbrink C. Cardiac resynchronization therapy improves central sleep apnea and Cheyne-Stokes respiration in patients with chronic heart failure. J Am Coll Cardiol. 2004;44:68–71.
86. Baruah R, Manisty CH, Giannoni A, Willson K, Mebrate Y, Baksi AJ, Unsworth B, Hadjiloizou N, Sutton R, Mayet J, Francis DP. Novel use of cardiac pacemakers in heart failure to dynamically manipulate the respiratory system through algorithmic changes in cardiac output. Circ Heart Fail. 2009;2:166–74.
87. Baruah R, Giannoni A, Willson K, Manisty CH, Mebrate Y, Kyriacou A, Yadav H, Unsworth B, Sutton R, Mayet J, Hughes AD, Francis DP. Novel cardiac pacemaker-based human model of periodic breathing to develop real-time, pre-emptive technology for carbon dioxide stabilisation. Open Heart. 2014;1(1), e000055.
88. Braver HM, Brandes WC, Kubiet MA, Limacher MC, Mills Jr RM, Block AJ. Effect of cardiac transplantation on Cheyne-Stokes respiration occurring during sleep. Am J Cardiol. 1995;76:632–4.
89. Murdock DK, Lawless CE, Loeb HS, Scanlon PJ, Pifarré R. The effect of heart transplantation on Cheyne-Stokes respiration associated with congestive heart failure. J Heart Transplant. 1986;5:336–7.
90. Mansfield DR, Solin P, Roebuck T, Bergin P, Kaye DM, Naughton MT. The effect of successful heart transplant treatment of heart failure on central sleep apnea. Chest. 2003;124:1675–81.
91. Collop NA. Cheyne-Stokes ventilation converting to obstructive sleep apnea following heart transplantation. Chest. 1993;104:1288–9.
92. Javaheri S, Abraham WT, Brown C, Nishiyama H, Giesting R, Wagoner LE. Prevalence of obstructive sleep apnoea and periodic limb movement in 45 subjects with heart transplantation. Eur Heart J. 2004;25:260–6.
93. Rubin AE, Gottlieb SH, Gold AR, Schwartz AR, Smith PL. Elimination of central sleep apnoea by mitral valvuloplasty: the role of feedback delay in periodic breathing. Thorax. 2004;59:174–6.
94. Yasuma F, Hayashi H, Noda S, Tsuzuki M, Tanaka M, Okada T. A case of mitral regurgitation whose nocturnal periodic breathing was improved after mitral valve replacement. Jpn Heart J. 1995;36:267–72.

95. Vermes E, Fonkoua H, Kirsch M, Damy T, Margarit L, Hillion ML, Hittinger L, d'Ortho MP. Resolution of sleep-disordered breathing with a biventricular assist device and recurrence after heart transplantation. J Clin Sleep Med. 2009;5:248–50.
96. Padeletti M, Henriquez A, Mancini DM, Basner RC. Persistence of Cheyne–Stokes breathing after left ventricular assist device implantation in patients with acutely decompensated end-stage heart failure. J Heart Lung Transplant. 2007;26:742.
97. Giannoni A, Emdin M, Poletti R, Bramanti F, Prontera C, Piepoli M, Passino C. Clinical significance of chemosensitivity in chronic heart failure: influence on neurohormonal derangement, Cheyne-Stokes respiration and arrhythmias. Clin Sci (Lond). 2008;114:489–97.
98. Ponikowski P, Chua TP, Anker SD, Francis DP, Doehner W, Banasiak W, Poole-Wilson PA, Piepoli MF, Coats AJ. Peripheral chemoreceptor hypersensitivity: an ominous sign in patients with chronic heart failure. Circulation. 2001;104:544–9.
99. Giannoni A, Emdin M, Bramanti F, Iudice G, Francis DP, Barsotti A, Piepoli M, Passino C. Combined increased chemosensitivity to hypoxia and hypercapnia as a prognosticator in heart failure. J Am Coll Cardiol. 2009;53:1975–80.
100. Schultz HD, Marcus NJ, Del Rio R. Role of the carotid body chemoreflex in the pathophysiology of heart failure: a perspective from animal studies. Adv Exp Med Biol. 2015;860: 167–85.
101. Marcus NJ, Del Rio R, Schultz EP, Xia XH, Schultz HD. Carotid body denervation improves autonomic and cardiac function and attenuates disordered breathing in congestive heart failure. J Physiol. 2014;592:391–408.
102. Del Rio R, Marcus NJ, Schultz HD. Carotid chemoreceptor ablation improves survival in heart failure: rescuing autonomic control of cardiorespiratory function. J Am Coll Cardiol. 2013;62:2422–30.
103. Giannoni A, Passino C, Mirizzi G, Del Franco A, Aimo A, Emdin M. Treating chemoreflex in heart failure: modulation or demolition? J Physiol. 2014;592:1903–4.
104. Prabhakar NR, Peng YJ. Peripheral chemoreceptors in health and disease. J Appl Physiol. 2004;96:359–66.
105. Del Rio R, Marcus NJ, Schultz HD, 1985. Inhibition of hydrogen sulfide restores normal breathing stability and improves autonomic control during experimental heart failure. J Appl Physiol. 2013;114:1141–50.
106. Piepoli M, Clark AL, Volterrani M, Adamopoulos S, Sleight P, Coats AJ. Contribution of muscle afferents to the hemodynamic, autonomic, and ventilatory responses to exercise in patients with chronic heart failure: effects of physical training. Circulation. 1996;93: 940–52.
107. Groehs RV, Toschi-Dias E, Antunes-Correa LM, Trevizan PF, Rondon MU, Oliveira P, Alves MJ, Almeida DR, Middlekauff HR, Negrão CE. Exercise training prevents the deterioration in the arterial baroreflex control of sympathetic nerve activity in chronic heart failure patients. Am J Physiol Heart Circ Physiol. 2015;308:H1096–102.
108. Li Y, Ding Y, Agnew C, Schultz HD. Exercise training improves peripheral chemoreflex function in heart failure rabbits. J Appl Physiol. 2008;105:782–90.
109. Zurek M, Corrà U, Piepoli MF, Binder RK, Saner H. Schmid JP Exercise training reverses exertional oscillatory ventilation in heart failure patients. Eur Respir J. 2012;40:1238–44.
110. Dall'Ago P, Chiappa GR, Guths H, Stein R, Ribeiro JP. Inspiratory muscle training in patients with heart failure and inspiratory muscle weakness: a randomized trial. J Am Coll Cardiol. 2006;47:757–63.
111. Bernardi L, Spadacini G, Bellwon J, Hajiric R, Roskamm H, Frey AW. Effect of breathing rate on oxygen saturation and exercise performance in chronic heart failure. Lancet. 1998;351:1308–11.
112. Bernardi L, Sleight P, Bandinelli G, Cencetti S, Fattorini L, Wdowczyc-Szulc J, Lagi A. Effect of rosary prayer and yoga mantras on autonomic cardiovascular rhythms: comparative study. BMJ. 2001;323:1446–9.
113. Spicuzza L, Gabutti A, Porta C, Montano N, Bernardi L. Yoga and chemoreflex response to hypoxia and hypercapnia. Lancet. 2000;356:1495–6.

114. Emdin M, Passino C, Giannoni A. After the SERVE-HF trial, is there still a need for treatment of central apnea? J Card Fail. 2015;21:903–5.
115. Poletti R, Passino C, Giannoni A, Zyw L, Prontera C, Bramanti F, Clerico A, Piepoli M, Emdin M. Risk factors and prognostic value of daytime Cheyne-Stokes respiration in chronic heart failure patients. Int J Cardiol. 2009;137:47–53.
116. Brack T, Tüer I, Clarenbach F, Senn O, Noll G, Russi EW, Bloch KE. Daytime Cheyne-Stokes respiration in ambulatory patients with severe congestive heart failure is associated with increased mortality. Chest. 2007;132:1463–71.
117. Corrà U, Pistono M, Mezzani A, Braghiroli A, Giordano A, Lanfranchi P, Bosimini E, Gnemmi M, Giannuzzi P. Sleep and exertional periodic breathing in chronic heart failure: prognostic importance and interdependence. Circulation. 2006;113:44e50.
118. Apostolo A, Agostoni P, Contini M, Antonioli L, Swenson ER. Acetazolamide and inhaled carbon dioxide reduce periodic breathing during exercise in patients with chronic heart failure. J Card Fail. 2014;20:278e88.
119. Emdin M, Passino C. Targeting periodic breathing in heart failure patients, and treating it – gently. J Card Fail. 2014;20:289–91.

Novel Tools for Treating Central Apneas

13

Stimulating the Phrenic Nerve

Maria Rosa Costanzo

Abbreviations

AHI	Apnea-hypopnea index
ASV	Adaptive servo-ventilation
CAI	Central apnea index
CANPAP	Continuous positive airway pressure for central sleep apnea in heart failure
CPAP	Continuous positive airway pressure therapy
CSA	Central sleep apnea
DSMB	Data safety and monitoring board
EPSS	Epworth sleepiness scale
GDMT	Guideline-based medical treatment
HF	Heart failure
hs-CRP	C-reactive protein
MLWHFQ	Minnesota living with heart failure questionnaire
OSA	Obstructive sleep apnea
PGA	Patient global assessment
PNS	ODI4% Oxygen desaturation index $\geq 4\%$ phrenic nerve stimulation
SERVE-HF	Treatment of sleep-disordered breathing with predominant central sleep apnea by adaptive servo-ventilation in patients with heart failure

M.R. Costanzo
Advocate Heart Institute, Naperville, IL, USA
e-mail: mariarosa.costanzo@advocatehealth.com

© Springer International Publishing Switzerland 2017
M. Emdin et al. (eds.), *The Breathless Heart*,
DOI 10.1007/978-3-319-26354-0_13

13.1   Introduction

Central sleep apnea (CSA) is distinguished by a temporary lack of neural output from the respiratory control center, which results in loss of respiratory stimulation and airflow cessation [1, 2]. CSA has a high prevalence across diverse populations [2], including the elderly [3] and patients with a broad range of cardiovascular (heart failure, atrial fibrillation, valvular disease, pulmonary hypertension) [4–9] and cerebrovascular (stroke, carotid stenosis) [10, 11] diseases.

Similar to obstructive sleep apnea (OSA), CSA also is associated with a pattern of hypoxia and surges in sympathetic activity, [12–14] which leads to increases in blood pressure, preload, and afterload [12] and promotes myocardial ischemia and arrhythmias [15, 16]. Hypoxia in the setting of sleep-disordered breathing has been associated with an increased risk of unfavorable outcomes [17]. CSA also enhances oxidative stress, causing endothelial dysfunction and inflammation and activating neurohormonal systems, which contribute to progression of underlying diseases [12]. This pathophysiology may explain the association between CSA and poor outcomes that has been observed in some populations [12].

Currently available treatment options for CSA are not widely accepted because of limited effectiveness data, poor patient adherence in some studies, and potential safety risks that currently are not well understood [18, 19].

Continuous positive airway pressure (CPAP) therapy has been the most common approach to the treatment of CSA. In contrast to treatment of OSA, where application of nasal CPAP consistently results in the virtual elimination of obstructive disordered breathing events, application of CPAP to the treatment of CSA in systolic heart failure (HF) has yielded variable results [20–24]. In one randomized trial of patients with HF and predominantly CSA, CPAP therapy failed to reduce mortality in its overall population [15], although survival improved in those patients in whom the apnea-hypopnea index (AHI) was reduced by CPAP to ≤15 events/h [20].

Another mask-based treatment, adaptive servo-ventilation (ASV), a therapy that delivers servo-controlled inspiratory pressure support on top of expiratory positive airway pressure, was studied in patients with predominantly CSA, left ventricular ejection fraction (LVEF) ≤45 %, and AHI ≥ 15 events/h. In the adaptive servo-ventilation for central sleep apnea in systolic heart failure (SERVE-HF) trial, 1325 patients were randomized to receive either guideline-based medical treatment (GDMT) with ASV (treatment) or GDMT alone (control). In the ASV group, 12-month AHI was reduced to a mean of 6.6 events/h. The primary end point of time to the first event of death from any cause, lifesaving cardiovascular intervention, or unplanned hospitalization for worsening HF, did not differ significantly between groups [54.1 % (ASV) and 50.8 % (control); HR = 1.13; 95 % CI: 0.97–1.31; $P = 0.10$]. Unexpectedly all-cause mortality and cardiovascular mortality were significantly higher in the ASV than in the control group ($p < 0.01$) [25].

The pathophysiological causes of the excess mortality remain unknown. The details of the debate on whether CSA is a compensatory mechanism or whether ASV may have detrimental hemodynamic effects in advanced HF patients are presented in Chap. 9. Nevertheless, based on the result of SERVE-HF, ASV is no longer recommended as an acceptable treatment of CSA in HF patients.

The lack of effective therapies for CSA and its serious adverse effects on underlying disease progression renders the pursuit of alternative treatments for this sleep-disordered breathing both attractive and compelling.

Phrenic nerve stimulation (PNS) offers an alternative means to regulate breathing by utilizing a physiological approach to initiate respiration. This therapy is currently used to provide respiratory support in select patients with respiratory paralysis from high cervical spinal cord injury and in patients with central alveolar hypoventilation syndrome (Ondine's curse) [26–29]. Given this experience, PNS to regulate breathing may also prove useful in HF for the treatment of CSA.

Until recently, chronic stimulation of the phrenic nerve required transthoracic surgical placement of cuff electrodes on the nerve itself. This surgical procedure was not well tolerated in patients with advanced HF and was complicated by instances of damage to the nerve either by direct surgical manipulation or by contact with the electrode [30]. A transvenous approach to the stimulation of the phrenic nerves has been developed, and it has been tested in the studies which are described below.

13.2 Feasibility Trial of Transvenous Phrenic Nerve Stimulation

The first study of transvenous unilateral PNS employed temporary venous access and compared patients' sleep variables during one night of therapy versus those of a control night [31]. Venous access was obtained via the axillary or subclavian veins. Based on the patient's anatomy and the implanting physician's preference, stimulation leads (Cardima catheter, Cardima Inc., Fremont, CA, USA, or proprietary stimulation leads, Respicardia Inc., Minnetonka, MN, USA) were placed in the right brachiocephalic vein, the left brachiocephalic vein, or the left pericardiophrenic vein to stimulate the adjacent phrenic nerve. An external pulse generator system (Respicardia Inc., Minnetonka, MN, USA) provided low-energy phrenic nerve stimulation. During the lead implantation procedure, capture was determined by external palpation of diaphragmatic contraction on the side of stimulation. The stimulation lead was then secured to the skin for the duration of the study. Additionally, two patients underwent optional temporary azygos lead implantation for sensing respiration by intrathoracic impedance [31]. Therapy period was (mean + SD) 251 + 71 min. Stimulation resulted in significant improvement in the AHI [median (inter-quartile range); 45 (39–59) vs. 23 (12–27) events/h, $P<0.002$], central apnea index (CAI) [27 (11–38) vs. 1 (0–5) events/h, $P\leq0.001$], arousal index [32 (20–42) vs. 12 (9–27) events/h, $P<0.001$], and oxygen desaturation index $\geq 4\%$ (ODI4%) [31 (22–36) vs. 14 (7–20) events/h, $P<0.002$]. No significant changes occurred in the obstructive AHI or hypopnea index [31] (Figs. 13.1 and 13.2).

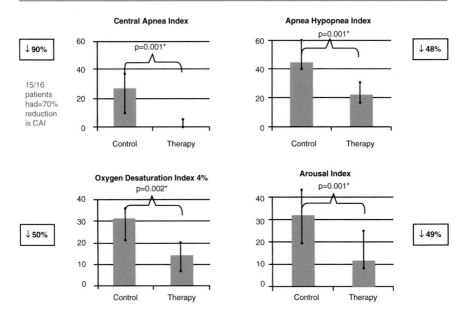

Fig. 13.1 Feasibility trial of phrenic nerve stimulation with the remedē® System. Compared to the control night, therapy resulted in a reduction of 90 % in central apnea events (*p* < 0.001), 48 % in apnea-hypopnea index (*p* = 0.002), 50 % in oxygen desaturation by ≥4 % index (*p* = 0.002), and 49 % in arousal index (*p* = 0.001) (Adapted with permission from Ref. [31])

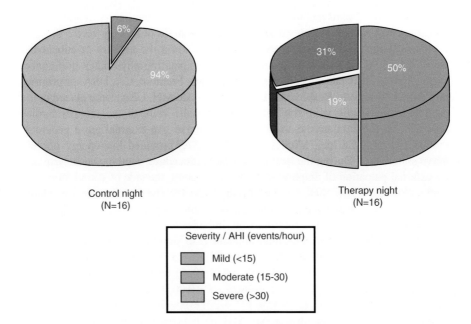

Fig. 13.2 Feasibility trial of phrenic nerve stimulation with the remedē® System. Change in the severity of sleep apnea, as measured by apnea-hypopnea events per hour during the treatment compared to the control night (Adapted with permission from Ref. [31])

Since the cardiovascular effects of CSA are thought to be largely mediated by intermittent hypoxia and arousal, the observed improvement in desaturations and arousals supports the potential beneficial clinical effects of unilateral transvenous PNS therapy. Notably, in both OSA and CSA, mortality is highest in those with the most severe sleep apnea, defined as an AHI ≥ 30 events/h [32, 33]. In the feasibility trial of unilateral transvenous PNS, the percentage of patients with severe sleep apnea decreased from 94 % to 19 % with therapy. This study had the expected limitations of an early phase feasibility trial. Although the study was nonrandomized and open label, the individuals scoring polysomnograms (PSGs) were blinded to whether the sleep variables were assessed during a treatment or control night. Admittedly the study's sample was small, and all subjects were male, a fact which may be due to the significantly higher frequency of CSA in male HF patients [5, 23]. The short duration of the study may have prevented the adequate assessment of potential complications of PNS, including possible interference with preexisting implanted cardiac rhythm devices. The authors of the study acknowledged that 15/31 patients could not be enrolled in the study due to the inability to obtain adequate venous access [31]. However, it should be recognized that this study represented the first experience with placement of leads in the brachiocephalic or pericardiophrenic veins and that achievement of adequate venous access improved throughout the course of the study. Due to the small sample size, it was impossible for the feasibility trial to evaluate the physiological mechanisms by which PNS provided the observed clinical benefits.

13.3   Description of the Fully Implantable remedē® System and Pilot Trial of Phrenic Nerve Stimulation

The encouraging results of the feasibility trial lead to the development of a fully implantable system for unilateral transvenous PNS (Respicardia Inc., Minnetonka, MN, USA). The remedē® System consists of a pulse generator, a stimulation lead, an optional sensing lead, and an external programmer used to adjust the settings on the pulse generator or to review diagnostic data via telemetry (Figs. 13.3 and 13.4). The remedē® pulse generator, similar in size and appearance to a standard pacemaker, is implanted in the right or left pectoral region (Fig. 13.3). The system uses a transvenous lead implanted in the left pericardiophrenic or right brachiocephalic vein to provide neurostimulation to the adjacent phrenic nerve, resulting in diaphragmatic contraction. Sensing of respiration is accomplished either by the stimulation lead or a separate lead inserted in the azygos vein. Device-based sensors detect patient position and activity, aiding the device in determining appropriate therapy delivery times per the algorithm described in Fig. 13.5. As shown in Fig. 13.6, phrenic neurostimulation enables the resumption of normal breathing. By stabilizing carbon dioxide, the remedē® System prevents apneic events and the subsequent periods of rapid breathing [19].

This PNS and subsequent diaphragmatic contraction create negative intrathoracic pressure so that airflow is augmented and cyclical periodic breathing and

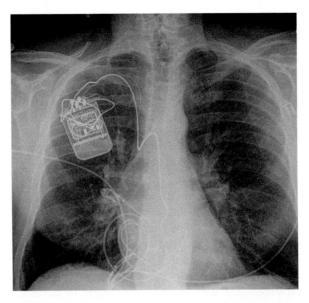

Fig. 13.3 Implanted remedē® System. In this patient, the neurostimulator was implanted in the right pectoral area. The right subclavian approach was used to place the stimulation lead in the left pericardiophrenic vein and to place the sensing lead in the azygos vein

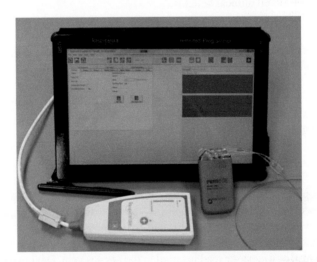

Fig. 13.4 The remedē® System consists of an implantable pulse generator, an implantable stimulation leads, and an external system programmer

blood gas alterations are prevented. In contrast, PAP therapy forces air into the lungs under pressure, thereby increasing intrathoracic pressure. Increased intrathoracic pressure adversely affects both right and left ventricular preload and afterload, which ultimately has detrimental effects on cardiac output. Negative pressure

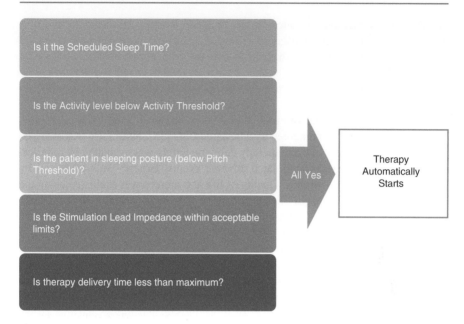

Fig. 13.5 The therapy algorithm used by the remedē® System to provide phrenic nerve stimulation during sleep. The system uses time of day, activity level, and body position (upright or recumbent) to determine a potential sleeping state and, therefore, if stimulation should occur. All of these parameters are adjustable and can be tailored to each patient's specific sleeping routine

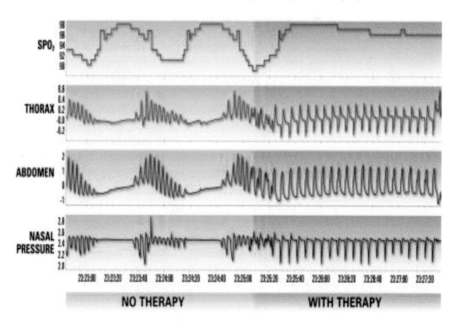

Fig. 13.6 Polysomnogram demonstrating the effects of phrenic nerve stimulation. The tracing shows respiratory stabilization of a patient with central sleep apnea with Cheyne-Stokes respiration after transvenous, unilateral phrenic nerve stimulation therapy

ventilation, such as that provided by the remedē® System, is similar to that of a cuirass ventilator, which is designed to prevent the adverse hemodynamic effects of positive pressure ventilation in lung injury patients and post-thoracic surgery patients [34]. Therefore, the remedē® System, designed to mimic this negative pressure ventilation, minimizes any negative hemodynamic effects in patients with cardiovascular diseases.

The pilot trial of transvenous unilateral PNS using the remedē® System enrolled 57 patients with CSA documented by a baseline PSG [35]. Feasibility was assessed by implantation success rate and therapy delivery. Safety was evaluated by monitoring of device- and procedure-related adverse events. Efficacy was evaluated by changes in the AHI at 3 months. Quality of life at 6 months was evaluated using the Epworth Sleepiness Scale (EPSS) questionnaire, patient global assessment (PGA), and, in patients with HF at baseline, the Minnesota Living with Heart Failure Questionnaire (MLWHFQ). The study met its primary end point, demonstrating a 55 % reduction in AHI from baseline to 3 months (49.5 ± 14.6 episodes/h vs. 22.4 ± 13.6 episodes/h of sleep; $p < 0.0001$; 95 % CI for change: -32.3 to -21.9). Central apnea index, oxygenation, and arousals significantly improved. Favorable effects on quality of life and sleepiness were noted. In patients with HF, the MLWHF score significantly improved. Device- or procedure-related serious adverse events occurred in 26 % of patients through 6 months after therapy initiation, predominantly due to the need to reposition the stimulating lead early in the study. Therapy was well tolerated and efficacy was maintained at 6 months [35]. This pilot study confirmed that the fully implantable remedē® System could achieve acutely improvement in sleep variables as significant as those observed in the feasibility trial with temporary venous access [31]. In addition, the pilot trial extended the findings of the earlier study by showing that improvement in AHI, central apnea index, arousals, sleep efficiency, and rapid eye movement (REM) sleep observed after 3 months of treatment was sustained at 6 months and was accompanied by alleviation of both sleepiness and HF symptoms. The mean obstructive apnea index was unchanged, suggesting that therapy neither induced nor contributed to upper airway obstruction. The fact that improvement in sleep variables was paralleled by improvement in quality-of-life measures lends credibility to the clinical significance of the benefit provided by PNS. Importantly, the 6-month improvement in the MLWHF score in the study's HF population was significant and comparable to that seen with cardiac resynchronization therapy [36]. Although quality-of-life indicators can be influenced by knowledge of the therapy applied, especially in an unblinded, open-label, uncontrolled study, the AHI is an unbiased end point lending credibility to the statistically significant amelioration of PGA and sleepiness. Reduction in AHI has been shown to improve outcomes for patients with OSA. In CSA there is a correlation between mortality and number of AHI [37, 38], making it plausible that a reduction in AHI by the remedē® System may also reduce mortality risk. System implantation was successful in 86 % of patients, which is similar to that seen in early trials of new transvenous lead technologies, such as cardiac resynchronization therapy at a similar stage of development [36]. The implantation success rate improved throughout the study, particularly with the introduction of a right brachiocephalic vein lead better suited for some anatomies and improved procedural techniques. In this pilot study of unilateral transvenous PNS, 26 % of patients had serious adverse events related to the device or procedure [39]. Coupled with a growing experience, advancements made to the implantation tools and techniques are expected to reduce the rate of device- and procedure-related adverse events in the future. The benefit of AHI improvement demonstrated by the remedē® System is clinically meaningful and may outweigh the risk for adverse events occurring in the pilot trial [35]. Given the prevalence of CSA and its association with increased morbidity and mortality in certain clinical disorders, the need for better therapies for this disease is obvious. The pilot trial with the remedē® System has the typical limitations of this study's type, including the small sample size, the diversity of the patient population, and the lack of a parallel control arm. Because of this latter limitation, some of the effect could be due to regression to the mean. However, longitudinal studies of CSA have shown that a significant improvement in sleep variable parameters does not occur without effective treatment [15]. Thus, the efficacy seen in the present study likely represents a treatment rather than a placebo effect. This hypothesis is strengthened by the results of the evaluation of the 12-month data from the subjects enrolled in the pilot trial of PNS with the remedē® System [40]. At 1 year, compared to baseline, there was sustained improvement in the AHI (49.9 ± 15.1 events/h vs. 32 27.5 ± 18.3 events/h, $P < 0.001$) and CAI (28.2 ± 15.0 events/h vs. 6.0 ± 9.2 33 events/h, $P < 0.001$). Sustained improvement in the ODI4 (46.1 ± 19.1 34 events/h vs. 26.9 ± 18.0 events/h, $P < 0.001$), REM sleep (11.4 ± 6.1 % vs. 35 17.1 ± 8.0 %, $P < 0.001$), and sleep efficiency (69.3 ± 16.9 % vs. 75.6 ± 17.1 %, $P = 0.024$) were also observed. Additionally, there were continued favorable effects on sleepiness and quality of life. Furthermore, patients with a history of symptomatic HF at baseline continued to show improvement in their MLWHF score at 12 months [Table]. Three deaths unrelated to remedē® System therapy and five serious adverse events occurred through 12 months of follow-up. The average hypopnea index was essentially unchanged (15.8–16.4 events/h) [40]. It should be noted that the majority of the residual apnea/hypopnea events seen in the pilot study were related to patient movement (such as turning or getting up to go to the bathroom). The residual events were primarily hypopneas and were associated with less oxygen desaturation than that measured during the patients' baseline PSGs. Residual apnea/hypopnea events occur primarily while the system is autotitrating treatment levels. The autotitration algorithms minimize patient awareness of the therapy during transitional sleep time periods allowing patients to be compliant with therapy all night, every night. Furthermore, hypopneas are treated by the proprietary algorithm, and the unchanged HI can be also be explained by the fact that therapy converts apneas into hypopneas, and these, in turn, can become normal breaths.

The significant reduction of the AHI to 27.5 events/h does leave the group as a whole with the presence of moderate sleep apnea at 12 months. However, it is important to recognize that the CSA patients enrolled in the remedē® System pilot trial had a baseline AHI of 49.9 events/h, a number higher than that of subjects enrolled in any other trial of therapies for CSA [35]. In addition, the absolute change in AHI of −22 events/h seen in this trial is similar to that seen in randomized trials of CPAP therapy and represents a statistically and clinically significant reduction in the number of events [15, 25]. Furthermore, in comparison to other therapies such as CPAP, the remedē® System therapy works throughout the night for all the hours the patient sleeps. Mask-based studies have documented that PAP users only wear the mask an average of 3.6 h per night [15, 25]. Thus, the remedē® System can be as effective, or more so, when the full apnea burden (total number of apnea and hypopnea events/night) of the entire night is taken into consideration. It is plausible that significant reduction, rather than complete elimination of the number of central apneas a patient experiences throughout the night, will provide some benefit, similar to that seen, for example, when previously poorly controlled comorbidities, such as diabetes, are adequately treated. The results of the 12-month follow-up study of the subjects enrolled in the remedē® System pilot trial confirmed that the device can be used chronically without significant complications. Furthermore, the improvements in sleep indices were maintained in a subset of patients who agreed to a later PSG performed at 18 months after implant [40].

Over 12 months of follow-up, only five serious adverse events related to the device or procedure occurred, and none of them resulted in death. There were no observed interactions between the remedē® System and concomitantly present cardiac rhythm devices which affected the function of either therapy. Additionally, three patients died during the 12 months of follow-up, and, based on the opinion of the Data Safety and Monitoring Board (DSMB), these deaths were not related to either the procedure or the remedē® System therapy [40]. Similar to the initial pilot trial, this 12-month follow-up study was nonrandomized, open label, and included a small number of subjects. Female patients were few, due to the predominance of CSA in men.

13.4   Design of the remedē® System Pivotal Trial

The limitations of the remedē® System's feasibility and pilot studies are acknowledged and have been noted earlier in this chapter [31, 35]. However, it is also true that the results of both studies consistently showed significant improvements in sleep variables in a population with moderate to severe CSA. In addition, the 3- and 6-month results of the pilot trial and the follow-up extended to 12 months show that the improvements in sleep variables are sustained over time and are associated with consistent and lasting amelioration of patients' reported measures of quality of life and sleepiness [40]. The consistency between improvement in sleep and quality-of-life measures lends support to the belief that the reduction in AHI produced by PNS is clinically relevant and may result in favorable outcomes. Furthermore, the strength of the findings was considered convincing enough to test the effectiveness and safety of unilateral transvenous PNS with the remedē® System in a prospective, controlled multicenter randomized clinical study [19]. This was designed as a prospective multicenter randomized trial with blinded end points to evaluate the safety and efficacy of the remedē® System. One hundred fifty-one patients with CSA were randomized 1:1 to remedē® System therapy initiated at 1 month after implantation (treatment) or to an implanted remedē® System that remained inactive for 6 months (control). Importantly, both qualifying and follow-up PSGs were scored by a core laboratory blinded to the patients' randomization assignment. Primary efficacy end point was the comparison of the percentage of patients who experienced a reduction in AHI by ≥50% at 6 months in the treatment versus the control group. Primary safety end point was freedom from SAE related to the device, procedure, or therapy through 12 months. Prespecified secondary end points (CAI, AHI, arousal index, REM, PGA, ODI4, and EPSS) were hierarchically assessed. Although the study included patients with CSA of different etiologies, an exploratory analysis was conducted to evaluate the effectiveness of PNS in the cohort of patients with underlying HF [41]. The selection of the primary end point was based on the understanding that 50% reduction in AHI is clinically meaningful and has been the efficacy criterion upon which other therapies for sleep-disordered breathing have been approved by the US Food and Drug Administration [42]. Prior to SERVE-HF small placebo-controlled randomized clinical trials in HF and CSA showed that attenuation of CSA/hypopnea by 50% had important cardiovascular advantages, such as a decrease in sympathetic activity and nocturnal minute ventilation (resulting in diaphragmatic rest) and improvement in quality of life [41–45]. To the extent that each central apnea results in oxygen desaturation and arousal, any reduction in the CAI should attenuate the detrimental consequences of these events.

Although the primary end point of remedē® System pivotal trial was a reduction in AHI, it was expected that the AHI reduction would be associated with improvements in other sleep variables, such as sleep quality, oxygenation, and arousals. Although the prevalence of central apnea events in HF patients is greater during the night than during the day, the central apnea and hypopnea events occurring during wakefulness cannot be ignored, particularly because the distribution of time of sleep and wakefulness is highly variable in the CSA population. It is hoped that PNS, by improving sleep duration and quality, may also attenuate the detrimental effects of daytime central apnea and hypopnea events [46]. This is important because, regardless of the status of consciousness during which they occur, episodes of oxygen desaturation and increase in carbon dioxide levels significantly contribute to enhance sympathetic activity via chemoreceptor stimulation [9]. Although both PAP and PNS are mechanical methods for the treatment of CSA, the two types of therapy have fundamental differences in their mechanism of action. The contraction of the diaphragm resulting from phrenic nerve stimulation, by creating a negative intrathoracic pressure similar to that produced by normal breathing, augments airflow and prevents the central apnea events that occur during sleep.

The remedē® System pivotal trial has enrolled patients with both reduced and preserved left ventricular ejection fraction. This is another important difference between the PNS pivotal trial and both the SERVE-HF and the continuous positive airway pressure for central sleep apnea and heart failure (CANPAP) studies, which enrolled only patients with systolic HF [9, 15, 16, 19]. The end points of the remedē® System pivotal trial were also designed to assess the safety and efficacy of transvenous PNS specifically for the treatment of individuals with moderate to severe CSA. The trial was not powered or designed as a morbidity/mortality trial. The assessment of safety was focused on serious adverse events associated with the implantation procedure, the remedē® System, or the delivered therapy. These safety events, along with events associated with morbidity and mortality, were closely monitored by an independent DSMB, which had access to all adverse event data. Efficacy was determined by comparing the proportion of subjects with ≥50% reduction in AHI at 6 months in patients treated with the remedē® System at 1 month after implant compared with that of patients receiving standard medical therapy alone.

Conclusions

Assuming that the results of the remedē® System pivotal study are favorable, a number of additional questions remain to be answered. The evaluation of the impact of the remedē® System on structural heart changes, symptoms (as measured by quality-of-life questionnaires), and exercise capacity (measured by peak oxygen consumption) will add important data regarding the potential long-term benefits of this therapy. Eventually, a trial powered to detect a difference in morbidity and mortality in treated versus untreated CSA in HF patients would support the growing evidence of the importance of eliminating CSA in this population. CSA is now recognized as a major comorbidity in multiple pathologic conditions and especially in HF, adversely affecting patients' quality of life and prognosis. Transvenous PNS is a novel approach to treating CSA, and small nonrandomized studies have demonstrated significant reduction in CSA episodes, restoration of a more natural breathing pattern throughout the sleep period, and improved quality of life. As an implanted device, the remedē® System requires no patient intervention to function effectively, eliminating the need for patient adherence to treatment. The remedē® System pivotal trial is the first large, prospective, randomized, sleep core laboratory-blinded study to evaluate the safety and effectiveness of PNS in the treatment of CSA over a 6-month follow-up period.

References

1. Eckert DJ, Jordan AS, Merchia P, Malhotra A. Central sleep apnea: pathophysiology and treatment. Chest. 2007;131:595–607.
2. Javaheri S, Dempsey JA. Central sleep apnea. Comp Physiol. 2013;3:141–63.
3. Minic M, Granton JT, Ryan CM. Sleep disordered breathing in group 1 pulmonary arterial hypertension. J Clin Sleep Med. 2014;10:277–83.
4. Linhart M, Sinning JM, Ghanem A, et al. Prevalence and impact of sleep disordered breathing in patients with severe aortic stenosis. PLoS One. 2015;10, e0133176.
5. Javaheri S. Sleep disorders in systolic heart failure: a prospective study of 100 male patients. The final report. Int J Cardiol. 2006;106:21–8.
6. Herrscher TE, Akre H, Overland B, Sandvik L, Westheim AS. High prevalence of sleep apnea in heart failure outpatients: even in patients with preserved systolic function. J Card Fail. 2011;17:420–5.
7. Arzt M, Woehrle H, Oldenburg O, et al. Prevalence and predictors of sleep-disordered breathing in patients with stable chronic heart failure: the SchlaHF registry. JACC Heart Fail. 2016;4:116–25.

8. Lavergne F, Morin L, Armitstead J, Benjafield A, Richards G, Woehrle H. Atrial fibrillation and sleep-disordered breathing. J Thorac Dis. 2015;7:E575–84.
9. Costanzo MR, Khayat R, Ponikowski P, et al. Mechanisms and clinical consequences of untreated central sleep apnea in heart failure. J Am Coll Cardiol. 2015;65:72–84.
10. Floras JS, Ponikowski P. The sympathetic/parasympathetic imbalance in heart failure with reduced ejection fraction. Eur Heart J. 2015;36:1974–82b.
11. Spaak J, Egri ZJ, Kubo T, et al. Muscle sympathetic nerve activity during wakefulness in heart failure patients with and without sleep apnea. Hypertension. 2005;46:1327–32.
12. Bitter T, Westerheide N, Prinz C, et al. Cheyne-Stokes respiration and obstructive sleep apnoea are independent risk factors for malignant ventricular arrhythmias requiring appropriate cardioverter-defibrillator therapies in patients with congestive heart failure. Eur Heart J. 2011;32:61–74.
13. Javaheri S, Shukla R, Wexler L. Association of smoking, sleep apnea, and plasma alkalosis with nocturnal ventricular arrhythmias in men with systolic heart failure. Chest. 2012;141:1449–56.
14. Oldenburg O, Wellmann B, Buchholz A, et al. Nocturnal hypoxaemia is associated with increased mortality in stable heart failure patients. Eur Heart J. 2015. doi:10.1093/eurheartj/ehv624.
15. Bradley TD, Logan AG, Kimoff RJ, et al. Continuous positive airway pressure for central sleep apnea and heart failure. N Engl J Med. 2005;353:2025–33.
16. Cowie MR, Wegscheider K, Teschler H. Adaptive servo-ventilation for central sleep apnea in heart failure. N Engl J Med. 2016;374:690–1.
17. Zhang XL, Ding N, Wang H, et al. Transvenous phrenic nerve stimulation in patients with Cheyne-Stokes respiration and congestive heart failure: a safety and proof-of-concept study. Chest. 2012;142:927–34.
18. Oldenburg O, Bitter T, Fox H, Horstkotte D, Gutleben KJ. Effects of unilateral phrenic nerve stimulation on tidal volume. First case report of a patient responding to remede(R) treatment for nocturnal Cheyne-Stokes respiration. Herz. 2014;39:84–6.
19. Costanzo MR, Augostini R, Goldberg LR, Ponikowski P, Stellbrink C, Javaheri S. Design of the remede system pivotal trial: a prospective, randomized study in the use of respiratory rhythm management to treat central sleep apnea. J Card Fail. 2015;21:892–902.
20. Arzt M, Floras JS, Logan AG, Kimoff RJ, Series F, Morrison D, CANPAP Investigators, et al. Suppression of central sleep apnea by continuous positive airway pressure and transplant-free survival in heart failure: a post hoc analysis of the Canadian Continuous Positive Airway Pressure for Patients With Central Sleep Apnea and Heart Failure Trial (CANPAP). Circulation. 2007;115:3173–80.
21. Javaheri S. Effects of continuous positive airway pressure on sleep apnea and ventricular irritability in patients with heart failure. Circulation. 2000;101:392–7.
22. Tkacova R, Liu PP, Naughton MT, Bradley TD. Effect of continuous positive airway pressure on mitral regurgitant fraction and atrial natriuretic peptide in patients with heart failure. J Am Coll Cardiol. 1997;30:739–45.
23. Sin DD, Logan AG, Fitzgerald FS, Liu PP, Bradley TD. Effects of continuous positive airway pressure on cardiovascular outcomes in heart failure patients with and without Cheyne-Stokes respiration. Circulation. 2000;102:61–6.
24. Naughton MT, Liu PP, Bernard DC, Goldstein RS, Bradley TD. Treatment of congestive heart failure and Cheyne-Stokes respiration during sleep by continuous positive airway pressure. Am J Respir Crit Care Med. 1995;151:92–7.
25. Cowie MR, Woehrle H, Wegscheider K, et al. Adaptive servo-ventilation for central sleep apnea in systolic heart failure. N Engl J Med. 2015;373:1095–105.
26. Glenn WWL, Holcomb WG, Gee JBL, Rath R. Central hypoventilation: long-term ventilator assistance by radiofrequency electrophrenic respiration. Ann Surg. 1970;172:755–73.
27. Glenn WWL, Phelps ML. Diaphragm pacing by electrical stimulation of the phrenic nerve. Neurosurgery. 1985;17:974–84.

28. DiMarco AF. Phrenic nerve stimulation in patients with spinal cord injury. Respir Physiol Neurobiol. 2009;169:200–9.
29. Chen ML, Tablizo MA, Kun S, Keens TG. Diaphragm pacers as a treatment for congenital central hypoventilation syndrome. Expert Rev Med Devices. 2005;2:577–85.
30. Glenn WW, Brouillette RT, Dentz B, et al. Fundamental considerations in pacing of the diaphragm for chronic ventilatory insufficiency: a multicenter study. Pacing Clin Electrophysiol. 1988;11:2121–7.
31. Ponikowski P, Javaheri S, Michalkiewicz D, et al. Transvenous phrenic nerve stimulation for the treatment of central sleep apnoea in heart failure. Eur Heart J. 2012;33:889–94.
32. Lanfranchi PA, Braghiroli A, Bosimini E, et al. Prognostic value of nocturnal Cheyne-Stokes respiration in chronic heart failure. Circulation. 1999;99:1435–40.
33. Young T, Finn L, Peppard PE, Szklo-Coxe M, Austin D, Nieto FJ, Stubbs R, Hla KM. Sleep disordered breathing and mortality. Sleep. 2008;31:1071–8.
34. Dempsey JA, Veasey SC, Morgan BJ, O'Donnell CP. Pathophysiology of sleep apnea. Physiol Rev. 2010;90:47–112.
35. Abraham WT, Jagielski D, Oldenburg O, et al. Phrenic nerve stimulation for the treatment of central sleep apnea. JACC Heart Fail. 2015;3:360–9.
36. McAlister FA, Ezekkowitz J, Hooton N, et al. Cardiac resynchronization therapy for patients with left ventricular systolic dysfunction. A systematic review. JAMA. 2007;297:2502–14.
37. Javaheri S, Shukla R, Zeigler H, Wexler L. Central sleep apnea, right ventricular dysfunction and low diastolic blood pressure are predictors of mortality in systolic heart failure. J Am Coll Cardiol. 2007;49:2028–34.
38. Jilek C, Krenn M, Sebah D, et al. Prognostic impact of sleep disordered breathing and its treatment in heart failure: an observational study. Eur J Heart Fail. 2011;13:68–75.
39. Alonso C, Leclercq C, d'Allones FR, et al. Six-year experience of transvenous left ventricular lead implantation for permanent biventricular pacing in patients with advanced heart failure: technical aspects. Heart. 2001;86:405–10.
40. Jagielski D, Ponikowski P, Augostini R, Kolodziej A, Khayat R, Abraham WT. Transvenous stimulation of the phrenic nerve for the treatment of central 1 sleep apnoea: 12 months' experience with the remedē® System. Eur J Heart Fail. 2016. doi:10.1002/ejhf593.
41. Weaver TE, Grunstein RR. Adherence to continuous positive airway pressure therapy: the challenge to effective treatment. Proc Am Thorac Soc. 2008;5:173–8.
42. Strollo Jr PJ, Soose RJ, Maurer JT, de Vries N, Cornelius J, Froymovich O, et al. Upper-airway stimulation for obstructive apnea. N Engl J Med. 2014;370:139–49.
43. Naughton MT, Benard DC, Liu PP, Rutherford R, Rankin F, Bradley TD. Effects of nasal CPAP on sympathetic activity in patients with heart failure and central sleep apnea. Am J Respir Crit Care Med. 1995;152:473–9.
44. Javaheri S. Acetazolamide improves central sleep apnea in heart failure. A double-blind, prospective study. Am J Respir Crit Care Med. 2006;173:234–7.
45. Naughton MT, Benard DC, Rutherford R, Bradley TD. Effect of continuous positive airway pressure on central sleep apnea and nocturnal PCO 2 in heart failure. Am J Respir Crit Care Med. 1994;150:1598–604.
46. Giannoni A, PassinoA MG, Del Franco A, Aimo A, Emdin M. Treating chemoreflex in heart failure: modulation or demolition? J Physiol. 2014;592:1903–4.

Breathless Heart: Final Remarks

14

Michele Emdin, Alberto Giannoni, and Claudio Passino

Whichever the initial *noxa* damaging the heart is, this elicits a remodeling process, leading to cardiac dysfunction and pump failure, as well as to an increasing arrhythmic burden. The abnormal hemodynamics, accompanied by a decrease in cardiac output, are sensed by visceral feedback systems, modulating autonomic tone. As a consequence, baroreflex is deactivated, while ergoreflex and chemoreflex are stimulated, inducing vagal withdrawal and eliciting adrenergic activation, with a net effect of sympathetic predominance on the neural drive to the heart and vessels. This may be considered an initial compensatory response, because of its effect on vasomotion and mean arterial pressure, on inotropism, and on water–salt retention and plasma volume, further becoming maladaptive, accelerating ventricular remodeling, causing peripheral and pulmonary edema, with accompanying dyspnea, and increasing the risk of sudden death. With time, the combined effect of delayed circulatory time and increased chemoreflex (together with other mechanisms) promotes a delayed robust ventilatory response and blood gas instability, thus favoring the occurrence of periodic breathing (PB) or Cheyne–Stokes respiration (CSR). PB/CSR can be therefore considered as a «marker of clinical severity» of heart failure and has been outlined as a «risk marker», i.e., as predictor of future fatal events.

Two centuries ago, Cheyne and Stokes first described that patients with heart failure present with PB/CSR, associated with waxing and waning of ventilation, with repetitive phases of apnea and hyperpnea [1]. Although this observation has been long overlooked in clinical practice, the recent guidelines on heart failure management [2] underscore the clinical significance of abnormal breathing in heart failure patients. PB/CSR, associated with sleep fragmentation, further sympathetic activation, and poor outcome, has then been considered a "risk factor," i.e., a

M. Emdin (✉) • C. Passino
Institute of Life Sciences, Scuola Superiore Sant'Anna, Pisa, Italy

Division of Cardiology and Cardiovascular Medicine, Fondazione Toscana G. Monasterio, Pisa, Italy
e-mail: emdin@ftgm.it; m.emdin@sssup.it; passino@ftgm.it

A. Giannoni
Division of Cardiology and Cardiovascular Medicine, Fondazione Toscana G. Monasterio, Pisa, Italy
e-mail: alberto.giannoni@ftgm.it

© Springer International Publishing Switzerland 2017
M. Emdin et al. (eds.), *The Breathless Heart*,
DOI 10.1007/978-3-319-26354-0_14

mediator of risk, per se by enhancing the sympathetic mediated facilitation of dys-rhythmias occurrence and worsening of hemodynamics in both pulmonary and systemic vascular beds [3].

Noninvasive mechanical ventilation has then been proposed as a treatment for PB/CSR in heart failure, but two multinational randomized controlled trials with either continuous positive airway pressure (CANPAP) or adaptive servoventilation (SERVE-CHF) failed to improve outcome in systolic heart failure [4–6]. They both revealed poor compliance to treatment and incremental mortality risk in treated patients.

This apparent paradox may be perhaps explained by study limitations related to inclusion criteria and technical features of mechanical ventilation applied, but may even point to the limited efficacy of therapeutic approaches targeting PB/CSR as the final event (namely) and not its pathophysiological triggers. In addition, noninvasive mechanical ventilation cannot abolish the daytime PB/CSR, but apneas did not occur only during sleep time [7]. In fact, the literature predominantly refers to "sleep apnea" in heart failure, but PB/CSR often occurs during awake hours, as demonstrated by several studies using laboratory or ambulatory polygraphic recordings, which outlined also an independent prognostic value of "awake apneas" [8, 9]. In addition, PB/CSR may be present even during effort, showing an independent and additive prognostic value compared with sleep apnea [9].

Naughton has proposed that PB/CSR "has physiological features more likely to be compensatory and beneficial than injurious in HF" and that "some aspects of CS apneas and CSR are similar to those seen with positive airway pressure." Naughton's elegant arguments focus on PB/CSR as a compensatory mechanism in heart failure. Naughton indicates as beneficial physiologic attributes of PB/CSR: gas exchange salutary effects of hyperventilation-associated increased end-expiratory lung volume; sympatholytic effects of the hyperpneic phases; beneficial effects on the myocardium of hyperventilation and associated alkalosis; improved bronchial patency associated with hyperpnea; relief of respiratory muscle fatigue associated with cyclic decreased work of breathing (apnea), reduced preload and afterload, as well as blunting of pulmonary vasoconstriction, all effects which have been postulated to have an analogy with positive airway pressure [10, 11].

This intriguing, yet not proven, hypothesis challenges the idea of "one-size-fit-all treatment," based on the mere presence of PB/CSR. Indeed, no study has actually identified whether either a single indicator (biohumoral, clinical, instrumental, or related with the severity of PB/CSR phenomenon) or a multimarker approach might identify a subset who could benefit from a therapy, which should preferably target pathophysiological triggers, and only when related symptoms impact on life quality or increase risk of death [12].

All these observations, which have been object of a thorough analysis throughout the chapters of this book, still generate more questions than answers: Does PB/CSR always negatively affect the evolution of heart failure disease or this may be true only in specific subset of patients? Will it be possible that future studies could investigate how we can identify those patients in whom PB/CSR is no more compensatory but detrimental? May we design an ideal, feasible diagnostic work-up, not only aimed to detect the presence or absence of periodic breathing phenomenon but considering also, as a guide to decision-making, its severity identified by polygraphy (e.g., by the evaluation of daytime occurrence and/or apnea/hypopnea index, morphology and duration of apnea/hyperpnea phase), the level of neurohormonal activation (e.g., by the assessment of plasma concentration of norepinephrine or B-type natriuretic peptides), the severity of background cardiac function, or a combination of all these?

Two centuries after the descriptions by Cheyne and Stokes, an effort is needed and much must be understood of the individual differential profile and of the noncardiovascular effects of PB/CSR.

References

1. Stokes W. The diseases of the heart and the aorta. Dublin: Hodges and Smith; 1854. p. 340.
2. Yancy CW, Jessup M, Bozkurt B, Butler J, Casey Jr DE, Drazner MH, et al. American College of Cardiology Foundation/American Heart Association Task Force on Practice Guidelines 2013 ACCF/AHA guideline for the management of heart failure: a report of the American College of Cardiology Foundation/American Heart Association Task Force on Practice Guidelines. Circulation. 2013;128:e240–327.
3. Oldenburg O, Lamp B, Faber L, Teschler H, Horstkotte D, Topfer V. Sleep-disordered breathing in patients with symptomatic heart failure: a contemporary study of prevalence in and characteristics of 700 patients. Eur J Heart Fail. 2007;9:251e7.
4. Bradley TD, Logan AG, Kimoff RJ, Sériès F, Morrison D, Ferguson K, Belenkie I, Pfeifer M, Fleetham J, Hanly P, Smilovitch M, Tomlinson G, Floras JS, CANPAP Investigators. Continuous positive airway pressure for central sleep apnea and heart failure. N Engl J Med. 2005;353:2025–33.
5. Cowie MR, Woehrle H, Wegscheider K, Angermann C, d'Ortho MP, Erdmann E, Levy P, Simonds AK, Somers VK, Zannad F, Teschler H. Adaptive servo-ventilation for central sleep apnea in systolic heart failure. N Engl J Med. 2015;373:1095–105.
6. Emdin M, Passino C, Giannoni A. After the SERVE-HF trial, is there still a need for treatment of central apnea? J Card Fail. 2015;21:903–5.
7. Poletti R, Passino C, Giannoni A, Zyw L, Prontera C, Bramanti F, Clerico A, Piepoli M, Emdin M. Risk factors and prognostic value of daytime Cheyne-Stokes respiration in chronic heart failure patients. Int J Cardiol. 2009;137:47–53.
8. Brack T, Thüer I, Clarenbach CF, Senn O, Noll G, Russi EW, Bloch KE. Daytime Cheyne-Stokes respiration in ambulatory patients with severe congestive heart failure is associated with increased mortality. Chest. 2007;132:1463–71.
9. Corrà U, Pistono M, Mezzani A, Braghiroli A, Giordano A, Lanfranchi P, Bosimini E, Gnemmi M, Giannuzzi P. Sleep and exertional periodic breathing in chronic heart failure: prognostic importance and interdependence. Circulation. 2006;113:44–50.
10. Naughton MT. Cheyne-Stokes respiration: friend or foe? Thorax. 2012;67:357–60.
11. Naughton MT. Respiratory sleep disorders in patients with congestive heart failure. J Thorac Dis. 2015;7:1298–310.
12. Emdin M, Passino C. Targeting periodic breathing in heart failure patients, and treating it gently. J Card Fail. 2014;20:289–91.

Printed in the United States
By Bookmasters